ATLAS OF
Interstitial Lung Disease Pathology

Pathology with High Resolution CT Correlations

Second Edition

Andrew Churg, MD
Professor of Pathology
The University of British Columbia
Pathologist, Vancouver General Hospital
Vancouver, British Columbia, Canada

Nestor L. Müller, MD
Professor Emeritus of Radiology
The University of British Columbia
Vancouver, British Columbia, Canada

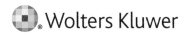 Wolters Kluwer

Philadelphia · Baltimore · New York · London
Buenos Aires · Hong Kong · Sydney · Tokyo

Acquisitions Editor: Nicole Dernoski
Development Editor: Ariel S. Winter
Editorial Coordinator: Julie Kostelnik
Marketing Manager: Julie Sikora
Production Project Manager: Bridgett Dougherty
Design Coordinator: Teresa Mallon
Senior Manufacturing Coordinator: Beth Welsh
Prepress Vendor: S4Carlisle Publishing Services

Second edition

9 8 7 6 5 4 3 2 1

Printed in China

Library of Congress Cataloging-in-Publication Data

ISBN-13: 978-1-9751-2467-0

ISBN-10: 1-975124-67-7

Library of Congress Control Number: 2019946526.

shop.lww.com

Dedicated to the late Drs. Charles Carrington
and William Thurlbeck

—ANDREW CHURG

To my wife Isabela and my children Noah, Phillip,
and Alison Müller

—NESTOR L. MÜLLER

In the 6 years since the publication of the first edition, there have been a number of important developments in the field of interstitial lung disease (ILD). The most dramatic of these is the demonstration that antifibrotic agents (pirfenidone, nintedanib) slow the course of, and may decrease mortality in, idiopathic usual interstitial pneumonia (idiopathic pulmonary fibrosis, IPF). These agents have become the standard of care for IPF, and this situation has made the clinical, radiologic, and pathologic separation of other types of ILD from IPF even more critical than in the past. For this same reason, accurate identification of chronic (fibrotic) hypersensitivity pneumonitis (HP) has become very important for the clinician, radiologist, and pathologist, because this disease can be difficult to separate from IPF, but is treated with immunosuppressive agents rather than antifibrotics. However, the exact features that allow a pathologic diagnosis of HP are controversial, as to a certain extent are the clinical and radiologic features, because it has become clear that there is poor agreement on the diagnosis of chronic HP among multidisciplinary discussion groups. Another problem in the area of fibrotic ILD is the presence of features suggesting an underlying collagen vascular disease in cases in which there is no clear clinical evidence of a rheumatologic condition; this idea has been formalized in the concept of interstitial pneumonia with autoimmune features. We devote considerable detail in this second edition to these three areas.

A variety of other new entities have been described in the pathology literature or clearly separated from other entities, including interstitial fibrosis related to cigarette smoking, a process notable for its numerous names, often dramatic morphology, but lack of adverse effects; fibrosing bronchiolitis; and cicatricial organizing pneumonia, and we illustrate and discuss them here. We have, in addition, expanded the discussion of ILD associated with granulomas, including newly described detail on primary biliary cholangitis in the lung. The pathologist may also have to deal with a new type of biopsy: transbronchial cryobiopsy. We review the limitations and diagnostic possibilities associated with such biopsies.

Although molecular diagnosis is well established for lung cancer, in the field of ILD, it is still in its infancy. We have added information on molecular diagnosis and molecular pathogenesis where this exists, particularly for Langerhans cell histiocytosis, Erdheim–Chester disease, pulmonary alveolar proteinosis, and lymphangioleiomyomatosis, and comment on possible applications of molecular testing in other diseases. We have also emphasized immunohistochemical tests that can be utilized to demonstrate molecular abnormalities and point to pathologic diagnosis or treatment, for example, BRAF V600E staining in Langerhans cell histiocytosis and Erdheim–Chester disease. In part because of demonstrated molecular abnormalities there is an emerging idea that Langerhans cell histiocytosis and lymphangioleiomyomatosis should be viewed as low-grade malignancies rather than non-neoplastic ILD, and we discuss the utility or lack thereof of this concept.

Lastly, we have expanded the details and provided more illustrations in a number of other areas where more information has emerged in the last 6 years.

Andrew Churg
Nestor L. Müller
Vancouver, British Columbia

Preface to the First Edition

Interstitial lung disease (ILD) is an extremely confusing topic, and this problem extends from clinicians to radiologists to pathologists. Confusion arises in part because of the sheer number of ILDs; clinicians can name more than 150 separate entities. From the point of view of the pathologist, there are many fewer diagnosable patterns, but this phenomenon immediately raises the question of how to make those patterns correspond to clinically defined diseases, particularly so because, at first glance, there appears to be considerable morphologic overlap among these various conditions. A further source of confusion is that much of what is called "interstitial" lung disease is really characterized by processes that take place largely in the airspaces—bronchiolitis obliterans organizing pneumonia (BOOP) is a good example—or those that affect primarily small airways, for example, constrictive bronchiolitis.

However, we believe that the biggest problem for pathologists trying to deal with ILD is that the nonlung specialist will see relatively few such cases in a year, and turning to standard textbooks provides only limited help because textbooks by their very nature can supply only a few illustrations of any particular condition.

This atlas is intended to address this problem by providing a large number of illustrations to give the practicing pathologist a feel for the morphologic spectrum of any given ILD and also to illustrate the various differential diagnoses of any particular condition, something that textbooks often do not provide. For this reason, we have included some uncommon variants of relatively common ILD, for example, fibrosis in chronic eosinophilic pneumonia and in BOOP, interstitial spread of Langerhans cell histiocytosis, and progression of desquamative interstitial pneumonia to a picture of fibrotic nonspecific interstitial pneumonia. We have also included some material on imaging in every chapter, because non-neoplastic lung disease in general and ILD in particular are very difficult to diagnose without clinical and especially radiologic information. Conversely, we hope that radiologists will find this volume to be helpful in understanding the pathologic changes behind the radiologic appearances. But this book is not intended as a general detailed text on clinical features, imaging, pathogenesis, treatment, and so on of ILD, and we have also purposely kept references to an absolute minimum. Rather, the book is meant as a quick reference whereby one can look at a set of pictures and get a reasonable idea of whether and how well a particular case shows the diagnostic features of a particular disease.

Andrew Churg
Nestor L. Müller

Contents

General Approach to Interstitial Lung Disease: Clinical, Radiologic, and Pathologic Considerations

Interstitial lung diseases (ILDs) constitute a very broad class of confusing entities. The number of possible pathologic patterns of ILD is far smaller than the number of corresponding clinical conditions, the latter estimated as 150 or greater.[1] Although some pathologic ILD patterns are morphologically specific, for example, lymphangioleiomyomatosis (LAM) or Langerhans cell histiocytosis (LCH), many are reaction patterns with a broad range of etiologies; thus, nonspecific interstitial pneumonia (NSIP) is an entity in itself, but a pattern of NSIP may be seen in collagen vascular diseases, hypersensitivity pneumonitis (HP), and drug reactions, to name just a few. A further confusing feature of ILD is that the pathologic features of one ILD can appear in another; thus, small foci of organizing pneumonia (OP, also called bronchiolitis obliterans organizing pneumonia, BOOP or cryptogenic organizing pneumonia, COP) are common in HP and in NSIP, whereas NSIP patterns can be seen focally in biopsies of usual interstitial pneumonia (UIP). Additional confusion is sown by the use of alphabetic abbreviations, sometimes referred to facetiously as "alphabet soup" (Table 1.1).

The relative nonspecificity of many pathologic ILD patterns mandates that the pathologist obtain some sort of clinical information, and, even more important, learn something about imaging of ILD. The use of high-resolution computed tomography (HRCT) has revolutionized the diagnosis of ILD. For some conditions such as sarcoid, UIP, LCH, or LAM, HRCT often provides a highly specific diagnosis. But even where HRCT is less specific, for example when the radiologist sees a pattern of ground-glass opacities (see Chapter 2 for definitions), this still provides important guidelines to pathologic diagnosis. For these reasons, we have written this atlas as a book primarily directed to pathologic diagnosis, but with an emphasis on HRCT correlations as well. It should be noted that in a sense the accuracy of HRCT makes the pathologist's job harder, because the combination of clinical findings and HRCT results will obviate biopsy in many cases, and cases that do get biopsied tend to be the nonobvious ones.

The most important conclusion from the above comments is that ILD usually cannot be diagnosed by sitting in one's office without any clinical and radiologic information, but the pathologist needs to get into the habit of

Table 1.1	
Commonly used abbreviations for ILDs	
AIP	Acute interstitial pneumonia
DAD	Diffuse alveolar damage
DIP	Desquamative interstitial pneumonia
HP	Hypersensitivity pneumonitis
IPAF	Interstitial pneumonia with autoimmune features
LAM	Lymphangioleiomyomatosis
LCH	Langerhans cell histiocytosis
NSIP	Nonspecific interstitial pneumonia
OP	Organizing pneumonia (when idiopathic called BOOP [bronchiolitis obliterans organizing pneumonia or COP, cryptogenic organizing pneumonia])
PAP	Pulmonary alveolar proteinosis
RBILD	Respiratory bronchiolitis with interstitial lung disease
RBF	Respiratory bronchiolitis with fibrosis, also called smoking-related interstitial fibrosis (SRIF)
UIP	Usual interstitial pneumonia
UIP/IPF	Idiopathic pulmonary fibrosis (idiopathic UIP)

talking to the clinician and radiologist about each case. Sometimes the clinician can only say that the patient has evidence of an ILD, but more often he or she can narrow the diagnosis to likely possibilities. Similarly, HRCT often allows the radiologist to narrow the diagnostic possibilities, and the pathologist should attempt to review the HRCT images with the radiologist.

The idea that many cases of ILD cannot be diagnosed on biopsy or imaging alone is now frequently translated into the concept of multidisciplinary discussion (MDD). MDD is a formal and typically a face-to-face (or video conference) meeting in which respiratory clinicians, radiologists, and pathologists discuss with ILD patients and try to arrive at a consensus diagnosis. Some MDD groups also include a rheumatologist because of the frequency of underlying connective tissue diseases in ILD patients (see Chapter 21).

MDD is most useful in fibrosing interstitial pneumonias, that is ILD in which various patterns of interstitial fibrosis/inflammation (rather than a single specific pathognomonic finding such as granulomas or LAM cells or aggregates of Langerhans cells) is the major pathology, because these entities share many overlapping features (see below). MDD evaluation of a given case not infrequently results in changes in clinical, radiologic, and sometimes pathologic impression and has been shown to improve diagnostic accuracy.[1,2] This is particularly important when dealing with fibrosing interstitial pneumonias because of distinctly different treatments for some of these conditions (see below).

MDD is not perfect and some diagnoses pose more problems than others. Walsh et al.[3] carried out an exercise in which seven experienced MDD groups reviewed the same 70 cases. There was overall good diagnostic agreement for a diagnosis of idiopathic pulmonary fibrosis (IPF, weighted kappa 0.71) and for connective tissue disease-associated ILD (weighted kappa 0.73), but poor agreement for chronic HP (weighted kappa 0.29). Nonetheless, MDD still offers much greater likelihood of achieving an accurate evaluation than does blind pathologic or radiologic diagnosis.

That said, there is a general pathologic approach, which is useful in dealing with a new case of ILD. As shown in Table 1.2, when there is no helpful clinical or radiologic information, the idea is to first eliminate things that are relatively easy for the pathologist to diagnose (tumors such as lymphangitic carcinomas or lymphomas that can mimic ILD pathologically or radiologically; infections such as cytomegalovirus [CMV] or pneumocystis that can produce a microscopic picture of interstitial inflammation), then to eliminate diseases with distinctive features such as granulomas, and then to consider diseases with fewer specific features and more low-power architectural patterns such as UIP or NSIP.

It is also useful to ask oneself if the biopsy could be a bad sample; sometimes biopsies pick up the edge of lesions or even misleading lesions and this can be very confusing;

Table 1.2
General morphologic approach to ILD and mimics of ILD
Is this a malignancy that mimics ILD; e.g., lymphangitic carcinoma, lymphoma?
Is this an infection that mimics ILD (PCP, CMV)?
Is this an ILD with a defined specific feature; e.g., sarcoid?
Is this a form of fibrosing interstitial pneumonia; e.g., UIP?
Is this a *localized* artifact (scar, edge of another lesion, etc.)?
Is this a drug reaction or a connective tissue disease?

for example, a biopsy taken at the edge of OP can look like cellular NSIP (see Fig. 5.11), and nonspecific scars can mimic UIP (see Figs. 6.37 and 6.38). OP itself can be seen around mass lesions (tumors, abscesses, and nodules of granulomatosis with polyangiitis [Wegener granulomatosis]) that are not ILD (see Fig. 5.22). As pathologists we get small samples to work with, whereas the radiologist has two whole lungs, and a radiologic consultation often solves those particular problems. Lastly, remember that when one encounters a strange ILD pattern, particularly a strange combination of patterns, drug reactions and collagen vascular diseases should be considered. Obviously within each of these categories there are lots of important details, and we will go through these details in this atlas.

CLINICAL FEATURES OF ILD

There are a general set of clinical signs and symptoms that suggest ILD. Most patients with ILD present with shortness of breath that is often slowly progressive and frequently have nonproductive cough as well. Physical examination often shows small lung volumes and so-called "velcro" rales (the sound of two pieces of velcro being ripped apart, also called crackles or dry rales) at the lung bases, the latter a finding characteristic of ILD.[4]

Pulmonary function tests in most forms of ILD demonstrate a restrictive impairment and impaired diffusing capacity, and in relatively early disease, only the diffusing capacity may be abnormal. However, some ILD also have airflow obstruction, for example in constrictive bronchiolitis (bronchiolitis obliterans, see Chapter 20).

Although these abnormalities are typical of ILD and are valuable to the clinician for following disease progression and determining prognosis, they are generally not useful by themselves for determining the underlying disease. For that reason, we will not emphasize signs, symptoms, or pulmonary function tests in the sections that follow, except where there are specific patterns that are helpful.

THE IDIOPATHIC INTERSTITIAL PNEUMONIAS

Anyone dealing with ILD will, sooner than later, encounter the term "idiopathic interstitial pneumonia (IIP)." This term refers to a set of different lesions that, partly for historic reasons and partly for reasons of nomenclature, are often grouped together. There is a standard classification of these entities promulgated by the American Thoracic Society and European Respiratory Society,[5] as shown in Table 1.3.

Although we discuss all the entities in Table 1.3, we are going to largely ignore the concept of IIP for several reasons: First, acute interstitial pneumonia (AIP) is idiopathic acute respiratory distress syndrome (ARDS) and ARDS is not generally viewed as an ILD; second, except for respiratory bronchiolitis with interstitial lung disease (RBILD) and desquamative interstitial pneumonia (DIP), these diseases have no relationship to each other, and, in fact, they tend to be both radiologically and pathologically quite different; third, RBILD and DIP are actually not idiopathic but rather are smoking-related diseases, as the updated classification now acknowledges; and fourth, because the clinical, radiologic, and pathologic features and treatment and prognosis are so different, a diagnosis of "IIP" has no meaning.

We believe it is much more useful to create other categories such as smoking-related diseases (RBILD, DIP, and LCH) where these exist as logical units or have some morphologic continuity, and to treat the remaining conditions as individual diseases.

FIBROSING INTERSTITIAL PNEUMONIAS, DIAGNOSTIC ONTOLOGY, AND TREATMENT

"Fibrosing interstitial pneumonia" is a general name for any kind of ILD in which the major pathologic finding is some pattern of dense old fibrosis with or without interstitial chronic inflammation; thus, UIP, fibrotic NSIP, and chronic HP all can be described as fibrosing interstitial pneumonias. The diagnosis of fibrosing interstitial pneumonias is primarily based on low-power architecture, although sometimes more or less specific features such as granulomas (chronic HP) or a high proportion of plasma cells (collagen vascular disease-associated ILD) may indicate the correct diagnosis. Some processes such as fibroblast foci or acute exacerbations (see Chapters 4 and 6 for detailed definitions of these terms) can be seen with any form of fibrosing interstitial pneumonia.

We reserve "fibrosing interstitial pneumonia" as a diagnostic term for situations where the combination of biopsy, imaging, and clinical features does not allow a more exact classification. Fibrosing interstitial pneumonias are consistently the most difficult problems in ILD, and in a significant proportion of such cases, even MDD fails to come up with a consensus diagnosis. Ryerson et al.[6] have recently proposed a diagnostic ontology to deal with this problem. This scheme is based on diagnostic confidence after MDD and runs from "confident diagnosis" (>90% likelihood) to "provisional diagnosis high-confidence" (70% to 89% likelihood), "provisional diagnosis low-confidence" (55%

Table 1.3

Classification of the IIPs

Category	Clinical-radiologic-pathologic diagnosis	Radiology and/or pathology pattern
Chronic fibrosing IP	Idiopathic pulmonary fibrosis (IPF)	Usual interstitial pneumonia (UIP)
	Idiopathic nonspecific interstitial pneumonia (NSIP)	Nonspecific interstitial pneumonia (NSIP)
Smoking-related IP	Respiratory bronchiolitis with Interstitial lung disease (RBILD)	Respiratory bronchiolitis
	Desquamative interstitial pneumonia (DIP)	Desquamative interstitial pneumonia (DIP)
Acute/subacute IP	Cryptogenic organizing pneumonia (COP, BOOP)	Organizing pneumonia (OP)
	Acute interstitial pneumonia (AIP)	Diffuse alveolar damage (DAD)
Rare IIPs	Idiopathic lymphocytic interstitial pneumonia (LIP)	Lymphocytic interstitial pneumonia (LIP)
	Pleuroparenchymal fibroelastosis	Pleuroparenchymal fibroelastosis
Unclassifiable IP	No clear diagnosis after MDD	Radiology/pathology patterns are conflicting

Modified from Travis WD, Costabel U, Hansell DM, et al.; ATS/ERS Committee on Idiopathic Interstitial Pneumonias. An official American Thoracic Society/European Respiratory Society statement: update of the international multidisciplinary classification of the idiopathic interstitial pneumonias. *Am J Respir Crit Care Med.* 2013;188:733–748. IP = interstitial pneumonia.

Table 1.4

Treatment of fibrosing interstitial pneumonias

Disease	Recommended therapy
Idiopathic pulmonary fibrosis (UIP/IPF)	Antifibrotic agents (pirfenidone, nintedanib)
Chronic (fibrotic) HP	Anti-inflammatory agents (steroids, mycophenolate, azathioprine)
Collagen vascular disease-associated ILD (including IPAF, see Chapter 21)	Anti-inflammatory agents (steroids, mycophenolate, azathioprine, cyclophosphamide, rituximab)
Unclassifiable fibrosing interstitial pneumonia	Case-by-case decision based on MDD Current clinical trial of antifibrotic agents

to 69% likelihood) to "unclassifiable ILD" (likelihood 50% or below). Although the exact separation of 51% to 69%, 70% to 89%, and greater than 90% confidence levels as proposed by Ryerson et al. in practice is likely to be a very rough approximation, especially for pathologic diagnoses, at least these approximations provide some guide to treatment and prognosis.

In the past, fibrosing interstitial pneumonias were typically treated with steroids, and exact diagnostic classification generally did not affect therapy. However, the situation has now changed, in part because of recognition that steroids are harmful in UIP/IPF,[7] and because antifibrotic therapy is now the preferred treatment for UIP/IPF (Table 1.4 and see Chapter 6), whereas most other fibrosing interstitial pneumonias are treated with some form of immunosuppression (Table 1.4). This situation makes accurate diagnosis much more critical.

Fibrosing interstitial pneumonia as a pathologic diagnosis in some senses corresponds to the clinical and radiologic notion of "unclassifiable ILD." However, this should always be a pathologic diagnosis of last resort because it provides little treatment and prognostic guidance to clinicians, and one should always try to provide a differential diagnosis when signing out a case as a "fibrosing interstitial pneumonia." For example, one might report a biopsy as "fibrosing interstitial pneumonia, favor chronic HP over UIP."

REFERENCES

1. Flaherty KR, Andrei AC, King TE Jr, et al. Idiopathic interstitial pneumonia: do community and academic physicians agree on diagnosis? *Am J Respir Crit Care Med.* 2007;175:1054–1060.
2. Flaherty KR, King TE Jr, Raghu G, et al. Idiopathic interstitial pneumonia: what is the effect of a multidisciplinary approach to diagnosis? *Am J Respir Crit Care Med.* 2004;170:904–910.
3. Walsh SLF, Maher TM, Kolb M, et al.; IPF Project Consortium. Diagnostic accuracy of a clinical diagnosis of idiopathic pulmonary fibrosis: an international case-cohort study. *Eur Respir J.* 2017;50. pii: 1700936.
4. Schwarz MI, King TE. *Interstitial Lung Disease.* 3rd ed. Hamilton, ON: BC Decker Inc; 1998.
5. Travis WD, Costabel U, Hansell DM, et al.; ATS/ERS Committee on Idiopathic Interstitial Pneumonias. An official American Thoracic Society/European Respiratory Society statement: update of the international multidisciplinary classification of the idiopathic interstitial pneumonias. *Am J Respir Crit Care Med.* 2013;188:733–748.
6. Ryerson CJ, Corte TJ, Lee JS, et al. A standardized diagnostic ontology for fibrotic interstitial lung disease. An International Working Group Perspective. *Am J Respir Crit Care Med.* 2017;196:1249–1254.
7. Idiopathic Pulmonary Fibrosis Clinical Research Network, Raghu G, Anstrom KJ, King TE Jr, et al. Prednisone, azathioprine, and N-acetylcysteine for pulmonary fibrosis. *N Engl J Med.* 2012;366:1968–1977.

Imaging in Interstitial Lung Disease

The two imaging modalities that are used almost routinely in the assessment of patients with interstitial lung disease (ILD) are the chest radiograph and high-resolution computed tomography (HRCT). The radiograph is inexpensive, has a very low radiation dose, and can provide useful information regarding the progression of disease and the presence of associated findings. In some cases, the presence of characteristic findings on the radiograph in the proper clinical context can be highly suggestive of a specific diagnosis. For example, in a patient with minimal or no symptoms and no exposure history, the presence of symmetric bilateral hilar and paratracheal lymphadenopathy with associated ILD in a predominantly upper lobe distribution is highly suggestive of sarcoidosis. In the majority of cases, however, because of the superimposition of shadows, the radiograph plays a limited role in the differential diagnosis of ILD.

HRCT can depict the normal and abnormal interstitium with anatomic detail similar to that of gross pathologic specimens and is the imaging modality of choice in the evaluation of patients with suspected ILD.[1] In some patients, in the proper clinical context and interpreted by experts, it can provide a highly specific diagnosis, as has been shown particularly in usual interstitial pneumonia (UIP), lymphangioleiomyomatosis, Langerhans cell histiocytosis, and sarcoidosis.[2] When the findings are less specific, it provides an overall view of the pattern and distribution of disease throughout both lungs and is therefore helpful to the pathologist to determine whether the findings seen on the biopsy specimen are truly representative of the overall process. HRCT is also helpful in determining the optimal surgical biopsy site. It is recommended that the surgeon discuss with the radiologist the best sites to be biopsied in order to sample active disease and to avoid areas of end-stage lung (honeycombing), which would be nondiagnostic.[3]

The two technical modifications of CT technique that are required to optimize the spatial resolution and that define HRCT are thin sections (typically on the order of 1 mm) and image reconstruction with a high-spatial-frequency (sharp) algorithm. The thinner the section, the greater the spatial resolution. Reconstruction of the image using a high-spatial-frequency algorithm, rather than a standard algorithm, reduces image smoothing, making structures appear sharper and increasing spatial resolution. Currently, the vast majority of CT scans of the chest are performed on multidetector scanners that provide a volumetric assessment of both lungs during a single breath hold. Although HRCT images can be obtained routinely in these scanners, in many centers, the radiologists elect to reformat the images using thicker sections (typically 3 to 5 mm) and standard algorithms. These thick sections can be helpful in the assessment of a variety of conditions, but they do not provide the spatial resolution necessary for the interpretation of findings in ILD.

The differential diagnosis of ILD on the chest radiograph and HRCT is based on the pattern and distribution of abnormalities and the presence of associated findings such as lymph node enlargement or pleural effusion.[4,5] ILD results in six distinct radiologic patterns of abnormality: interlobular septal thickening, reticulation, cystic pattern, nodular pattern, ground-glass opacities, and consolidation. Each of these patterns can be visualized on HRCT and correlated with specific histopathologic findings. The appearances on the chest radiograph, on the other hand, are frequently nonspecific and sometimes misleading.[6] For example, a reticular pattern on the radiograph may result from summation of smooth or irregular linear opacities, cystic spaces, or both. Furthermore, in approximately 10% of patients with ILD, the chest radiograph is normal.[7] Because of the limitations of the radiograph, the discussion of imaging findings in ILD will focus on HRCT.

PATTERNS OF ABNORMALITY AND DIFFERENTIAL DIAGNOSIS OF ILD ON HRCT

INTERLOBULAR SEPTAL THICKENING

Normally, only a few interlobular septa can be seen on HRCT. The presence of numerous visible interlobular septa almost always indicates the presence of septal thickening by interstitial fluid, cellular infiltration, or fibrosis.

On HRCT, thickened interlobular septa are most readily seen in the lung periphery as lines 1 to 2 cm in length

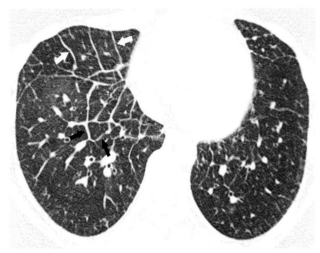

FIGURE 2.1. Interlobular septal thickening—HRCT shows thickened interlobular septa as lines 1 to 2 cm in length, separated by 1 to 2 cm, extending to the pleura (*white arrows*) and as polygonal arcades (*black arrows*) outlining secondary pulmonary lobules. The patient had interstitial pulmonary edema due to fluid overload. Lymphangitic carcinoma can also produce thickened interlobular septa (compare Fig. 2.2).

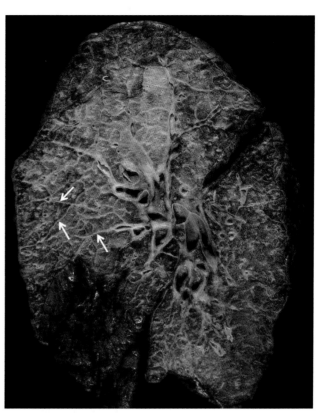

FIGURE 2.2. Interlobular septal thickening. Gross photograph of thickened interlobular septa (*arrows*) in a case of lymphangitic carcinoma.

outlining part of or an entire pulmonary lobule and extending to the pleura roughly perpendicular to the pleural surface (Fig. 2.1). Within the central lung, thickened septa outlining lobules appear as polygonal arcades (Fig. 2.1).

The most common conditions in which interlobular septal thickening is the predominant or only interstitial abnormality evident on HRCT are interstitial pulmonary edema and lymphangitic carcinomatosis (Fig. 2.2). In interstitial pulmonary edema, the septal thickening is typically smooth, whereas in lymphangitic carcinomatosis, it may be smooth or nodular. It should be noted, however, that septal thickening is also frequently seen in association with other findings. In these cases, the differential diagnosis is more complex and influenced by the pattern and distribution of the septal thickening and of the associated findings and, most importantly, by the clinical history. For example, at least some thickening of the interlobular septa is commonly evident in patients with interstitial fibrosis. In these patients, the septal thickening is typically irregular and tends to be a minor finding, the predominant abnormality being a reticular pattern.

RETICULAR PATTERN (= RETICULATION)

A reticular pattern is characterized by innumerable, interlacing linear opacities that suggest a mesh (Fig. 2.3).[8] In ILD, it usually results from irregular thickening of the interlobular septa and the presence of irregular intralobular linear opacities separated by only a few millimeters. Reticulation typically reflects thickening of the interstitium within the secondary pulmonary lobule. It is most commonly caused by fibrosis but may also be seen in a variety of other conditions. In order to suggest the presence of

fibrosis, it must be associated with distortion of the parenchymal architecture, traction bronchiectasis, and traction bronchiolectasis. Architectural distortion is characterized by abnormal displacement of bronchi, vessels, interlobar fissures, or interlobular septa. Traction bronchiectasis and bronchiolectasis, respectively, represent irregular bronchial and bronchiolar dilatation caused by surrounding retractile pulmonary fibrosis (Figs. 2.4 and 2.5).[8]

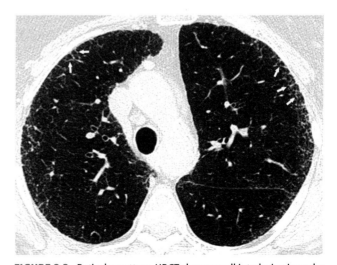

FIGURE 2.3. Reticular pattern. HRCT shows small interlacing irregular lines (*arrows*) separated by only a few millimeters in the periphery of both lungs. The patient had mild UIP.

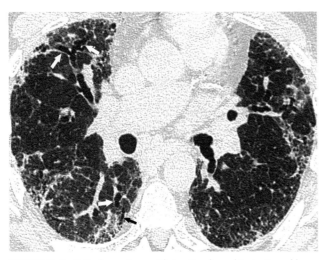

FIGURE 2.4. Reticular pattern with traction bronchiectasis and bronchiolectasis—HRCT demonstrates small interlacing irregular lines forming a reticular pattern mainly in the peripheral lung regions associated with irregular dilatation of the bronchi within areas of fibrosis (traction bronchiectasis) (*white arrows*). Dilated airways within a few millimeters from the pleura represent traction bronchiolectasis (*black arrow*). The patient had idiopathic pulmonary fibrosis with extensive interstitial fibrosis.

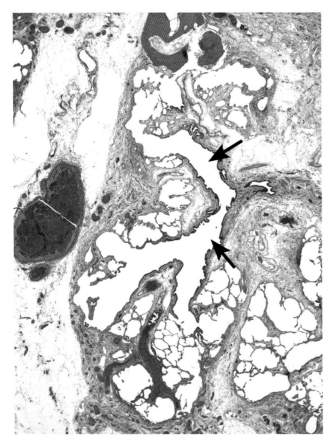

FIGURE 2.5. Microscopic appearance of traction bronchiolectasis (*arrows*) in a case of UIP. The dilated bronchioles are held open by surrounding fibrous tissue and do not narrow toward the periphery.

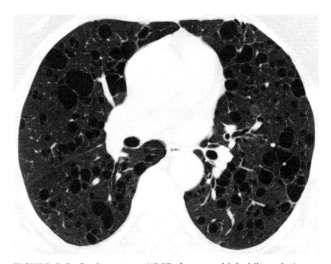

FIGURE 2.6. Cystic pattern. HRCT shows multiple bilateral circumscribed air-containing spaces ranging from a few millimeters to approximately 2 cm in diameter with fine smooth walls. The patient was a 55-year-old woman with lymphangioleiomyomatosis.

CYSTIC PATTERN AND HONEYCOMBING

A cystic pattern on HRCT refers to the presence of multiple round, air-containing parenchymal spaces with well-defined walls (Fig. 2.6).[8] The definition on CT is therefore distinct from the histologic definition of a cyst as any round circumscribed space that is surrounded by an epithelial or fibrous wall. The HRCT term is commonly used to describe enlarged thin-walled airspaces seen in patients with lymphangioleiomyomatosis (Fig. 2.7) or

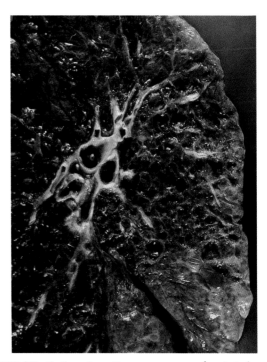

FIGURE 2.7. Cystic pattern. Gross appearance of cysts in lymphangioleiomyomatosis.

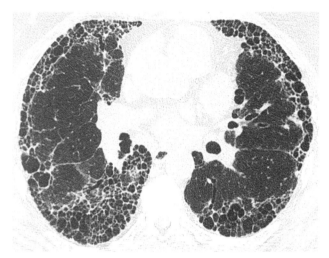

FIGURE 2.8. Honeycombing. HRCT demonstrates multiple clustered cystic air spaces with well-defined walls in the subpleural regions of both lungs. The patient had end-stage idiopathic pulmonary fibrosis.

Langerhans cell histiocytosis and to the thicker-walled honeycomb cysts seen in patients with end-stage fibrosis.

Honeycombing is characterized on HRCT by the presence of clustered cystic air spaces with thick walls and usually measuring 3 to 10 mm in diameter (Figs. 2.8 and 2.9).[8] It is usually predominantly subpleural and associated with other findings of fibrosis including reticulation, traction bronchiectasis, and traction bronchiolectasis.

NODULAR PATTERN

A nodular pattern in ILD is characterized by the presence of numerous round opacities measuring less than 1 cm in diameter. It results from expansion of the parenchymal interstitium by a roughly spherical cellular infiltrate, fibrous tissue, or both. On HRCT, the distribution of the nodules can be classified into three types: perilymphatic, centrilobular, and random.[8]

A perilymphatic distribution on HRCT is characterized by a predominance along the lymphatic route in lungs, that is, along the pleura, interlobular septa, airways, and vessels (Fig. 2.10). ILDs characterized by a perilymphatic distribution include sarcoidosis (Fig. 2.11) and lymphangitic spread of cancer.

Centrilobular nodular opacities are recognized on HRCT by their typical location a few millimeters away from the pleura, interlobar fissures, interlobular septa, major vessels, and bronchi (Fig. 2.12). They reflect the presence of bronchiolocentric ILD or bronchiolitis. Centrilobular nodules are typically seen in hypersensitivity pneumonitis and in various forms of bronchiolitis including respiratory bronchiolitis (RB), RB-ILD, and infectious bronchiolitis.

Randomly distributed nodules are those with a haphazard distribution in relation to structures of the lung and secondary lobule. Small nodules in a random distribution

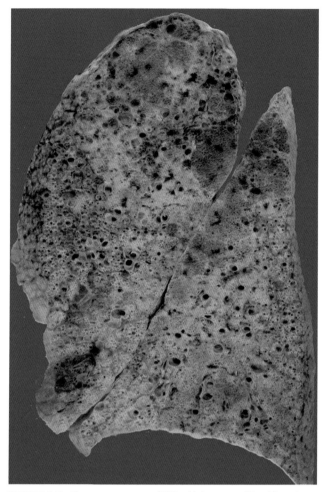

FIGURE 2.9. Gross appearance of UIP with honeycombing. There is extensive peripheral honeycombing appearing as fibrous-walled cysts under the pleura and in some areas extending deep into the lung parenchyma.

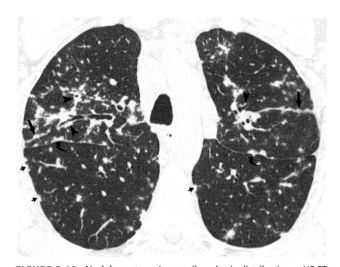

FIGURE 2.10. Nodular pattern in a perilymphatic distribution—HRCT shows bilateral small irregular nodules. The nodules are distributed mainly along the interlobular septa (*straight arrows*), interlobar fissures (*curved arrows*), costal pleura (*small arrows*), and the bronchi (*arrowheads*), characterizing a perilymphatic distribution.

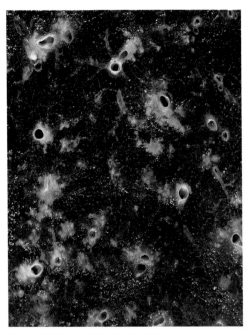

FIGURE 2.11. Gross appearance of sarcoid. Granulomas appear as small white nodules around the bronchovascular bundles.

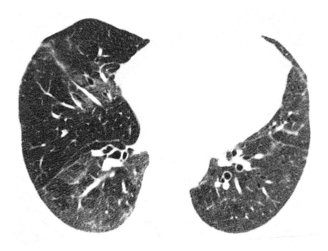

FIGURE 2.13. Ground-glass pattern—HRCT shows asymmetric bilateral areas of hazy increased opacity without obscuration of the underlying vascular margins. The patient was a 49-year-old woman with collagen vascular disease and nonspecific interstitial pneumonia.

are seen most commonly in miliary tuberculosis, miliary fungal infections, and hematogenous metastases.

GROUND-GLASS PATTERN

A ground-glass pattern consists of a hazy increase in opacity without obscuration of the underlying vascular margins (Fig. 2.13).[8] If the vessels are obscured, the term consolidation is used. Ground-glass opacity reflects the presence

of abnormalities below the resolution limit of CT. It is a common and nonspecific pattern that can result from partial filling of airspaces, interstitial thickening (due to fluid, cells, or fibrosis), partial atelectasis of alveoli, increased capillary blood volume, or a combination of these.

CONSOLIDATION

Consolidation on HRCT refers to a homogeneous increase in pulmonary parenchymal attenuation that obscures the margins of vessels and airway walls (Fig. 2.14).[8] Usually it reflects histopathologic consolidation, that is, presence of exudate or material that replaces alveolar air, rendering

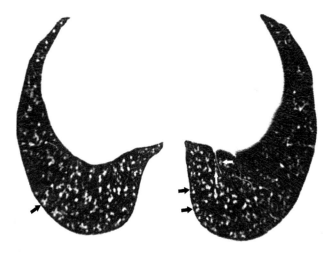

FIGURE 2.12. Nodular pattern in a centrilobular distribution—HRCT demonstrates small bilateral nodules that are clustered a few millimeters away from the pleura (*black arrows*) and the interlobular septa (*white arrows*) characterizing a centrilobular distribution. The patient was a 20-year-old woman with infectious bronchiolitis.

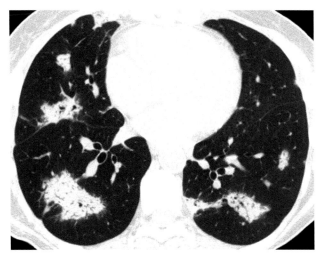

FIGURE 2.14. Consolidation—CT image demonstrates bilateral patchy areas of homogeneous increase in attenuation with obscuration of the underlying vessels. The patient was a 49-year-old woman with organizing pneumonia.

the lung solid. However, it may occasionally also result from severe interstitial disease such as may occur in sarcoidosis (pseudoalveolar sarcoid).

REFERENCES

1. Walsh SL, Hansell DM. High-resolution CT of interstitial lung disease: a continuous evolution. *Semin Respir Crit Care Med.* 2014;35:129–144.
2. Sundaram B, Chughtai AR, Kazerooni EA. Multidetector high-resolution computed tomography of the lungs: protocols and applications. *J Thorac Imaging.* 2010;25:125–141.
3. Quigley M, Hansell DM, Nicholson AG. Interstitial lung disease—the new synergy between radiology and pathology. *Histopathology.* 2006;49:334–342.
4. Jawad H, Chung JH, Lynch DA, et al. Radiological approach to interstitial lung disease: a guide for the nonradiologist. *Clin Chest Med.* 2012;33:11–26.
5. Nishino M, Itoh H, Hatabu H. A practical approach to high-resolution CT of diffuse lung disease. *Eur J Radiol.* 2014;83:6–19.
6. Grenier P, Valeyre D, Cluzel P, et al. Chronic diffuse interstitial lung disease: diagnostic value of chest radiography and high-resolution CT. *Radiology.* 1991;179:123–132.
7. Epler GR, McLoud TC, Gaensler EA, et al. Normal chest roentgenograms in chronic diffuse infiltrative lung disease. *N Engl J Med.* 1978;298:934–939.
8. Hansell DM, Bankier AA, MacMahon H, et al. Fleischner society: glossary of terms for thoracic imaging. *Radiology.* 2008;246:697–722.

Biopsy Choices and Handling in Interstitial Lung Disease

TYPES OF BIOPSIES SUITABLE FOR EVALUATING INTERSTITIAL LUNG DISEASE

Video-assisted thoracoscopic (VATS) and open lung biopsy: Low-power architecture is the key to diagnosis in many interstitial lung diseases (ILD), and the diagnostic features of ILD may be scattered within the parenchyma. This combination mandates a large biopsy, and thus the gold standard for ILD is the VATS or open lung biopsy (together often referred to as "surgical lung biopsies") because these specimens provide large areas to examine. But to be of any use, VATS and open biopsies must be of an adequate size; we suggest that the smallest diameter of an adequate biopsy should be at least 4 cm in length and 2 cm in depth. With the use of modern surgical staplers, it is common to obtain biopsies of 7 or 8 cm in length.

Core needle biopsy: Core needle biopsies are intended for the diagnosis of *mass* lesions and because, with the exceptions of nodular organizing pneumonia (OP, bronchiolitis obliterans organizing pneumonia [BOOP], cryptogenic organizing pneumonia) and Langerhans cell histiocytosis, ILDs are never mass lesions, core biopsies are generally not suitable for diagnosing ILD. Core biopsy is occasionally successful in Langerhans cell histiocytosis.[1]

Patterns that look like OP (Fig. 3.1, and see Chapter 5) can sometimes be found in core biopsies but should be reported as nonspecific because it is impossible to determine whether OP is the only lesion or represents a reaction around some other process such as a tumor or an abscess; the latter is statistically much more likely than the former (see Chapter 5).

Similarly, fibrosing interstitial pneumonias such as usual interstitial pneumonia (UIP), chronic hypersensitivity pneumonitis (HP), or fibrotic nonspecific interstitial pneumonia (NSIP) do not form masses and patterns that look like fibrotic NSIP, chronic HP, or UIP (Figs. 3.2 and 3.3, and see Chapters 6, 7, 12) should be reported as nondiagnostic. As is true of core biopsies showing OP, a core biopsy showing only old dense fibrosis might have sampled a scar but equally might well represent a fibrotic

reaction around a tumor. We advise against reporting these patterns as OP or "interstitial fibrosis" because such diagnoses are easily misinterpreted as being specific.

Transbronchial forceps biopsy: Transbronchial forceps biopsies (which we shall refer to as simply "transbronchial biopsies") in patients with putative ILD are a frequent cause of conflicts between clinicians and pathologists. Transbronchial biopsies have a limited role in this setting[2,3] and can be divided into categories of high reliability-high yield (i.e., the diagnosis made on a transbronchial biopsy is accurate and the features of interest are sufficiently frequent in the lung that they are likely to be picked up on transbronchial biopsy); high reliability-low yield (i.e., the features of interest are specific if seen but are scattered in the lung [Figs. 3.4 and 3.5] and probably will not be picked up on a transbronchial biopsy); and low reliability (i.e., the features seen in the transbronchial biopsy are probably misleading).[3] These categories are summarized in Tables 3.1 to 3.3 and Figures 3.4 to 3.9.

These rules are not absolute and need to be interpreted in context. A pattern of OP is not unusual in transbronchial biopsies (Figs. 3.6 and 3.7), but OP is seen in many settings, and whether it has any clinical meaning in a transbronchial biopsy requires consultation between the clinician, pathologist, and radiologist,[2-4] and see Chapter 5 for further information. Occasionally, subacute HP can be diagnosed on transbronchial biopsy (see Figs. 12.44 and 12.45), but only if there are classic pathologic features and the clinical and radiologic features fit HP. The finding of diffuse alveolar damage similarly may be useful in cases of acute interstitial pneumonia (AIP), but again must be viewed cautiously because a sample showing OP or diffuse alveolar damage in a transbronchial biopsy may have missed an adjacent important lesion.

In our view, transbronchial biopsies that show just interstitial inflammation (Fig. 3.8) and/or interstitial fibrosis (Fig. 3.9) have no specificity[3,4] and may be very misleading (e.g., Fig. 3.8). The problem is exacerbated by the collapse artifacts usually present in transbronchial biopsies, artifacts that can produce a false impression of interstitial

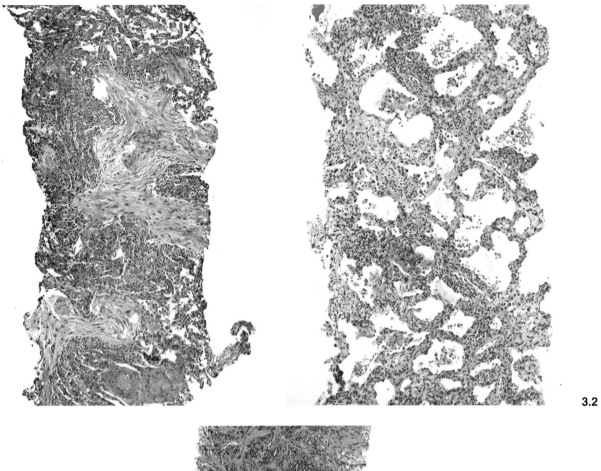

3.1

3.2

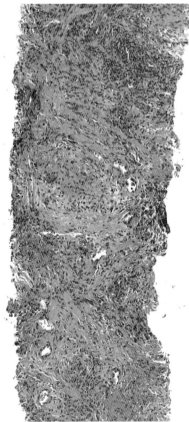

3.3

FIGURES 3.1 to 3.3. Mimics of ILD in core needle biopsies. **Figure 3.1** shows a pattern of OP, **Figure 3.2** shows a pattern mimicking cellular NSIP, and **Figure 3.3** shows dense fibrosis with chronic inflammation. Core needle biopsies are designed for the diagnosis of mass lesions, and none of the patterns illustrated here has any significance. We advise reporting these patterns as "nonspecific findings" to avoid misinterpretation.

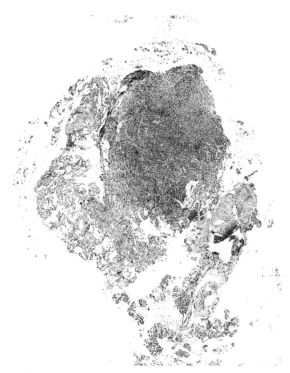
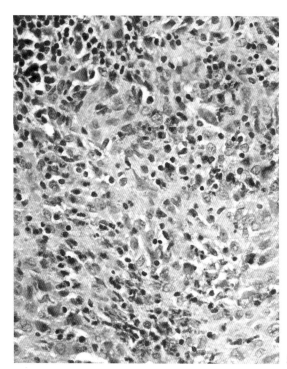

3.4

3.5

FIGURES 3.4 and 3.5. Low- and high-power views of Langerhans cell histiocytosis in a transbronchial biopsy. Transbronchial biopsy occasionally works for ILD when as here, a specific lesion is diagnostic if found.

fibrosis, and by inclusion of bronchial wall, which, depending on the cut, may also mimic interstitial fibrosis.

We recommend reporting such biopsies as nondiagnostic and we advise against putting terms such as "chronic interstitial inflammation" or "interstitial fibrosis"

in the diagnosis line because these words tend to be interpreted by clinicians as diagnostic of an ILD.

The 2011 UIP/idiopathic pulmonary fibrosis (IPF) guidelines[5] made a general recommendation against the use of transbronchial biopsy for diagnosing UIP/IPF,

Table 3.1
High reliability-high yield diagnoses on transbronchial biopsy

Malignancies

Transplant rejection

Sarcoid

Infections (with culture results)

Table 3.2
High reliability-low yield diagnoses on transbronchial biopsy

Langerhans cell histiocytosis

Alveolar proteinosis

Lymphangioleiomyomatosis

Chronic eosinophilic pneumonia

Any process in which a small but very specific feature is diagnostic

Table 3.3
Low reliability diagnoses on transbronchial biopsy

1. Idiopathic interstitial pneumonias
   - UIP
   - Desquamative interstitial pneumonia/respiratory bronchiolitis with interstitial lung disease/RBF (Respiratory bronchiolitis with fibrosis)
   - NSIP
   - OP (occasionally accurate in correct clinical/radiologic setting)
2. Processes resembling idiopathic interstitial pneumonias
   - Some pneumoconioses such as asbestosis
   - Interstitial pneumonia-like drug reactions
3. HP
   - Occasionally diagnosis can be made on transbronchial biopsy in correct clinical/radiologic setting
4. ARDS/AIP
   - Occasionally diagnosis can be made on transbronchial biopsy in correct clinical/radiologic setting
5. Any process that depends on a low-power architectural diagnosis

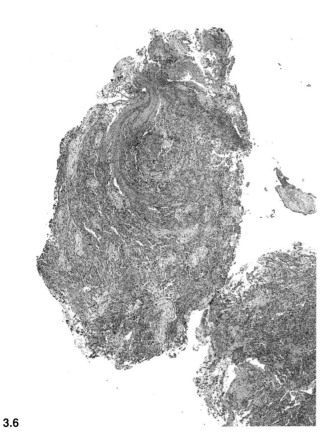

3.6

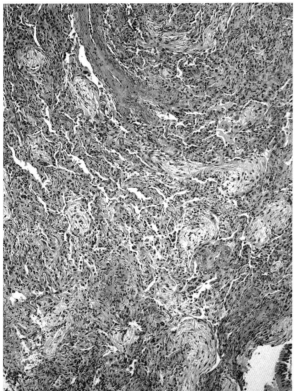

3.7

FIGURES 3.6 and 3.7. Low- and high-power views of OP in a transbronchial biopsy. OP in a transbronchial biopsy may be diagnostic if the clinical and imaging findings fit, but more often it is a nonspecific reaction pattern that can be found as a part of other lesions.

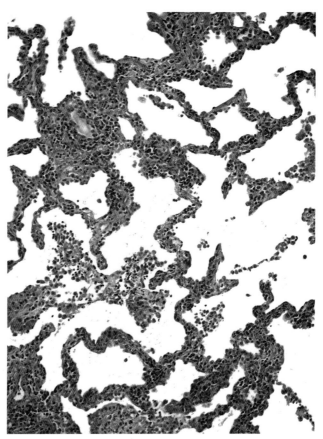

FIGURE 3.8. Chronic interstitial inflammation in a transbronchial biopsy. This finding is almost always nonspecific and should not be diagnosed as chronic interstitial inflammation. The present example is taken from the edge of a nodular lesion of Wegener granulomatosis, a condition that is not any form of ILD.

and this recommendation has been maintained in the 2018 guidelines.[6] Nonetheless, there are some who believe that transbronchial biopsies can be used, at least occasionally, to diagnose UIP/IPF[7] in the context of a conclusion from multidisciplinary discussion that the patient probably has UIP on clinical and radiologic criteria. However, even in this setting, transbronchial biopsy is very unlikely to allow separation of UIP from chronic HP[8] (see Chapters 5 and 12), diseases that can be morphologically, clinically, and radiologically similar but which require different treatments.

It has also been proposed[9] that transbronchial biopsies can be used to provide material for classification of ILD, and particularly UIP versus other ILD, by genomic analysis. This approach may become useful in the future, but, at present, is only an investigational tool.

Transbronchial cryobiopsy: Transbronchial cryobiopsy is performed by inserting a flexible cryoprobe of about 2 mm diameter through a bronchoscope. The probe is rapidly cooled for a few seconds and then withdrawn with any attached tissue.[10]

The potential advantages of cryobiopsy are as follows: (1) The tissue sample can be much larger than can

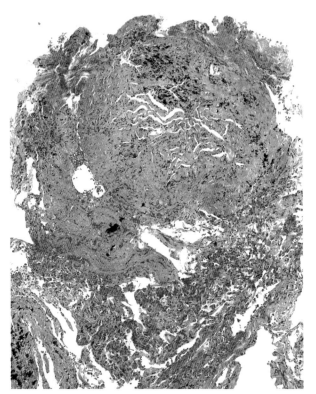

FIGURE 3.9. Fibrosis in a transbronchial biopsy. This finding is always nonspecific and should not be called "interstitial fibrosis" least it be misinterpreted as a form of ILD. In this case, deeper sections showed that the fibrosis is actually part of the bronchial wall.

be obtained by conventional forceps transbronchial biopsy (Fig. 3.10). Pieces with diameters larger than 0.5 cm and areas as high as 64 mm^2 have been reported, although there is considerable operator variability, and, in practice, pieces

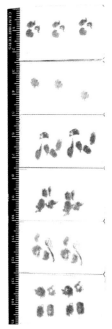

FIGURE 3.10. Size comparison of a series of successive cryobiopsies. (Courtesy Dr. Thomas Colby.)

are often much smaller than these numbers.[10] (2) Unlike conventional forceps biopsy, the tissue is not collapsed and is therefore often much easier to interpret (Fig. 3.11). (3) If accurate, cryobiopsy may avoid a VATS biopsy, a procedure that has a low but real risk of mortality. The procedural disadvantage of cryobiopsy is the relatively high frequency of significant pulmonary hemorrhage that may be life-threatening and also a fairly high incidence of pneumothorax.[11]

A recent review claims that cryobiopsy in ILD has a diagnostic yield of around 80% in ILD,[12] but this number is probably misleading. For some diseases where a specific lesion is diagnostic, for example, OP, amyloidosis, or Langerhans cell histiocytosis, cryobiopsy can certainly provide an accurate diagnosis if the lesion of interest is sampled.[13] However, when it comes to diseases defined largely by low-power architecture (Fig. 3.11), the existing data are problematic (reviewed in Johannson et al.[11]). For example, Fruchter et al.[14] reported a specific diagnosis in 73 of 75 patients, but in 22 of them the cryobiopsy was reported as "interstitial fibrosis" and in another 2 as normal, so that the actual specific diagnosis rate was 68%.

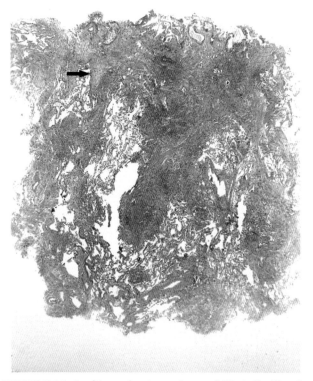

FIGURE 3.11. Cryobiopsy showing a picture of UIP. A fibroblast focus is present at the *arrow*. Note relatively well inflated parenchyma. Although this image looks like UIP, it is not clear how accurate cryobiopsies may be in separating UIP from chronic HP with a UIP pattern. (Reprinted from Colby TV, Tomassetti S, Cavazza A, et al. Transbronchial cryobiopsy in diffuse lung disease: update for the pathologist. *Arch Pathol Lab Med.* 2017;141:891–900 with permission from Archives of Pathology & Laboratory Medicine. Copyright 2017 College of American Pathologists.)

In addition, claims about the diagnostic accuracy for fibrosing interstitial pneumonias such as UIP are largely unproven. One small study[15] directly compared cryobiopsy and VATS biopsy in the same patient with a reported concordance in 12/13 cases. However, a more recent report examining cryobiopsy and VATS biopsy in 21 patients with ILD found pathologic agreement between the two types of specimen in only 38% of cases, and the agreement rate between the biopsy diagnosis and the multidisciplinary discussion diagnosis was considerably higher for VATS biopsy than cryobiopsy; in fact in 11 of 21 patients, the VATS biopsy diagnosis lead to a different treatment than would have been applied on the basis of the cryobiopsy.[16]

For some architectural problems such as separating UIP from chronic HP, where there can be considerable morphologic overlap and the presence of peribronchiolar fibrosis is important (see Chapter 12), cryobiopsies may still be too small to be useful. We suggest that considerable caution should be exercised in reporting cryobiopsies when low-power architecture is the major diagnostic criterion.

HANDLING VATS AND OPEN LUNG BIOPSIES

Collapsed lung parenchyma makes interpretation of surgical lung biopsies difficult (Figs. 3.12 and 3.13) and produces a false appearance of interstitial inflammation or can even mimic diffuse interstitial fibrosis (see Figs. 24.30 to 24.33). As noted above, collapse cannot be avoided in transbronchial biopsies, which is another reason that such biopsies are often unsuitable for diagnosing interstitial lung disease. However, misinterpretation related to parenchymal collapse can be avoided by inflating VATS and open biopsies (Fig. 3.14), and we recommend that all such biopsies should be routinely inflated with fixative using a small syringe[17] (Table 3.4). Inflation of VATS biopsies has been explicitly recommended in the latest American Thoracic Society/European Respiratory Society UIP guidelines.[6] The needle can be pushed through the pleura anywhere; if the biopsy encompasses an interlobular septum, only a portion of the specimen may inflate, but simply moving the needle solves this problem. After inflation, the whole specimen is put into fixative.

To use this technique, the specimen must be received *fresh* from the operating room because even short fixation will prevent subsequent inflation. After inflation, the fixation time can be of any duration, from 1 hour to overnight. Because low-power architecture is the key to the diagnosis of many ILDs, the biopsy should be cut to give the largest face that can be blocked and cut; avoid mincing the biopsy into small fragments because small fragments obscure low-power architecture.

Although the number/site and size of VATS biopsies is not, *per se*, within the purview of the pathologist, it is worth discussing this topic with the thoracic surgeon.

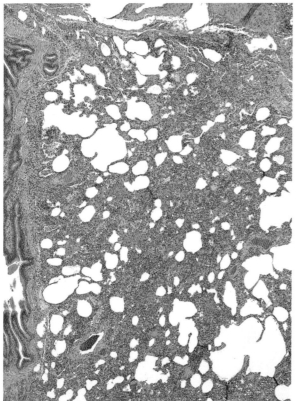
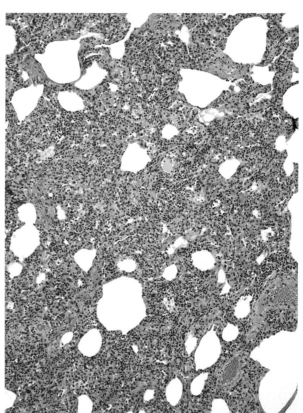

3.12

3.13

FIGURES 3.12 and 3.13. A completely collapsed surgical lung biopsy. The circular airspaces are a hint that the biopsy is collapsed (see Chapter 24). The biopsy is uninterpretable. We advise inflating all surgical lung biopsies using the method described in the text to avoid this problem.

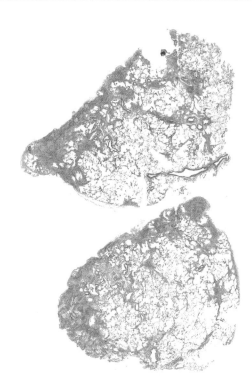

FIGURE 3.14. An inflated surgical lung biopsy. The diagnosis of UIP is readily apparent, even at scanning power.

VATS biopsies should be of an adequate size, at a minimum around 4 cm in length and 2 cm in depth.[6] A single VATS biopsy may well sample only honeycombing and thus prevent definitive diagnosis; as well, biopsies from different lobes may show different patterns, for example in chronic HP where one lobe may look like UIP but another lobe has characteristic peribronchiolar fibrosis (see Figs. 12.33 and 12.34). The solution to this problem is to routinely biopsy two or three different lobes if not contraindicated by the clinical situation, and biopsy of more than one site is recommended in the latest IPF guidelines.[6]

HANDLING FROZEN SECTIONS OF ILD BIOPSIES

In general, we advise against frozen sections of ILD because interpretation of collapsed lung in frozen sections is extremely difficult; the two exceptions to this rule are patients

Table 3.4
Procedure for inflating VATS and open lung biopsies
Specimen must be received fresh from the operating room.
Inflate gently with fixative using a small syringe and small (20G or smaller) needle.
Put inflated specimen into fixative for 1 hour minimum.
Cut to give the largest blockable face.

with AIP/ARDS and very fibrotic ILD, since in both of those conditions the parenchyma tends not to collapse. However, if a frozen section is absolutely necessary, the wedge should be inflated in a fashion similar to that described in Table 3.4, but with a 50:50 mixture of OCT™ or similar frozen section medium and saline (straight OCT will not go through a needle).[18] A portion of the specimen can then be frozen and cut and the remainder is put directly into fixative. This approach avoids collapse artifacts, which are even more difficult to interpret in frozen sections than in paraffin sections.

HANDLING WEDGES AND WHOLE LOBES/LUNGS

Most large wedge biopsies are intended for the diagnosis of neoplasms, as are most lobectomies and pneumonectomies, except, of course, explanted lungs from transplantation. Such specimens may harbor an ILD, and we believe that all should be inflated, whether for neoplastic or nonneoplastic lung disease, because collapse artifacts produce just as many interpretation problems in large as in small specimens. Where a suitable bronchus is present, inflation through the bronchus with a tube and plastic nipple connected to a tank of fixative works well; after inflation, the bronchus is clamped and the whole specimen is put into fixative. For wedges without a bronchus, a 50-cc syringe and a large bore (14G to 18G) needle can be used, putting the needle through the pleura in as many places as necessary to get the whole specimen inflated. No specific inflation pressure is required. Resected specimens generally should be fixed overnight and then breadloafed (see Figs. 2.2 and 2.9).

REFERENCES

1. Mukhopadhyay S, Eckardt SM, Scalzetti EM. Diagnosis of pulmonary Langerhans cell histiocytosis by CT-guided core biopsy of lung: a report of three cases. *Thorax*. 2010;65:833–835.
2. Raghu G, Rochwerg B, Zhang Y, et al.; American Thoracic Society; European Respiratory society; Japanese Respiratory Society; Latin American Thoracic Association. An Official ATS/ERS/JRS/ALAT Clinical Practice Guideline: treatment of idiopathic pulmonary fibrosis. An update of the 2011 clinical practice guideline. *Am J Respir Crit Care Med*. 2015;192:e3–e19.
3. Churg A. Lung biopsy, lung resection, and autopsy lung specimens: handling and diagnostic limitations. In: Churg A, Myers J, Tazelaar H, Wright JL, eds. *Thurlbeck's Pathology of the Lung*. 3rd ed. New York, NY: Thieme Medical Publishers; 2005:95–108.
4. Wall CP, Gaensler EA, Carrington CB, et al. Comparison of transbronchial and open biopsies in chronic infiltrative lung diseases. *Am Rev Respir Dis*. 1981;123:280–285.
5. Raghu G, Collard HR, Egan JJ, et al.; ATS/ERS/JRS/ALAT Committee on Idiopathic Pulmonary Fibrosis. An official ATS/ERS/JRS/ALAT statement: idiopathic pulmonary fibrosis:

evidence-based guidelines for diagnosis and management. *Am J Respir Crit Care Med.* 2011;183:788–824.

6. Raghu G, Remy-Jardin M, Myers JL, et al. American Thoracic Society, European Respiratory Society, Japanese Respiratory Society, and Latin American Thoracic Society. Diagnosis of idiopathic pulmonary fibrosis. An Official ATS/ERS/JRS/ALAT Clinical Practice Guideline. *Am J Respir Crit Care Med.* 2018;198:e44–e68.

7. Sheth JS, Belperio JA, Fishbein MC, et al. Utility of transbronchial vs surgical lung biopsy in the diagnosis of suspected fibrotic interstitial lung disease. *Chest.* 2017;151:389–399.

8. Wells AU, Antoniou KM. The genomic detection of usual interstitial pneumonia from transbronchial biopsy tissue: a dress rehearsal for the future? *Ann Am Thorac Soc.* 2017;14:1632–1633.

9. Pankratz DG, Choi Y, Imtiaz U, et al. Usual interstitial pneumonia can be detected in transbronchial biopsies using machine learning. *Ann Am Thorac Soc.* 2017;14:1646–1654.

10. Colby TV, Tomassetti S, Cavazza A, et al. Transbronchial cryobiopsy in diffuse lung disease: update for the pathologist. *Arch Pathol Lab Med.* 2017;141:891–900.

11. Johannson KA, Marcoux VS, Ronksley PE, et al. Diagnostic yield and complications of transbronchial lung cryobiopsy for interstitial lung disease. A systematic review and meta-analysis. *Ann Am Thorac Soc.* 2016;13:1828–1838.

12. Iftikhar IH, Alghothani L, Sardi A, et al. Transbronchial lung cryobiopsy and video-assisted thoracoscopic lung biopsy in the diagnosis of diffuse parenchymal lung disease. A meta-analysis of diagnostic test accuracy. *Ann Am Thorac Soc.* 2017;14:1197–1211.

13. Ussavarungsi K, Kern RM, Roden AC, et al. Transbronchial cryobiopsy in diffuse parenchymal lung disease: retrospective analysis of 74 cases. *Chest.* 2017;151:400–408.

14. Fruchter O, Fridel L, El Raouf BA, et al. Histological diagnosis of interstitial lung diseases by cryo-transbronchial biopsy. *Respirology.* 2014;19:683–688.

15. Hagmeyer L, Theegarten D, Treml M, et al. Validation of transbronchial cryobiopsy in interstitial lung disease—interim analysis of a prospective trial and critical review of the literature. *Sarcoidosis Vasc Diffuse Lung Dis.* 2016;33:2–9.

16. Romagnoli M, Colby TV, Berthet JP, et al. Poor concordance between sequential transbronchial lung cryobiopsy and surgical lung biopsy in the diagnosis of diffuse interstitial lung diseases. *Am J Respir Crit Care Med.* 2019;199(10):1249–1256.

17. Churg A. An inflation procedure for open lung biopsies. *Am J Surg Pathol.* 1983;7:69–71.

18. Gianoulis M, Chan N, Wright JL. Inflation of lung biopsies for frozen section. *Mod Pathol.* 1988;1:357–358.

Acute Interstitial Pneumonia

NOMENCLATURE ISSUES

To a clinician "acute lung injury" is a mild form of acute respiratory distress syndrome (ARDS), although this terminology is now obsolete (Table 4.1 and see below). However, "acute lung injury" had also been proposed by Katzenstein[1] as a way of referring to both diffuse alveolar damage (DAD), the pathologic finding in acute interstitial pneumonia (AIP) and many cases that are clinically ARDS, and organizing pneumonia (OP, also called bronchiolitis obliterans organizing pneumonia [BOOP] or cryptogenic organizing pneumonia [COP], see Chapter 5).

Some pathologists diagnose "acute lung injury" on biopsies, but we advise avoiding "acute lung injury" as a pathologic term for two reasons: (1) it confuses the clinicians and (2) the clinical and radiologic features as well as the prognosis and treatment of ARDS/AIP/DAD and OP are quite different. Although there are morphologic overlaps sometimes, for the most part DAD and OP can be separated microscopically (see below). In a relatively rare situation where the separation is unclear on biopsy, consultation with a radiologist usually solves the problem because OP tends to appear as predominately peribronchovascular and peripheral consolidation (see Figs. 5.1 and 5.2), whereas DAD on imaging typically results in widespread ground-glass opacities and dependent consolidation (see section Imaging Features). As well the clinical story is different: DAD usually has a very acute course, abrupt onset, and severe hypoxemia, whereas BOOP typically has a time course of a few weeks to a few months and usually is accompanied by systemic symptoms such as fever but modest levels of hypoxemia.

The older clinical term "acute lung injury" has now been replaced by a grading scheme[2] in which the severity of ARDS is determined by the ratio of PaO_2/FiO_2 (partial pressure of O_2 in arterial blood/fraction of inspired O_2), and these definitions can be applied to AIP as well (Table 4.1).

DEFINITION

Historically, AIP was first described by Hamman and Rich in the 1930s and for many years there was confusion between what was called "Hamman-Rich syndrome" and UIP.[3] The modern term "acute interstitial pneumonia" was coined by Katzenstein et al.[4]

At the simplest level, AIP is just idiopathic ARDS; that is ARDS (specifically pathologic DAD) in a patient who has no known predisposing cause. However, many patients ultimately diagnosed as AIP present with a history of a preceding upper respiratory infection (URI), and it is likely that most cases of AIP are manifestations of a respiratory viral infection. Apart from the history, AIP cannot be separated on clinical, radiologic, or pathologic grounds from ARDS/DAD of any other cause (Table 4.2).

In recent years, there has been a tendency to use the term AIP for disease in patients who develop a typical clinical picture of ARDS/DAD but have a known cause such as licit or illicit drugs,[5,6] exposure to environmental agents,[7] and even in catastrophic antiphospholipid antibody syndrome with pulmonary involvement.[8] In our view, this usage invalidates the whole idea of AIP as an idiopathic process (i.e., there is no longer a distinction between AIP

Table 4.1
Past and current definitions of severity of ARDS by PaO_2/FiO_2
American European Consensus Conference 1994 Acute lung injury: $PaO_2/FiO_2 < 300$ mm Hg ARDS: $PaO_2/FiO_2 < 200$ mm Hg
Berlin Criteria 2012[2] Mild ARDS: PaO_2/FiO_2 200 to ≤ 300 mm Hg Moderate ARDS: PaO_2/FiO_2 100 to ≤ 200 mm Hg Severe ARDS: $PaO_2/FiO_2 \leq 100$ mm Hg

Table 4.2

Causes of a pathologic picture of DAD

Idiopathic = "acute interstitial pneumonia"
Infections
  • Sepsis (usually Gram negative bacteria)
  • Viral, fungal, pneumocystis pneumonias
  • Severe bacterial pneumonia
Aspiration of gastric contents (acid)
Inhalation of toxic gases
  • Smoke, oxygen, many fumes, and chemicals
Shock
Lung trauma, head trauma
Metabolic disorders
  • Pancreatitis, uremia
High exposure to a sensitizing agent
  • Acute eosinophilic pneumonia
Drug reactions
Fat and amniotic fluid emboli
Connective tissue disease (e.g., "lupus pneumonitis")
Near drowning
IV or lymphatic contrast material
Diffuse pulmonary hemorrhage (sometimes associated
  with a clinical picture of ARDS)

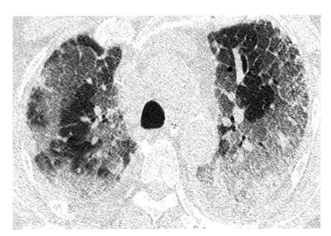

FIGURE 4.1. Acute interstitial pneumonia. HRCT image at the level of the upper lobes demonstrates almost complete whiteout of both lungs. The abnormalities consist of extensive bilateral ground-glass opacities and patchy areas of consolidation involving mainly the dependent lung regions. The patient was an 86-year-old man.

and ARDS) and may be detrimental to patient care, because discontinuance of the drug or removal from exogenous exposure is clearly important in preventing recurrent disease in such patients. When DAD is present in a biopsy and the etiology is known, such cases should instead be labeled "diffuse alveolar damage secondary to...."

CLINICAL FEATURES

Patients with AIP present with severe hypoxemic respiratory failure, sometimes developing over a few weeks after a URI; however, the severe shortness of breath typically develops over a few days. By definition, such patients neither have evidence of a (provable) infection nor do they have any other condition that would predispose to ARDS.[9]

IMAGING FEATURES

The findings are those of DAD.[10] The acute or exudative phase is characterized on high-resolution computed tomography (HRCT) by the presence of extensive bilateral ground-glass opacities and progressive consolidation (Fig. 4.1). There is often a sharp demarcation between areas of involved and apparently normal lung resulting in a geographic appearance.[10] The consolidation may be patchy or confluent and tends to involve mainly the

dependent regions of the lower lobes (Fig. 4.1). Distortion of bronchovascular bundles and bronchial dilatation develop in the organizing phase. The fibrotic phase is characterized by the presence of reticulation, architectural distortion, traction bronchiectasis, and, in some cases, honeycombing.

PATHOLOGIC FEATURES

Although the original description of AIP[4] illustrated a pattern that mimicked an interstitial process (hence the name, and hence also the inclusion of AIP in publications on idiopathic interstitial pneumonias, see Chapter 1), cases of AIP can show any pathologic pattern seen in ordinary ARDS/DAD, and in this chapter we have illustrated both AIP and ARDS cases because they are morphologically indistinguishable.

At autopsy, lungs from cases of AIP are typically very heavy, often over 1,000 g each, very firm, and demonstrate effacement of the normal, finely granular surface seen in fixed inflated and cut lungs (Fig. 4.2).

Microscopically, AIP/DAD can be divided into acute or exudative phase, organizing or proliferative phase, and fibrotic phase (Table 4.3). The acute phase is characterized by hyaline membranes (Figs. 4.3 and 4.4) and is readily recognized, but the organizing phase shows a large number of different patterns (Figs. 4.5 to 4.17) and can be confused with OP when the picture is one of granulation tissue plugs in respiratory bronchioles and alveolar ducts (Fig. 4.7). Table 4.4 offers some clues to separating DAD and OP in the equivocal case (Figs. 4.7 to 4.10). One helpful point is that in OP the granulation tissue plugs tend to have distinct borders and are usually separated from the underlying parenchyma, whereas in

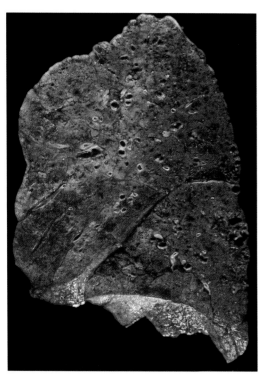

FIGURE 4.2. Gross appearance of DAD at autopsy. Note the effacement of the normal surface granularity. This lung weighed more than 1,000 g—a common finding in DAD.

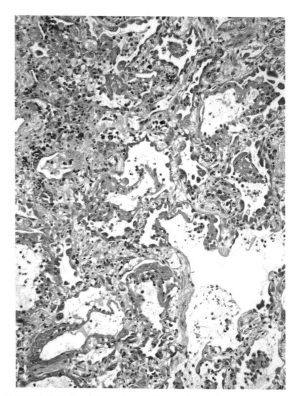

FIGURE 4.3. Exudative phase of DAD from the same case of AIP shown in Figure 1. Note the hyaline membranes and the very large reactive alveolar lining cells. There is parenchymal collapse. All the microscopic appearances illustrated in this chapter can be seen in DAD of any cause, including ARDS and AIP.

Table 4.3
Microscopic features of AIP (DAD)

Acute (exudative) phase (1–6 days after injury)
Necrosis of pneumocytes, endothelial cells
Hyaline membranes in alveolar ducts
Collapse of alveolar parenchyma
Diffuse alveolar hemorrhage in some cases
Organizing (proliferative) phase (as early as 2–3 days after injury but usually later)
Numerous morphologic patterns
Early
  • Organization of hyaline membranes
  • Formation of airspace granulation tissue
  • Squamous metaplasia
Late
  • Dense collagenization of airspace granulation tissue
  • Alveolar duct ("ring") fibrosis
  • "Interstitial pneumonia" pattern = interstitial-appearing granulation tissue secondary to parenchymal collapse
Fibrotic phase (usually after several weeks on respirator)
Cystic spaces with densely fibrotic walls

DAD the granulation tissue plugs often blend into the surrounding parenchyma (Figs. 4.8 and 4.9). However, organizing DAD can have areas that are indistinguishable from OP (Fig. 4.7).

Despite the name, the granulation tissue in AIP/ DAD is never really interstitial, but rather this appearance is an artifact caused by parenchymal collapse (Figs. 4.11 to 4.13). Squamous metaplasia is rare in OP and is a good clue that one is dealing with organizing DAD (Fig. 4.18), as is collapse of the parenchyma leaving only the respiratory bronchioles and alveolar ducts open (Fig. 4.11).

The fibrotic phase appears grossly as lungs with fibrotic but fairly thin-walled cysts (Fig. 4.19) and microscopically as cysts with fibrotic but fairly thin walls (Fig. 4.20). This pattern is only seen after weeks on a respirator and is uncommon with modern respirator settings.

DETERMINATION OF ETIOLOGY

Frequently, the clinician has a very good idea that the process in question is clinically AIP/ARDS and a biopsy

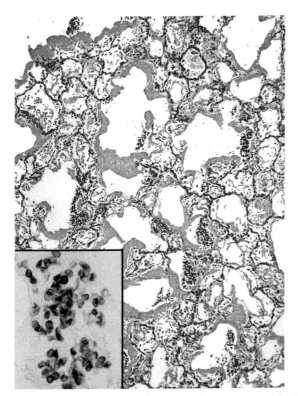

FIGURE 4.4. Early exudative phase of DAD with prominent hyaline membranes but no parenchymal collapse. This case was actually caused by pneumocystis (*inset*). We recommend staining all DAD cases with silver methenamine because pneumocystis produces no hint of its presence on hematoxylin and eosin stain.

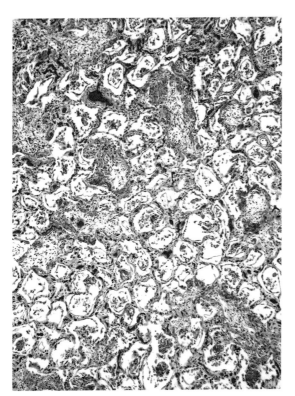

FIGURE 4.5. Early organizing phase of DAD with granulation tissue plugs in airspaces.

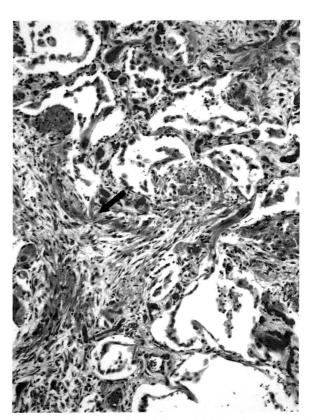

FIGURE 4.6. High-power view of Figure 4.5. Note the remnants of hyaline membranes in the granulation tissue (*arrow*).

is performed in an attempt to find a specific and hopefully treatable etiology. It should be noted that the clinical entity of ARDS encompasses more than just DAD pathologically; some cases turn out to be severe pneumonia or diffuse hemorrhage or occasionally some other process.[11] However, AIP by definition always shows DAD.[9]

Table 4.5 provides a list of pathologic findings that may indicate etiology when a biopsy shows DAD. Because pneumocystis can hide in DAD (Fig. 4.4), we suggest staining for fungal/pneumocystis in all cases, even in patients who are not known to be immunocompromised.

DIAGNOSTIC MODALITIES

Hyaline membranes may be picked up in transbronchial biopsies. Given a clinical and imaging setting of ARDS/AIP, a diagnosis of DAD is allowable, but there is always a danger that such biopsies miss evidence of an etiologic agent. Organizing DAD can be very difficult to recognize in a transbronchial biopsy and the distinction from OP may be impossible. Cryobiopsy has been reported to provide diagnostic tissue,[12] but whether cryobiopsies are large enough to identify etiologic agents is not known. Video-assisted thoracoscopic biopsies remain the gold standard.

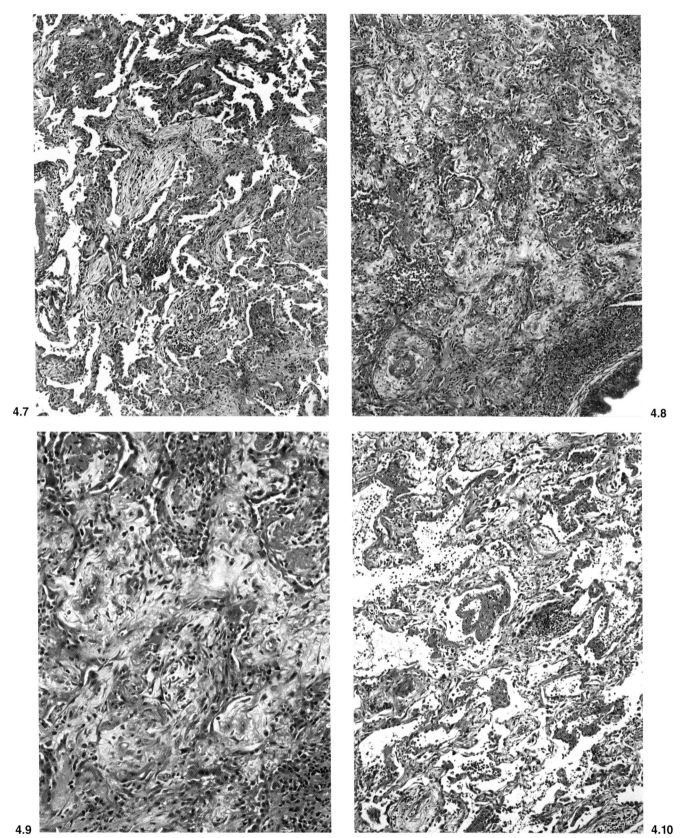

FIGURES 4.7 to 4.10. All images from the same case. **Figure 4.7**: Organizing DAD with granulation tissue plugs in alveolar ducts. Figure 4.7 is indistinguishable from OP (see Chapter 5) but **Figures 4.8 and 4.9** show a pattern of organization (granulation tissue that fades off into the surrounding parenchyma) not seen in OP, and **Figure 4.10** shows hyaline membranes. Finding areas such as Figure 4.8 or Figure 4.10 is a useful way to sort out OP from organizing DAD.

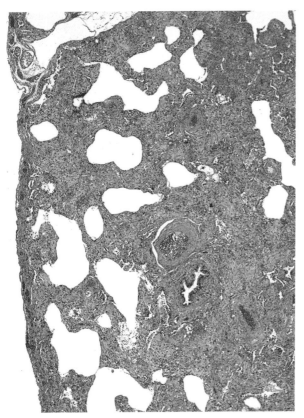

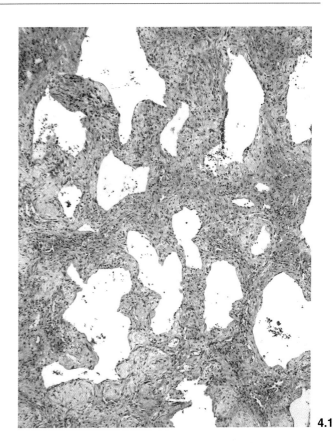

4.12

FIGURE 4.11. Parenchymal collapse in organizing DAD. This pattern is typical of DAD and helps separate organizing DAD from OP.

DIFFERENTIAL DIAGNOSIS

The differential diagnosis of AIP/ARDS/DAD is shown in Table 4.6. Acute exacerbation of UIP is the development of acute (typically within 30 days) worsening of dyspnea and the development of new diffuse pulmonary infiltrates consistent with ARDS/DAD[13,14] (Fig. 4.21), not fully explained by heart failure or fluid overload. In the past, infection and other specific etiologies such as aspiration were specifically excluded from the definition of acute exacerbation, but a more recent paradigm suggests that all etiologies should be included, in part because infection is often difficult to prove and in part because the clinical scenario is similar, no matter what the etiology.[13,14] On imaging, acute exacerbations show diffuse ground-glass opacities and/or consolidation with evidence of underlying fibrosis (Fig. 4.21). Microscopically, the acute process looks like DAD or OP superimposed on UIP[15] (Figs. 4.22 to 4.25).

In most cases of acute exacerbation, the patient is known to have underlying UIP, but sometimes UIP presents for the first time as an acute exacerbation. An important microscopic clue to the diagnosis is the presence of underlying old dense fibrosis (Figs. 4.22 and 4.24), something that is never part of DAD or OP. In a series of 58 cases of DAD on surgical lung biopsy, 12 turned out to be AIP and 7 acute exacerbations of UIP.[16]

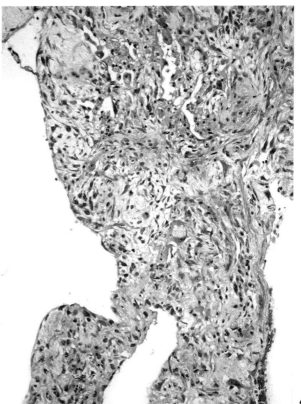

4.13

FIGURES 4.12 and 4.13. "Interstitial" pattern in a case of organizing DAD. This is the pattern originally described by Katzenstein in AIP. The interstitial pattern is actually an artifact caused by parenchymal collapse.

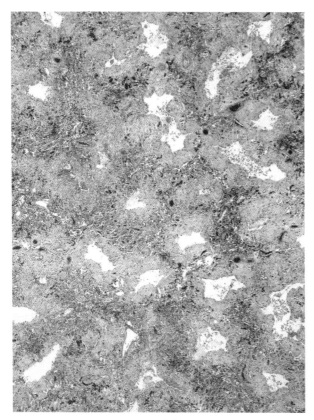

FIGURE 4.14. Organizing DAD with fibrosis of alveolar ducts. This is one of many patterns of organization of DAD.

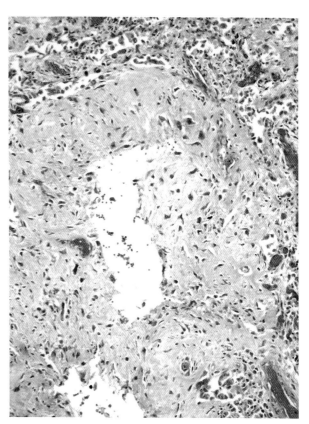

FIGURE 4.15. High-power view of Figure 4.14 showing dense fibrous tissue forming a ring around an alveolar duct. This process represents organization of hyaline membranes.

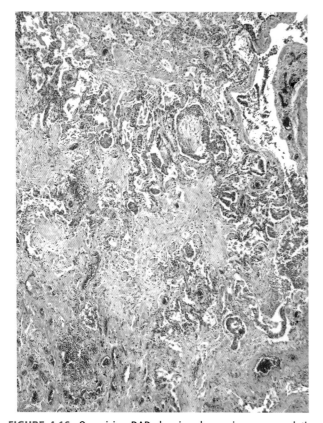

FIGURE 4.16. Organizing DAD showing dense airspace granulation tissue.

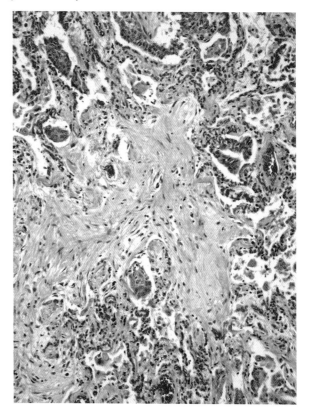

FIGURE 4.17. High-power view of Figure 4.13. Dense airspace granulation tissue is a pattern of organization of DAD and is rare in OP where the granulation tissue is typically much looser (see Chapter 5).

Table 4.4

Separation of organizing DAD (AIP/ARDS) from OP (BOOP, COP)

Organizing DAD	OP
Parenchymal collapse with dilated respiratory bronchioles and alveolar ducts	No parenchymal collapse
Hyaline membranes or remnants often present	Hyaline membranes never present
Granulation tissue may merge into surrounding parenchyma	Granulation tissue usually separated from parenchyma
Granulation tissue may appear to be interstitial	Granulation tissue always purely in alveolar ducts and respiratory bronchioles
Granulation tissue may appear dense	Granulation tissue always loose
Granulation tissue may form dense rings around alveoli ducts	Alveolar duct rings never present
Squamous metaplasia often present	Squamous metaplasia rarely present

Acute exacerbations also occasionally occur in other forms of fibrosing interstitial pneumonia, including chronic hypersensitivity pneumonitis (see Chapter 12), asbestosis (see Chapter 22), fibrotic nonspecific interstitial pneumonia (see Chapter 7), and desquamative interstitial pneumonia (see Chapter 8).[17] Additional discussion of acute exacerbations is provided in Chapter 6.

Diffuse hemorrhage is occasionally seen as part of acute DAD. However, it can also be a manifestation of vasculitis and the DAD may be secondary to the hemorrhage. The presence of hemosiderin-laden macrophages, indicating that hemorrhage has been present for several days, is suggestive of vasculitis, and the presence of capillaritis is diagnostic.

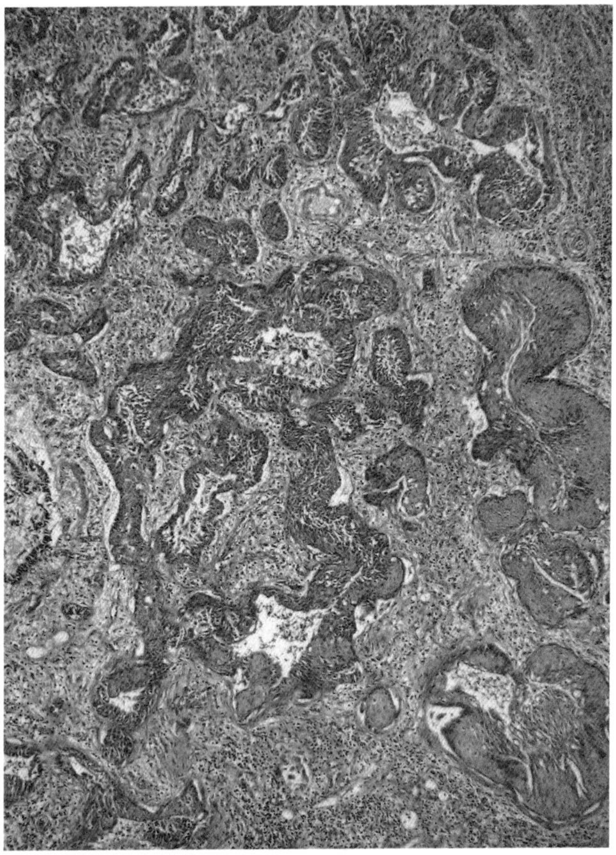

FIGURE 4.18. Extensive squamous metaplasia in organizing DAD. Squamous metaplasia in this setting can be cytologically very atypical, but the fact that metaplastic epithelium follows the outline of alveolar ducts and does not form a mass lesion is evidence against a neoplastic process.

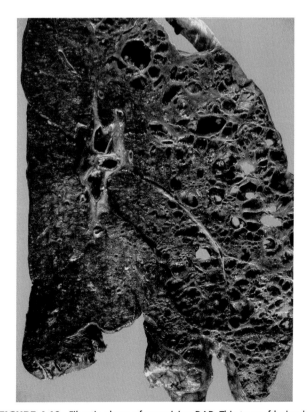

FIGURE 4.19. Fibrotic phase of organizing DAD. This type of lesion is only seen after weeks on a respirator and is rare in modern practice.

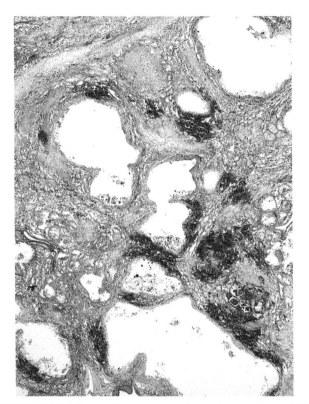

FIGURE 4.20. Microscopic appearance of case shown in Figure 4.16. Cystic spaces with dense fibrous walls somewhat mimic fibrotic nonspecific interstitial pneumonia (NSIP, see Chapter 7) but the spaces are much larger than one finds in fibrotic NSIP.

Eosinophils are ordinarily not seen in DAD, and their presence should raise a question of acute eosinophilic pneumonia (see Chapter 15) (Figs. 4.26 and 4.27). This diagnosis is important because acute eosinophilic pneumonia is the only form of DAD that responds to steroids.[17]

Table 4.5

Morphologic findings that suggest a specific etiology of DAD

Visible infectious organisms (pneumocystis, viral inclusions)

Neutrophil collections (implication: infection)

Granulomas (implication: infection, aspiration, drug reaction)

Aspirated food particles

Fat or amniotic fluid emboli

Drug-associated changes (see Chapter 18)

Foamy macrophages of amiodarone

Granulomas: methotrexate, anti-TNF agents

Eosinophils = acute eosinophilic pneumonia (see Chapter 15)

Diffuse hemorrhage plus capillaritis (implication: vasculitis)

Table 4.6

Differential diagnosis of AIP/ARDS/DAD and features that help in diagnosis

Acute stages

Acute exacerbation of UIP (presence of underlying old fibrosis) (see Chapter 6)

Connective tissue disease-associated ARDS (history/serology) (see Chapter 21)

Drug-induced ARDS (history, occasional specific morphology) (see Chapter 18)

Acute eosinophilic pneumonia (presence of eosinophils) (see Chapter 15)

Infections (infectious agent by morphology, culture, or nucleic acid amplification techniques) (Fig. 4.4)

Diffuse hemorrhage (may be part of DAD, but presence of capillaritis implies underlying vasculitis)

Fibrotic stage

Fibrotic NSIP (see Chapter 7)

PROGNOSIS

Early studies of AIP[4] indicated a very poor prognosis. Occasional reports[18] suggest that survival may be as good as 80%, but a recent review[9] concluded that the overall mortality is around 50% in the first 2 months. For ARDS, prognosis depends on the underlying condition and is worse with increasingly low PaO_2/FiO_2; the overall survival is currently 60% to 70%, but patients with sepsis, advanced age, and multiorgan failure have a worse prognosis.

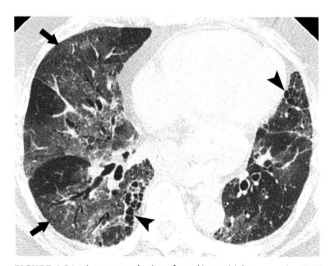

FIGURE 4.21. Acute exacerbation of usual interstitial pneumonia. HRCT shows extensive bilateral ground-glass opacities, patchy mild reticulation, and focal areas of honeycombing (*arrowheads*). Note that there is no definite evidence of fibrosis in the right middle lobe and lateral segment of the right lower lobe (*arrows*). A biopsy of these regions may therefore only show DAD without old fibrosis. The patient had acute exacerbation of usual interstitial pneumonia secondary to rheumatoid arthritis.

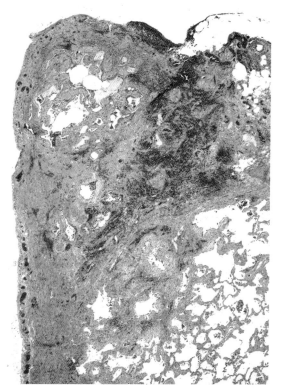

FIGURE 4.22. Acute exacerbation of UIP. This portion of the biopsy shows dense old fibrosis with honeycombing typical of UIP.

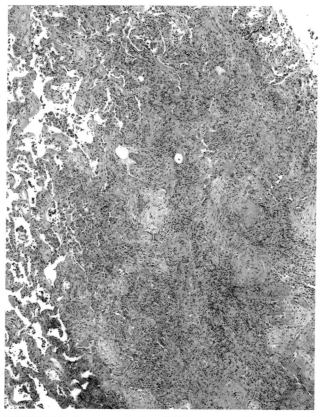

FIGURE 4.23. Acute exacerbation of UIP. Same case as Figure 4.22. This portion of the biopsy shows organizing DAD. The combination of features in Figures 4.21 and 4.22 allows a diagnosis of acute exacerbation of UIP.

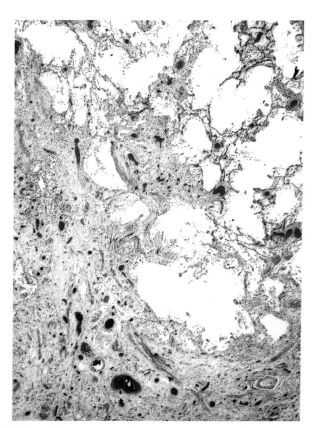

FIGURE 4.24. Acute exacerbation of UIP. Autopsy lung. This area shows a UIP pattern.

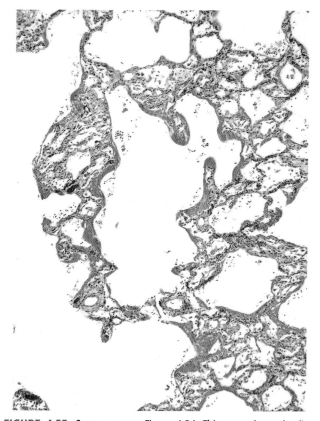

FIGURE 4.25. Same case as Figure 4.24. This area shows hyaline membranes. The combination of features in Figures 4.24 and 4.25 indicates a diagnosis of acute exacerbation of UIP.

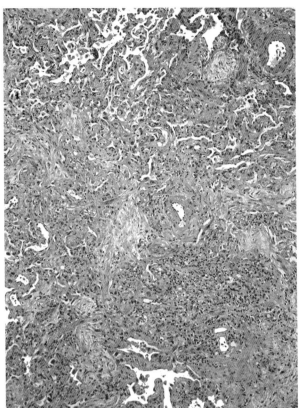

4.26

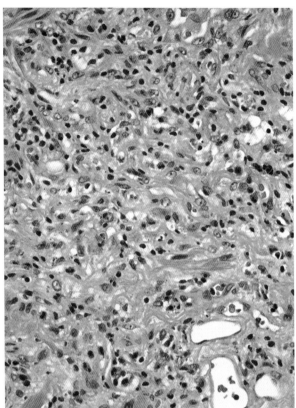

4.27

FIGURES 4.26 and 4.27. Acute eosinophilic pneumonia. Clinically the patient appeared to have ARDS. At low-power view (Fig. 4.26), the appearance is that of organizing DAD, but high-power view shows numerous eosinophils, indicating that the correct diagnosis is acute eosinophilic pneumonia. Additional images of acute eosinophilic pneumonia can be found in Chapter 15.

REFERENCES

1. Katzenstein ALA. Acute lung injury patterns: diffuse alveolar damage and bronchiolitis obliterans organizing pneumonia. In: *Katzenstein and Askin's Surgical Pathology of Non-Neoplastic Lung Disease*. 4th ed. Philadelphia, PA: Saunders Elsevier; 2006:17–50.
2. ARDS Definition Task Force, Ranieri VM, Rubenfeld GD, Thompson BT, et al. Acute respiratory distress syndrome: the Berlin definition. *JAMA*. 2012;307:2526–2533.
3. Olson J, Colby TV, Elliott CG. Hamman-Rich syndrome revisited. *Mayo Clin Proc*. 1990;65:1538–1548.
4. Katzenstein AL, Myers JL, Mazur MT. Acute interstitial pneumonia. A clinicopathologic, ultrastructural, and cell kinetic study. *Am J Surg Pathol*. 1986;10:256–267.
5. Deroux A, Buisson TT, Bernard C, et al. Acute interstitial pneumonia following heroin inhalation. *Presse Med*. 2015;44:119–121.
6. Fenocchio E, Depetris I, Campanella D, et al. Successful treatment of gemcitabine-induced acute interstitial pneumonia with imatinib mesylate: a case report. *BMC Cancer*. 2016;16:793.
7. Ohkouchi S, Ebina M, Kamei K, et al. Fatal acute interstitial pneumonia in a worker making chips from wooden debris generated by the Great East Japan earthquake and tsunami. *Respir Investig*. 2012;50:129–134.
8. Kameda T, Dobashi H, Susaki K, et al. A case of catastrophic antiphospholipid syndrome, which presented an acute interstitial pneumonia-like image on chest CT scan. *Mod Rheumatol*. 2015;25:150–153.
9. Mukhopadhyay S, Parambil JG. Acute interstitial pneumonia (AIP): relationship to Hamman-Rich syndrome, diffuse alveolar damage (DAD), and acute respiratory distress syndrome (ARDS). *Semin Respir Crit Care Med*. 2012;33:476–485.
10. Sverzellati N, Lynch DA, Hansell DM, et al. American Thoracic Society-European Respiratory Society classification of the idiopathic interstitial pneumonias: advances in knowledge since 2002. *Radiographics*. 2015;35:1849-71.
11. Thille AW, Esteban A, Fernβndez-Segoviano P, et al. Comparison of the Berlin definition for acute respiratory distress syndrome with autopsy. *Am J Respir Crit Care Med*. 2013;187:761–767.
12. Ussavarungsi K, Kern RM, Roden AC, et al. Transbronchial cryobiopsy in diffuse parenchymal lung disease: retrospective analysis of 74 cases. *Chest*. 2017;151:400–408.
13. Ryerson CJ, Cottin V, Brown KK, et al. Acute exacerbation of idiopathic pulmonary fibrosis: shifting the paradigm. *Eur Respir J*. 2015;46:512–520.
14. Collard HR, Ryerson CJ, Corte TJ, et al. Acute exacerbation of idiopathic pulmonary fibrosis. An international working group report. *Am J Respir Crit Care Med*. 2016;194:265–275.
15. Churg A, Wright JL, Tazelaar HD. Acute exacerbations of fibrotic interstitial lung disease. *Histopathology*. 2011;58:525–530.
16. Parambil JG, Myers JL, Aubry MC, et al. Causes and prognosis of diffuse alveolar damage diagnosed on surgical lung biopsy. *Chest*. 2007;132:50–57.
17. Tazelaar HD, Linz LJ, Colby TV, et al. Acute eosinophilic pneumonia: histopathologic findings in nine patients. *Am J Respir Crit Care Med*. 1997;155:296–302.
18. Suh GY, Kang EH, Chung MP, et al. Early intervention can improve clinical outcome of acute interstitial pneumonia. *Chest*. 2006;129:753–761.

Organizing Pneumonia

NOMENCLATURE ISSUES

The subject of this chapter is variably referred to as organizing pneumonia (OP), bronchiolitis obliterans organizing pneumonia (BOOP), and cryptogenic organizing pneumonia (COP). Although OP/BOOP/COP is morphologically identical to organizing bacterial pneumonia, none of these terms is entirely satisfactory, in part because currently OP/BOOP/COP only occasionally represents organization of a bacterial pneumonia, and in part because in many cases the etiology is known or suspected and is not at all related to a bacterial pneumonia.

The name "bronchiolitis obliterans organizing pneumonia" was popularized by Epler et al.[1] in their report and is itself a modification of the term "bronchiolitis obliterans with interstitial pneumonia" proposed by Liebow in the 1970s. The "bronchiolitis obliterans" portion stems from the presence of granulation tissue plugs in the lumens of respiratory bronchioles, a process originally, but no longer, thought to be part of true bronchiolitis obliterans (obliterative bronchiolitis, now called constrictive bronchiolitis, see Chapter 20).

The 2002 ATS/ERS (American Thoracic Society/European Respiratory Society) classification of the idiopathic interstitial pneumonias[2] suggested the term "organizing pneumonia" for the pathologic pattern, and "cryptogenic organizing pneumonia (COP)" rather than BOOP for the idiopathic disease. This terminology was maintained in the 2013 ATS/ERS update of the classification.[3] Although COP is more accurate in regard to idiopathic cases, our experience is that COP has not caught on, and currently there appears to be more of a tendency to simply call all such cases "organizing pneumonia." In practice, OP, BOOP, and COP often are used interchangeably and generally understood, but when reporting a biopsy, it may be advisable to use all three terms to be sure that the reader realizes that this is not actually an infectious pneumonia; for example, "Surgical lung biopsy showing organizing pneumonia (BOOP/COP)." If an etiology is known, then that etiology can be included in the pathologic diagnosis line, and the term COP can be excluded. For example, "organizing pneumonia (BOOP) secondary to aspiration" or "organizing pneumonia (BOOP) most likely representing a reaction to cyclophosphamide."

We advise against reporting OP/BOOP/COP as "acute lung injury" because this term is confusing to clinicians and conveys no prognostic or treatment information (see Chapter 4 for a discussion of this issue).

CLINICAL FEATURES

Idiopathic OP often mimics the signs and symptoms of a community-acquired pneumonia with fever, fatigue, cough, and shortness of breath and sometimes weight loss as well, but very high fevers and chills are not usually present.[4–6] Often there is a history of a preceding upper respiratory tract infection. In the majority of patients, symptoms are present for less than 2 months and sometimes for only a few weeks. Patients are usually not hypoxic and pulmonary function tests show mild to moderate restriction.

OP that is part of another pathologic process is usually overshadowed by the primary lesion; for example, OP around an abscess will typically appear clinically as an abscess.

IMAGING FEATURES

The characteristic high-resolution computed tomography (HRCT) findings of OP consist of areas of consolidation that are usually bilateral and in 60% to 80% of cases have a predominately peribronchial and/or subpleural distribution[7] (Fig. 5.1). The subpleural predominance can mimic that of chronic eosinophilic pneumonia (CEP), but

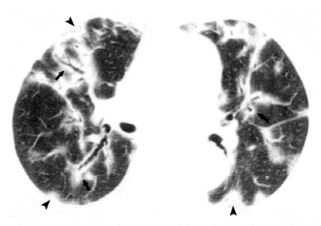

FIGURE 5.1. OP. HRCT demonstrates bilateral areas of consolidation in a peribronchial (*arrows*) and subpleural (*arrowheads*). The patient was an 81-year-old woman.

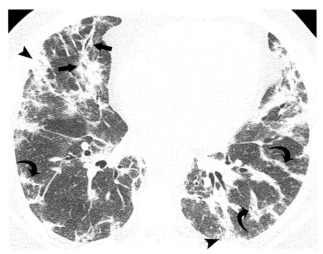

FIGURE 5.2. OP. HRCT shows bilateral areas of consolidation that involve mainly the subpleural (*arrowheads*), peribronchial (*straight arrows*), and perilobular (*curved arrows*) regions. The patient had OP secondary to polymyositis.

consolidation in a peribronchial distribution is highly suggestive of OP.[8] The consolidation often also has a characteristic perilobular distribution, that is along the periphery of the secondary lobules adjacent to the interlobular septa, resulting in a polygonal appearance[7,8] (Fig. 5.2). Although ground-glass opacities are present in the majority of cases, they usually occur in association with areas of consolidation and are seldom the predominant finding.

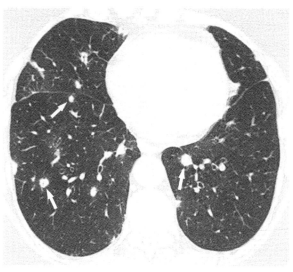

FIGURE 5.4. Nodular OP. HRCT demonstrates several bilateral nodules (*arrows*) and minimal areas of peribronchial and subpleural consolidation.

PATHOLOGIC FEATURES

Grossly OP appears as raised gray areas of lung that are more or less contiguous (Fig. 5.3) or less commonly as nodules on imaging and pathologic examination (Figs. 5.4 and 5.5). The microscopic features of OP are summarized in Table 5.1 and illustrated in Figures 5.6 to 5.11. The fundamental finding is granulation tissue plugs in the lumens

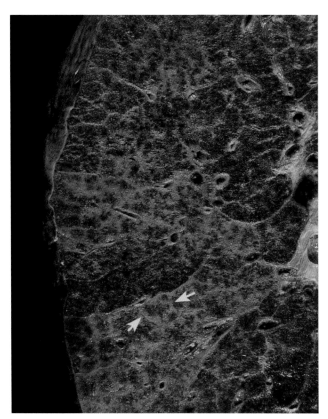

FIGURE 5.3. Gross appearance of OP. Note sparing of some lobules (*arrows*), the same pattern as may be seen on CT.

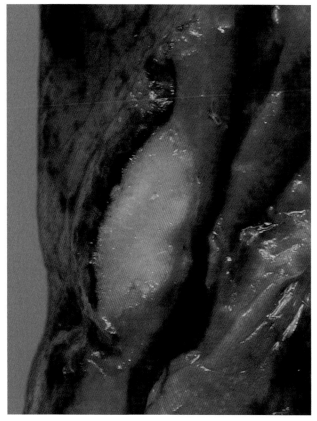

FIGURE 5.5. Gross appearance of nodular OP. (Case courtesy Dr. John English.)

Table 5.1

Pathologic features of OP

Granulation tissue plugs in respiratory bronchioles and alveolar ducts

Granulation tissue plugs typically are separated from the underlying lung tissue

Process often appears to spread from respiratory bronchioles

Variable interstitial infiltrate of chronic inflammatory cells

Reactive alveolar lining cells usually present

Process is temporally homogeneous

Underlying lung architecture preserved

No true old fibrosis or honeycombing

---

of respiratory bronchioles and alveolar ducts with a variable but typically mild accompanying chronic interstitial inflammatory infiltrate.

Two points that are important to note in OP are the homogeneity of the process and the absence of underlying old fibrosis or architectural distortion. Idiopathic OP by definition cannot have another lesion present. If extensive old dense fibrosis is present, then OP has been superimposed on some pre-existing fibrotic process. However, OP can occasionally organize to dense collagen in various patterns, a process that has been termed cicatricial OP (see below).

Small foci of OP are common in many types of interstitial lung disease (ILD) such as nonspecific interstitial pneumonia (NSIP, see Chapter 7) and hypersensitivity pneumonitis (HP, see Chapter 12), and in these settings the presence of OP is ignored when making a diagnosis. However, if large amounts of OP are present along with another defined ILD, then both components should be diagnosed; for example, the combination of OP plus NSIP is common in patients with collagen vascular disease (see Chapter 21). OP superimposed on usual interstitial pneumonia (UIP) frequently represents an acute exacerbation of UIP (see Chapters 4 and 6).

PATHOLOGIC VARIANTS OF OP

Nodular OP

Most cases of OP have irregular margins when viewed grossly (Fig. 5.3) and microscopically, but occasionally OP is distinctly nodular on imaging, grossly, and microscopically (Figs. 5.4, 5.5, and 5.8). Nodular OP can present as a solitary or multiple nodules on imaging.[9]

Biopsies at the Edge of OP Lesions

Biopsies that sample the edge of a lesion of OP can be very confusing pathologically, because OP is always associated with some degree of chronic interstitial inflammation

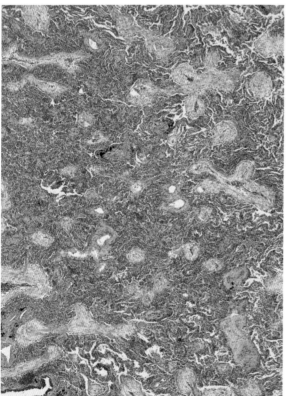
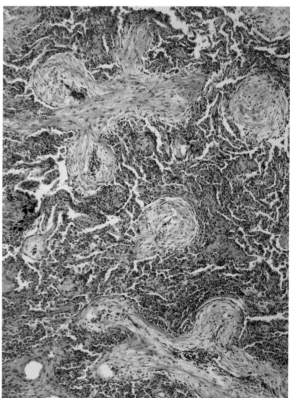

5.6   5.7

FIGURES 5.6 and 5.7. Low- and high-power microscopic views of OP. Note the absence of old fibrosis or architectural distortion. The high-power view shows the typical branching appearance of the granulation tissue plugs and the mild interstitial inflammatory infiltrate, something that is invariably present in OP.

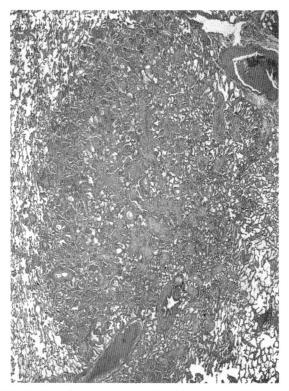

FIGURE 5.8. A low-power view of nodular OP. In nodular OP, the process is sharply circumscribed and can appear as a nodule on imaging, whereas in most examples of OP, the process fades off into the surrounding parenchyma.

(Figs. 5.7, 5.10, and 5.11), and at the edge of OP lesions the interstitial process sometimes spreads further than the granulation tissue plugs. This can produce an appearance mimicking cellular NSIP (Fig. 5.12, and see Chapter 7). However, reference to imaging will usually sort this out because NSIP and OP are radiologically distinct.

Acute Fibrinous and Organizing Pneumonia Pattern

It is not unusual to find small amounts of fibrin mixed in with the granulation tissue in OP, but occasionally the granulation tissue plugs are composed predominantly of fibrin (Figs. 5.13 to 5.15). This lesion has been called "acute fibrinous and organizing pneumonia (AFOP)"[10] but it really is just a reaction pattern that may be seen in OP, diffuse alveolar damage, eosinophilic pneumonias, and in restrictive lung allograft syndrome.[11] We advise against using AFOP as a diagnosis because it is not a specific entity and clinicians will not know what is meant, but rather we simply diagnose the underlying lesion (OP, diffuse alveolar damage, eosinophilic pneumonia) and ignore the fibrin.

SECONDARY OP

A pathologic picture of OP can be seen as part of many other processes in the lung, sometimes in conjunction with another lesion (Table 5.2), but sometimes producing

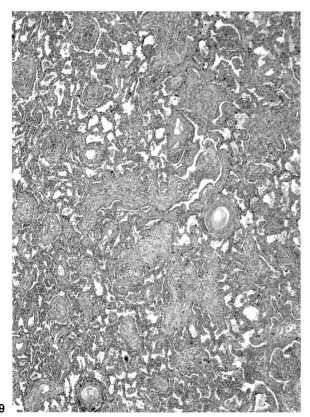

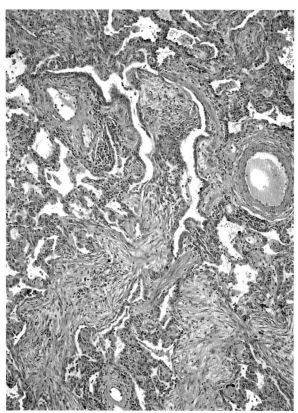

5.9   5.10

FIGURES 5.9 and 5.10. Medium- and high-power views the lesion shown in Figure 5.8. The microscopic appearance of OP is stereotypic. In **Figure 5.9**, a granulation tissue plug is seen in the lumen of a respiratory bronchiole.

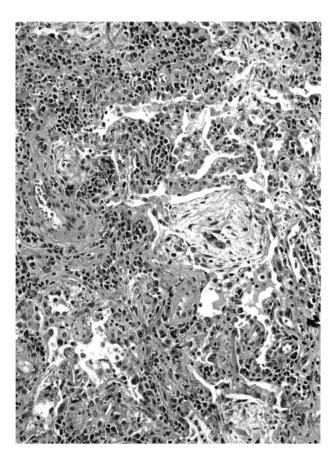

FIGURE 5.11. Appearance of a granulation tissue plug in cross section. In OP, the granulation tissue plugs tend to be separated from the underlying lung tissue, as here, whereas in fibroblast foci (see Chapter 6), the granulation tissue is closely applied to the underlying lung tissue. Note also the chronic interstitial inflammation.

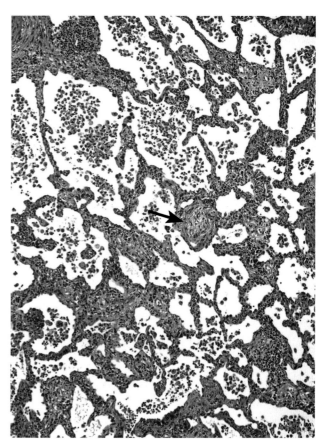

FIGURE 5.12. Edge of a lesion of OP mimicking NSIP (see Chapter 7). When a biopsy samples the edge of an OP lesion, the interstitial inflammatory infiltrate may predominate and granulation tissue plugs (*arrow*) may be few or absent, as here. If the morphology is equivocal, the nature of the lesion can almost always be sorted out by examining the CT scan.

a picture of pure OP; for example, post-viral or mycoplasma infection (Figs. 5.16 to 5.18) or as a drug reaction (Figs. 5.19 and 5.20).

The proper pathologic diagnosis in this situation depends on the clinical situation, imaging, and pathologic findings. For example, with an abscess (Figs. 5.21 and 5.22) or tumor (Figs. 5.23 and 5.24) that has surrounding or distal OP, the OP can be ignored and only the lesion of interest should be diagnosed. As noted above, occasional small foci of OP can be seen in HP or NSIP, but need not be diagnosed because the presence or absence of OP does not change prognosis or therapy.

OP is extremely common in eosinophilic pneumonias and may be the predominant microscopic pattern (Figs. 5.25 and 5.26, and see below), but the diagnosis remains CEP (see below).

OP is a very common drug reaction pattern (Figs. 5.19 and 5.20, and see Chapter 18), and in this situation, a diagnosis of "OP, consistent with reaction to [drug]" is actually useful to the clinician because it implies reversibility and suggests treatment with steroids as well as discontinuance of the drug. Similarly, a diagnosis of "OP secondary to previous mycoplasma infection" (Figs. 5.16 to 5.18) implies a process that should be responsive to steroids.

In addition to being a response to a previous infection, OP can be a reaction to an active infection. Pneumocystis is a particular problem in this regard, because the organism often produces no clues to its presence on hematoxylin and eosin stain (Fig. 5.27). For this reason, we routinely do silver stains for pneumocystis in all cases of OP (Fig. 5.28) unless there is another known cause for the process.

OP is a very common reaction to aspiration.[12] Clues to the correct diagnosis are the presence of individual giant cells or foreign body granulomas, or acute bronchiolitis, or occasionally necrotizing granulomas, along with the OP, and foreign material, most commonly vegetable particles (Figs. 5.29 and 5.30) or birefringent material. Even if foreign material is not visible, the combination of OP and giant cells is strongly suggestive of aspiration.

OP can be a reaction to acute or chronic hemorrhage. With hemorrhage, hemosiderin may be found in the granulation tissue tufts (Fig. 5.31), and this is a useful clue that the OP is a secondary process. The presence of ferruginated elastic fibers is also an indicator of chronic hemorrhage (see Chapter 24). Some patients with chronic hemorrhage will develop interstitial fibrosis (see Figs. 24.3 and 24.4); the most common settings are in patients with

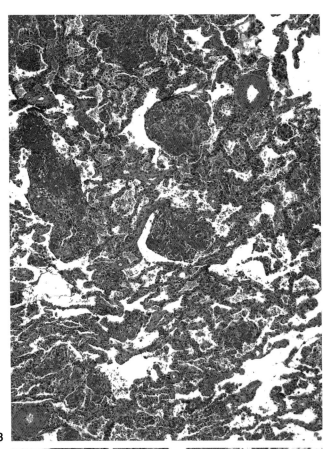

5.13

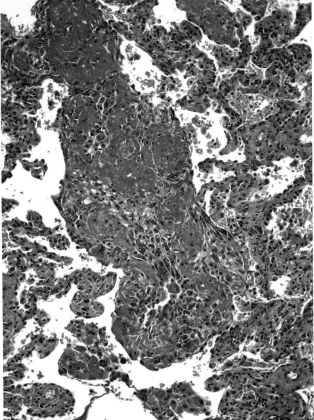

5.14

microscopic polyangiitis, where the fibrosis is diffuse, and in pulmonary veno-occlusive disease, where the fibrosis is localized to the subpleural regions. Care should be taken in such cases to look for capillaritis, as this would indicate that the patient has an active vasculitis.

DIFFERENTIAL DIAGNOSIS, OP MIMICKING FIBROBLAST FOCI, AND CICATRICIAL OP

The differential diagnosis of OP tends to reflect the presence of other morphologic features; for example, if an abscess with surrounding OP is present, the diagnosis is "abscess" rather than OP (Figs. 5.21 and 5.22).

An important differential of OP is CEP. As noted above, OP and CEP can be radiologically very similar (see Chapter 15). At a microscopic level, some cases of CEP look mostly like OP, but with numerous eosinophils (Figs. 5.25 and 5.26 and see Figs. 15.14 and 15.15). Occasional eosinophils are common in OP, but when eosinophils become easy to find in what at first glance looks like OP, the diagnosis of CEP should be entertained. Clinical features can be helpful. A history of asthma or allergic rhinitis or blood eosinophilia makes the diagnosis of eosinophilic pneumonia much more likely. In an equivocal case, we recommend at least raising the possibility of eosinophilic

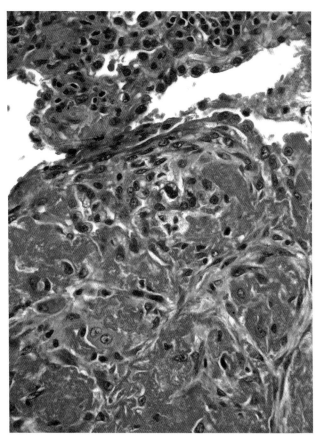

5.15

FIGURES 5.13 to 5.15. AFOP pattern. In AFOP, fibrin replaces much of the granulation tissue of OP, although some granulation tissue still remains, as is clear from **Figure 5.14**. AFOP pattern may be seen in OP, DAD (see Chapter 4), and CEP (see Chapter 15). AFOP is not a specific entity and should not be diagnosed.

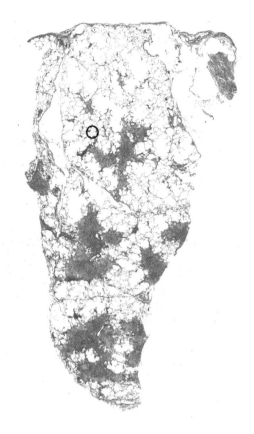

5.16

Table 5.2

Causes of secondary OP

Aspiration (look for giant cells/granulomas and foreign material)

Drug reactions (see Chapter 18)

Infections
  Bacterial infections (many species but especially *Streptococcus pneumoniae*)
  Fungal infections including pneumocystis
  Viral infections

Reactions to inhaled toxins, especially noxious gases

CEP (look for eosinophils) (see Chapter 15)

As a minor part of HP (see Chapter 12)

As a minor part of NSIP (see Chapter 6)

Collagen vascular disease (see Chapter 21)

Distal to airway obstruction (especially by slow growing tumors)

Inflammatory bowel disease involving the lung (see Chapter 14)

Primary biliary cholangitis involving the lung (see Chapter 14)

Postradiation therapy for breast cancer

Associated with acute or chronic hemorrhage

Around other inflammatory or mass lesions (tumors, abscesses, infarcts)

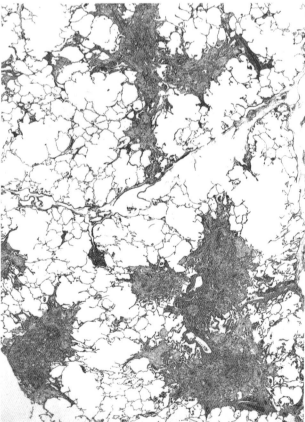

5.17

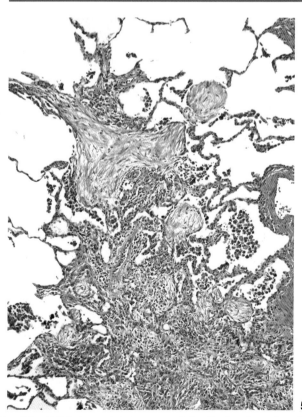

5.18

FIGURES 5.16 to 5.18. OP post-mycoplasma infection. The low-power view (**Fig. 5.16**) shows that the process is localized to the region of the bronchovascular bundles and reflects damage to the respiratory bronchioles during the acute phase of the infection (see Chapter 20). However, the morphology is simply that of OP and only the history indicates etiology.

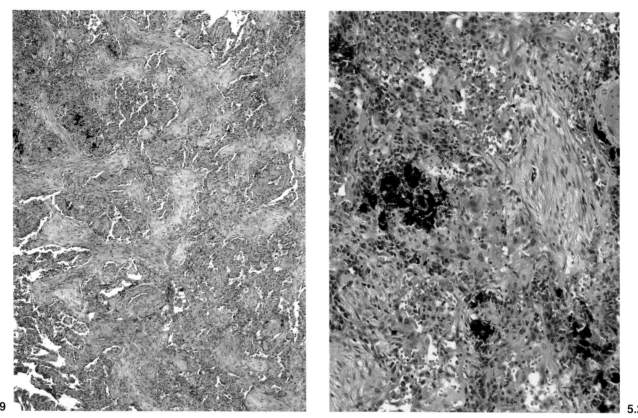

5.19   5.20

FIGURES 5.19 and 5.20. Two examples of OP as drug reaction: **Figure 5.19** is from a patient given cyclophosphamide for glomerulonephritis and **Figure 5.20** is from a crack cocaine smoker (note the extensive dense black crack pigment).

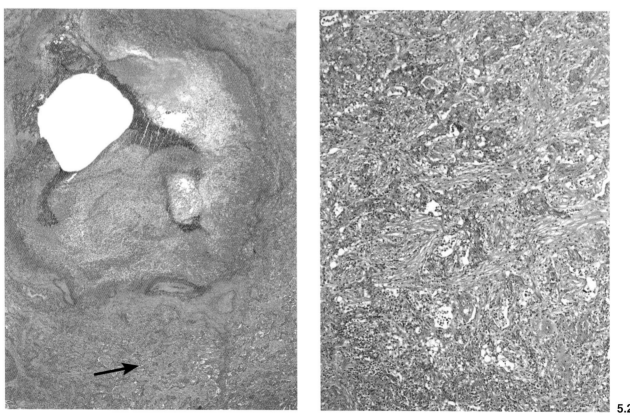

5.21   5.22

FIGURES 5.21 and 5.22. OP around an abscess. The low-power view (**Fig. 5.21**) shows an abscess. The region marked by the *arrow* is shown in **Figure 5.21** and is OP. In this setting, the proper diagnosis is lung abscess and the OP can be ignored.

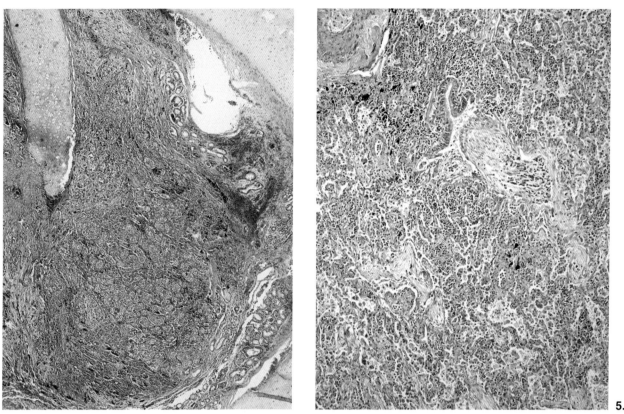

5.23   5.24

FIGURES 5.23 and 5.24. OP behind a carcinoid tumor. The tumor completely obstructs the bronchus of origin (**Fig. 5.23**) and there is OP (**Fig. 5.24**) distal to the tumor.

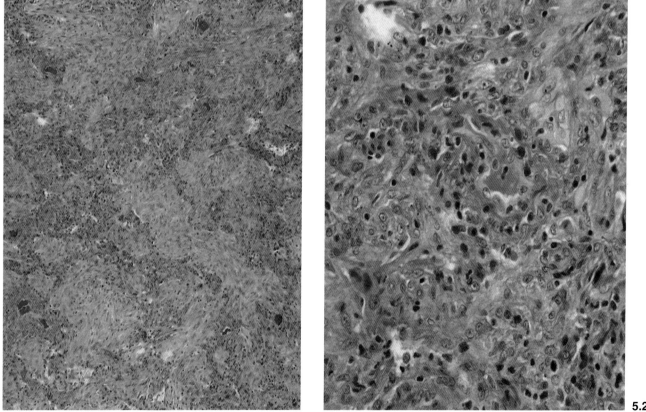

5.25   5.26

FIGURES 5.25 and 5.26. CEP disguised as OP. The medium-power view (**Fig. 5.25**) looks like OP, but the high-power view (**Fig. 5.26**) shows numerous eosinophils. OP is a very common pattern in CEP (see Figs. 15.14 and 15.15 for additional examples).

Table 5.3

Separation of OP from fibroblast foci

OP

Granulation tissue clearly in alveolar ducts or lumens of respiratory bronchioles

Granulation tissue largely separate from underlying lung

Granulation tissue fibroblasts randomly oriented vis-à-vis underlying lung

No dense fibrosis in surrounding lung

OP foci usually not covered by epithelium

OP foci usually much more numerous than fibroblast foci

OP rarely shows signs of organization (all the granulation tissue is the same age)

FIBROBLAST FOCI

A background fibrosing process always present (e.g., UIP, chronic HP, collagen vascular disease-associated ILD)

Granulation tissue always tightly attached to underlying lung

Granulation tissue typically applied to fibrotic lung

Granulation tissue fibroblasts oriented parallel to the underlying lung

Granulation tissue frequently re-epithelialized

Granulation tissue typically shows various degrees of organization (some granulation tissue is loose, but some is partly collagenized)

pneumonia so that the clinician is alerted to look for an offending antigen.

Another differential is the separation of OP from fibroblast foci because both are composed of granulation tissue. Details for this separation are listed in Table 5.3. Fibroblast foci are typically seen in fibrosing interstitial pneumonias such as UIP (see Chapter 6) and chronic HP (see Chapter 12), but can be found in any process characterized by actively developing dense fibrosis, whereas OP typically is usually not part of a fibrosing lung disease. Useful features to bear in mind are that fibroblast foci typically show granulation tissue with various degrees of organization from very loose to nearly completely collagenized, and fibroblast foci are always tightly applied to the underlying lung tissue (see Figs. 6.27 to 6.35), whereas in OP all the granulation is loose and is the same age and most often is separated from the underlying lung tissue.

There are rare cases in which these rules are violated. Occasionally, OP in the very periphery of the lung shows granulation tissue tightly apposed to underlying somewhat fibrotic tissue (Fig. 5.32). This situation can be confusing,

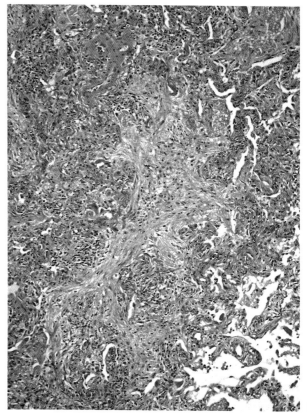
5.27

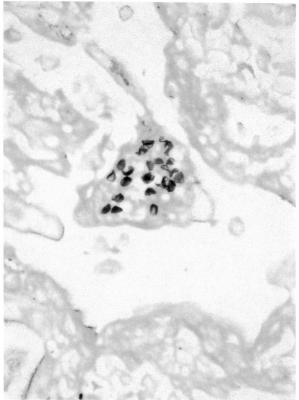
5.28

FIGURES 5.27 and 5.28. OP caused by pneumocystis infection. The hematoxylin and eosin stain (H&E) view (**Fig. 5.27**) is indistinguishable from idiopathic OP but the Grocott stain (**Fig. 5.28**) shows pneumocystis organisms. Because pneumocystis can hide in OP without any clue to its presence on H&E, we advise staining all cases of OP for pneumocystis unless there is another good reason for OP to be present.

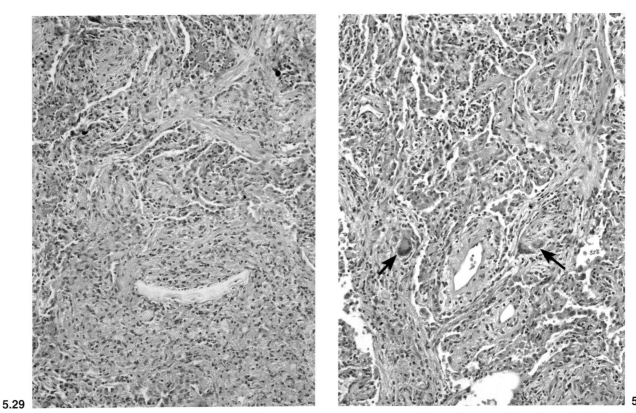

5.29

5.30

FIGURES 5.29 and 5.30. OP caused by aspiration. OP is a common response to aspiration. Clues to the correct diagnosis are the finding of food particles (in this case a fragment of a yellow vegetable wall in **Fig. 5.29**) and/or giant cells/granulomas (*arrows* in **Fig. 5.30**).

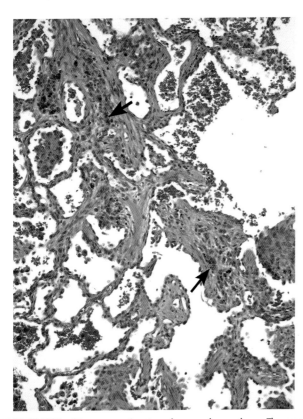

FIGURE 5.31. OP as a reaction to pulmonary hemorrhage. The presence of hemosiderin in the granulation tissue plugs (*arrows*) is a clue to the correct diagnosis.

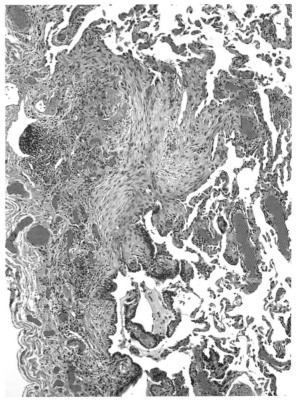

FIGURE 5.32. Unusual pattern of OP occasionally encountered in the periphery of the lung where granulation tissue plugs are applied directly to underlying tissue, mimicking fibroblast foci (see Chapter 6). This case had ordinary OP elsewhere and was probably secondary to aspiration.

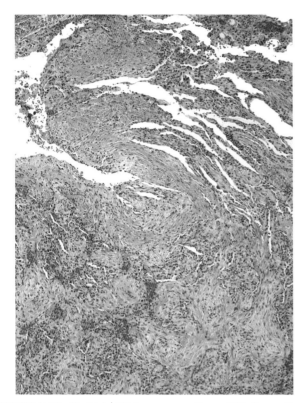

FIGURE 5.33. Cicatricial OP. Same case as Figure 5.32. Conventional OP at bottom and beginning organization into fibrotic bands at top.

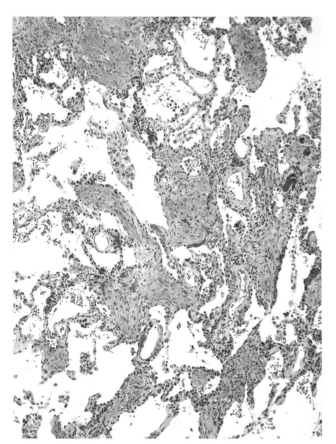

FIGURE 5.34. Cicatricial OP. Same case as Figure 5.32. Developing irregular bands of fibrous tissue.

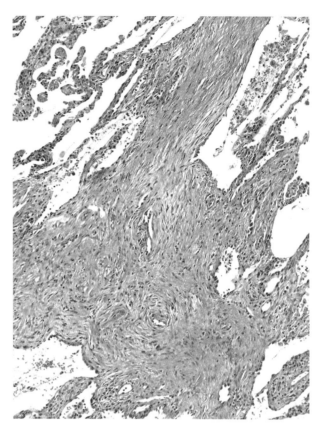

FIGURE 5.35. Cicatricial OP. Same case as Figure 5.32. High-power view of a developing band of fibrous tissue in cicatricial OP. The lighter granulation tissue is not a fibroblast focus; rather the previous loose granulation tissue of typical OP is now becoming collagenized. (Reproduced by permission from Churg A, Wright JL, Bilawich A. Cicatricial organising pneumonia mimicking a fibrosing interstitial pneumonia. *Histopathology.* 2018;72:846–854.)

but if there is OP elsewhere and no evidence of an underlying fibrosing interstitial pneumonia, then the process is probably all OP; this process may be a variant of cicatricial OP (see below).

The granulation tissue plugs of OP are ordinarily quite loose and disappear with therapy. However, occasionally the granulation tissue of OP does not disappear but instead becomes collagenized. This process has been termed "fibrosing OP,"[13] "collagenized OP,"[14] and "cicatricial OP"[15,16] (Figs. 5.33 to 5.41). In some instances, this form of OP has the same location within the alveolar parenchyma and same morphologic profile as ordinary OP (Fig. 5.41), but in other cases, the cicatricial process forms bands of variably dense fibrous tissue (Figs. 5.33 to 5.37); the bands may have looser granulation tissue at the edges and somewhat mimic fibroblast foci (Fig. 5.35), and the low-power appearance, at least locally, can resemble fibrotic NSIP (Figs. 5.36 and 5.37). Many such cases have areas of conventional OP, and the finding of changes that cover the spectrum from loose granulation tissue to dense fibrous tissue (such as Fig. 5.33) is helpful in arriving at the correct diagnosis.

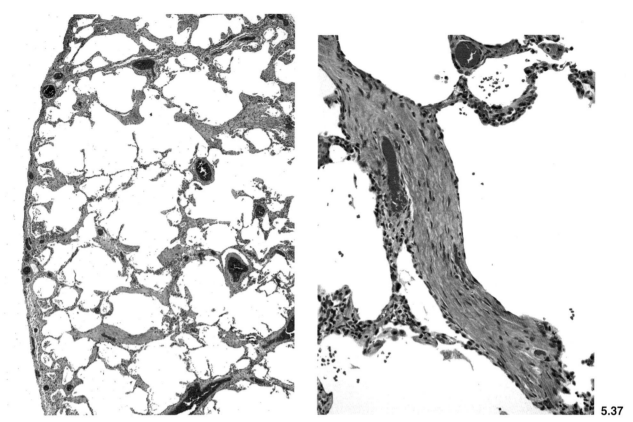

5.36   5.37

FIGURES 5.36 and 5.37. Cicatricial OP. Same case as Figures 5.32 to 5.35. In this area only fine bands of organized fibrous tissue remain. If this were the only pattern seen, it would mimic fibrotic NSIP, and some cases of fibrotic NSIP may represent organized OP. However, the fibrous tissue is much denser than one usually sees in NSIP and the fibroblasts all are aligned in the same direction. This is very typical of cicatricial OP.

In other cases, cicatricial OP appears as irregular densely fibrotic intraparenchymal nodules that may be ossified (Figs. 5.39 and 5.40), and areas of conventional OP can be sparse. What has been reported as the characteristic pattern of vascular Ehlers–Danlos syndrome in the

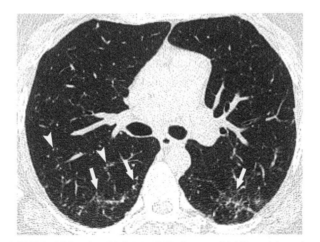

FIGURE 5.38. Cicatricial OP. HRCT shows mild bilateral irregular linear opacities and minimal ground-opacities, more severe on the left (*arrows*). Also noted are multiple small nodules (*arrowheads*). The nodules have a lower lung zone predominance and many are calcified consistent with dendritic ossification.

lung actually appears to be cicatricial OP with this pattern, with the OP probably secondary to recurrent hemorrhage (see Figs. 23.30 and 23.31).

On HRCT, fibrosis associated with OP commonly manifests as peribronchial or perilobular thickening with traction bronchiectasis and reticulation.[7] The findings of fibrosis becomes more evident as the consolidation resolves.[7] Therefore, cicatricial OP may be present histologically without evidence of fibrosis on computed tomography (CT).[17] However, in some patients initial CT findings typical of OP progress to lower lobe predominant ground-glass opacities, reticulation, traction bronchiectasis and, commonly, subpleural sparing characteristic of fibrotic NSIP.[7,17] In some patients with cicatricial OP, CT shows only patchy bilateral peripheral irregular linear and reticular opacities, occasionally associated with small calcified nodules due to dendritic ossification[16] (Fig. 5.38).

DIAGNOSTIC MODALITIES

An OP pattern is fairly common in transbronchial biopsies (see Figs. 3.6 and 3.7) and even in core needle biopsies (see Fig. 3.1). A diagnosis of OP in a transbronchial biopsy may be morphologically accurate, but whether that morphology is relevant will depend on clinical and imaging findings, and a comment to that effect should be

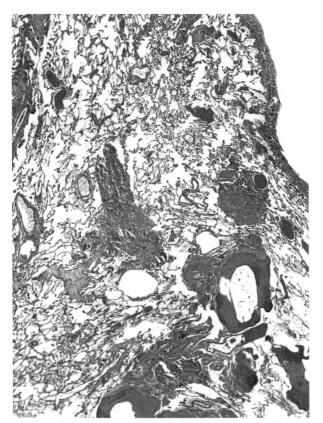

FIGURE 5.39. Cicatricial OP. Low-power view of cicatricial OP showing collagenized nodules, some of them ossified. (Reproduced by permission from Churg A, Wright JL, Bilawich A. Cicatricial organising pneumonia mimicking a fibrosing interstitial pneumonia. *Histopathology.* 2018;72:846–854.)

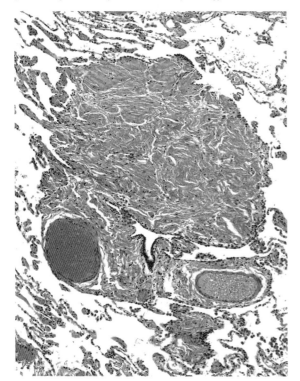

FIGURE 5.40. Cicatricial OP. High-power view of a collagenized nodule. Note the very dense paucicellular appearance; this is typical of some cases of cicatricial OP.

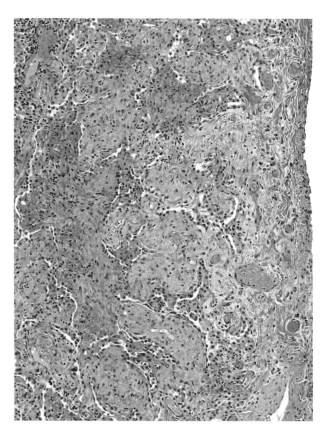

FIGURE 5.41. Cicatricial OP. An area with a residual ordinary OP pattern, but here the granulation tissue is also collagenized.

included when diagnosing OP in a transbronchial biopsy. OP can also be diagnosed by cryobiopsy[18] with the same caveats. However, a large video-assisted thoracoscopic biopsy is more accurate in ensuring that some other lesion is not present.

Because core needle biopsies are usually utilized for mass lesions, OP in a core needle biopsy (see Fig. 3.1) can be misleading since there is no way of knowing whether one is dealing with nodular OP (relatively uncommon) or OP around some other lesion such as a tumor, a much more common scenario. It has been reported[19] that core needle biopsy can be used to diagnose radiologically typical OP (i.e., with a pattern of peribronchial consolidation), but it is unclear what the advantage of a core needle biopsy would be over a less invasive transbronchial biopsy in this setting and this approach is not generally used.

PROGNOSIS

The prognosis in idiopathic OP overall is reasonably good, with 70% to 90% long-term survival in different series.[4,6,20,21] Steroids are the usual treatment, but responses have also been described with macrolide therapy and some patients have spontaneous remissions.[5,22] Relapses of idiopathic OP are common when steroids are tapered (50% of cases in some series), but the process generally responds to reinstitution of steroids and relapses do not affect overall mortality.[20] It has been suggested that OP with prominent fibrin on biopsy is more likely to recur or progress.[23]

The prognosis of secondary OP depends on the underlying condition,[21] but as noted above, the usual absence of dense fibrosis means that any lesion that has a pure OP pattern is potentially completely reversible.

Yousem[15] and Beardsley et al.[13] reported that patients with cicatricial OP have persisting infiltrates on imaging and in some cases a poor prognosis, but in our experience,[16] such cases behave like ordinary OP; the important point is not to confuse cicatricial OP with a fibrosing interstitial pneumonia.

REFERENCES

1. Epler GR, Colby TV, McLoud TC, et al. Bronchiolitis obliterans organizing pneumonia. *N Engl J Med*. 1985;312:152–158.
2. ATS/ERS International Multidisciplinary consensus classification of the idiopathic interstitial pneumonias. *Am J Respir Crit Care Med*. 2002;165:277–304.
3. Travis WD, Costabel U, Hansell DM, et al. ATS/ERS Committee on idiopathic interstitial pneumonias. An official American Thoracic Society/European Respiratory Society statement: update of the international multidisciplinary classification of the idiopathic interstitial pneumonias. *Am J Respir Crit Care Med*. 2013;188:733–748.
4. Cordier JF. Cryptogenic organizing pneumonia. *Eur Resp J*. 2006;28:422–446.
5. Cordier JF, Cottin V, Lazor R, et al. Many faces of bronchiolitis and organizing pneumonia. *Semin Respir Crit Care Med*. 2016;37:421–440.
6. Epler GR. Bronchiolitis obliterans organizing pneumonia, 25 years: a variety of causes, but what are the treatment options? *Expert Rev Respir Med*. 2011;5:353–361.
7. Kligerman SJ, Franks TJ, Galvin JR. From the radiologic pathology archives: organization and fibrosis as a response to lung injury in diffuse alveolar damage, organizing pneumonia, and acute fibrinous and organizing pneumonia. *Radiographics*. 2013;33:1951–1975.
8. Arakawa H, Kurihara Y, Niimi H, et al. Bronchiolitis obliterans with organizing pneumonia versus chronic eosinophilic pneumonia: high-resolution CT findings in 81 patients. *AJR Am J Roentgenol*. 2001;176:1053–1058.
9. Torrealba JR, Fisher S, Kanne JP, et al. Pathology-radiology correlation of common and uncommon computed tomographic patterns of organizing pneumonia. *Hum Pathol*. 2018;71:30–40.
10. Beasley MB, Franks TJ, Galvin JR, et al. Acute fibrinous and organizing pneumonia: a histological pattern of lung injury and possible variant of diffuse alveolar damage. *Arch Pathol Lab Med*. 2002;126:1064–1070.
11. von der Thüsen JH, Vandermeulen E, Vos R, et al. The histomorphological spectrum of restrictive chronic lung allograft dysfunction and implications for prognosis. *Mod Pathol*. 2018;31:780–790.
12. Mukhopadhyay S, Katzenstein AL. Pulmonary disease due to aspiration of food and other particulate matter: a clinicopathologic study of 59 cases diagnosed on biopsy or resection specimens. *Am J Surg Pathol*. 2007;31:752–759.
13. Beardsley B, Rassl D. Fibrosing organising pneumonia. *J Clin Pathol*. 2013;66:875–881.
14. Mengoli MC, Colby TV, Cavazza A, et al. Incidental iatrogenic form of collagenized organizing pneumonia. *Hum Pathol*. 2017;73:192–193.
15. Yousem SA. Cicatricial variant of cryptogenic organizing pneumonia. *Hum Pathol*. 2017;64:76–82.
16. Churg A, Wright JL, Bilawich A. Cicatricial organising pneumonia mimicking a fibrosing interstitial pneumonia. *Histopathology*. 2018;72:846–854.
17. Lee JW, Lee KS, Lee HY, et al. Cryptogenic organizing pneumonia: serial high-resolution CT findings in 22 patients. *AJR Am J Roentgenol*. 2010;195:916–922.
18. Ussavarungsi K, Kern RM, Roden AC, et al. Transbronchial cryobiopsy in diffuse parenchymal lung disease: retrospective analysis of 74 cases. *Chest*. 2017;151:400–408.
19. Miao L, Wang Y, Li Y, et al. Lesion with morphologic feature of organizing pneumonia (OP) in CT-guided lung biopsy samples for diagnosis of bronchiolitis obliterans organizing pneumonia (BOOP): a retrospective study of 134 cases in a single center. *J Thorac Dis*. 2014;6:1251–1260.
20. Lazor R, Vandevenne A, Pelletier A, et al. Cryptogenic organizing pneumonia. Characteristics of relapses in a series of 48 patients. *Am J Respir Crit Care Med*. 2000;162:571–577.
21. Lohr RH, Boland BJ, Douglas WW, et al. Organizing pneumonia. Features and prognosis of cryptogenic, secondary, and focal variants. *Arch Intern Med*. 1997;157:1323–1329.
22. Pathak V, Kuhn JM, Durham C, et al. Macrolide use leads to clinical and radiological improvement in patients with cryptogenic organizing pneumonia. *Ann Am Thorac Soc*. 2014;11:87–91.
23. Nishino M, Mathai SK, Schoenfeld D, et al. Clinicopathologic features associated with relapse in cryptogenic organizing pneumonia. *Hum Pathol*. 2014;45:342–351.

Usual Interstitial Pneumonia

NOMENCLATURE ISSUES AND CONCEPTUAL ISSUES

The term "usual interstitial pneumonia" (UIP) was coined by Liebow and dates back to the 1970s, whereas the British used "cryptogenic fibrosing alveolitis" for the same process, but the latter name has disappeared. In the 2002 and 2013 American Thoracic Society/European Respiratory Society classifications of idiopathic interstitial pneumonias and subsequent practice guidelines,[1-4] UIP is viewed as the pathologic pattern of a disease that, when combined with appropriate clinical and radiologic findings, is called "idiopathic pulmonary fibrosis" (IPF).[1-4]

The original Liebow term UIP was intended to replace some of the entities labeled "pulmonary fibrosis" with a more specific disease, but there is still clinical inconsistency in the use of "pulmonary fibrosis," which sometimes is meant to indicate IPF and sometimes simply some form of fibrosing lung disease. Because UIP is widely recognized by clinicians, radiologists, and pathologists as a reasonably specific name, we shall generally use UIP to refer to IPF, and UIP/IPF or IPF when we wish to emphasize the distinction from other forms of interstitial lung disease (ILD) or discuss purely clinical points. This distinction is particularly important when dealing with entities that microscopically can look like UIP, particularly chronic hypersensitivity pneumonitis (chronic HP) (Chapter 12) and connective tissue disease (CTD)-associated ILD (Chapter 21).

Because of its poor prognosis, accurate pathologic diagnosis of UIP has always been important, but rather than becoming clearer, the last few years have seen arguments in the pathology literature about the spectrum of morphologic findings that support or deny a diagnosis of UIP, particularly UIP as compared to chronic HP[5,6] (see section Differential Diagnosis and Controversies in the Pathologic Diagnosis of UIP). This issue is particularly crucial because IPF is now treated with antifibrotic agents and most other fibrosing interstitial pneumonias are treated with immunosuppressive agents, whereas immunosuppressive agents are contraindicated in IPF (see section Treatment and Prognosis).

ETIOLOGIES OF A UIP PATTERN

There are a number of different etiologies of a pathologic and to a lesser extent a radiologic picture of UIP (Table 6.1). Most cases of diffuse fibrotic lung disease that look like UIP on imaging or biopsy are idiopathic (i.e., IPF), a pulmonary manifestation of an underlying collagen vascular disease (CVD), or chronic HP. Some cases of CVD or chronic HP are indistinguishable from UIP on biopsy, although even in this situation there frequently are differences between UIP and chronic HP on imaging (Figs. 6.1 and 6.2 and see Chapters 12 and 21). Drug reactions can produce a UIP picture (Chapter 18). Asbestosis occasionally looks very much like UIP with the addition of asbestos bodies, but most cases of asbestosis are pathologically distinct[7] (see Chapter 22), and asbestosis frequently is accompanied by marked visceral pleural fibrosis, something that is not a feature of idiopathic UIP. IPF in two or more close relatives or IPF in the proband and ILD of other sorts in close relatives are labeled familial IPF. Although some of these cases look like UIP microscopically, a very large proportion either resemble another type of ILD or are morphologically unclassifiable.[8]

Table 6.1

Etiologies of a radiologic and morphologic picture of UIP

Idiopathic UIP
- Equivalent to clinical IPF

CVD
- Especially common in rheumatoid arthritis and scleroderma, but can be seen in any form of CVD

Drug reactions
- For example, amiodarone, nitrofurantoin, chemotherapeutic agents (see Chapter 18)

Familial UIP

UIP with specific genetic abnormalities

Some cases of chronic HP

Some pneumoconioses such as asbestosis (but usually not great microscopic mimics)

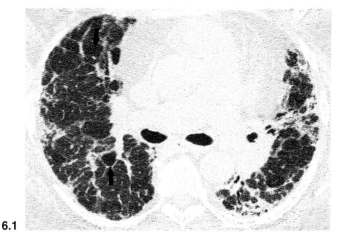

6.1

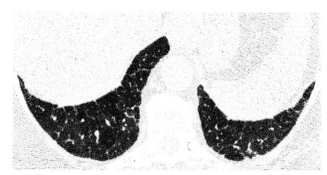

6.2

FIGURES 6.1 and 6.2. Chronic hypersensitivity pneumonitis. **Figure 6.1:** HRCT at the level of the upper lobes demonstrates dense subpleural reticulation that is suggestive of UIP. Findings that favor the diagnosis of chronic HP in this image include diffuse inhomogeneity of the lung parenchyma and lobular areas of decreased attenuation and vascularity (*arrows*). **Figure 6.2:** HRCT at the level of the lung bases in the same case as **Figure 6.1** shows minimal fibrosis. The predominant middle and upper lung zone distribution of the fibrosis with relative sparing of the lung bases is another feature that favors chronic HP over UIP. The patient was a 65-year-old woman with chronic HP because of mold exposure.

GENETIC FACTORS AND ILD

Around 20% of IPF patients have a family history of ILD, and there is considerable evidence that at least some forms of ILD, particularly IPF, have a genetic basis.

A body of literature now exists that has investigated the role of single nucleotide polymorphisms (SNPs) on the risk of ILD and to a lesser extent in the progression and diagnosis of ILD. The most extensively investigated SNP is the minor allele of *MUC5B* (rs35705950_T). This allele is present in around 10% of the non-Hispanic white population of North America, and its frequency is increased in patients with what are known as interstitial lung abnormalities (ILAs), that is, a variety of ILD-type high-resolution computed tomography (HRCT) changes in patients who do not have clinical ILD but may be at risk of progression to overt ILD. The *MUC5B* SNP is particularly associated with peripheral reticulation, in this context meaning underlying fibrosis, and not with centrilobular abnormalities on HRCT.[9]

There are numerous SNPs associated with IPF, but most have very low risk effects (see Adegunsoye et al.[10] for a listing). However, patients who are heterogeneous for the *MUC5B* minor allele have a 6- to 8-fold chance of developing clinical IPF compared to the general population, and patients who are homozygous have a 20-fold increased risk. Overall, the *MUC5B* minor allele is believed to account for around 35% of IPF risk. However, the *MUC5B* minor allele is also increased in frequency in patients with chronic HP,[11] and in some patients with CVD-associated ILD, particularly patients with rheumatoid arthritis–associated UIP,[12] suggesting that *MUC5B* acts as a broad effect profibrogenic factor rather than a disease-specific factor (Fig. 6.3). How this occurs is not known. Patients with the minor allele have greatly increased mucin (specifically MUC5B) production in the lung, and it has been suggested that excess mucus

either leads to aberrant repair of lung injury or increases the susceptibility to infection[13]; the amount of mucus production itself appears to be important because the more copies of the minor allele a patient carries, the greater the risk of progression of ILA or development of IPF.

Some investigators report that SNPs in *TOLLIP*, a gene that is related to immune function, are also common in IPF but are more complex because rs111521887 and rs5743894

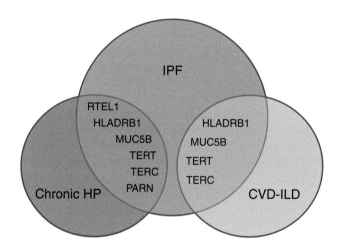

MUC5B (rs35705950): airway mucus, airway defense
TERT (rs2736100): maintenance of telomere length
HLADRB1 (rs2395655): critical to immune system function
RTEL1: DNA helicase activity
PARN: stability of mRNA
TERC: maintenance of telomere length

FIGURE 6.3. Overlapping SNPs in IPF, chronic HP, and CVD-associated ILD. Many SNPs appear to confer a propensity to fibrotic lung disease rather than a specific diagnosis. The function of the specific genes is also indicated. DNA, deoxyribonucleic acid; mRNA, messenger ribonucleic acid.

increase IPF risk by about 50%, whereas rs2743890 decreases the risk by about the same amount,[14] although not all studies have supported these associations.[11] SNPs that cause telomere maintenance dysfunction, typically leading to shortening of telomere length, such as *TERT* (rs2736100), are thought to account for up to 10% of sporadic IPF cases and 25% of familial IPF cases and are also seen in CVD-ILD[15] (Fig. 6.3). There are a number of rare variants that have very large effects on IPF risk, including SNPs in *TERC, RTEL1,* and *PARN* (see Adegunsoye et al.[10] for a detailed listing of common and rare genetic abnormalities in IPF); some of these variants are also seen in chronic HP and CTD-ILD (Fig. 6.3). Failure to maintain telomere length appears to be particularly associated with fibrotic ILD, and the shortest telomeres are found in patients with IPF; of interest, in situ studies have shown that the cells in the fibrotic regions of UIP/IPF lungs have much shorter telomeres than the cells in the unaffected regions.

The potential utility of the *MUC5B* SNP as a diagnostic tool for IPF has been proposed in the literature but is limited by the fact that the same minor allele is present in a portion of the general population as well as in non-IPF forms of fibrotic ILD. However, the progression of IPF is slower in patients with the *MUC5B* minor allele than in those without.[13]

EPIDEMIOLOGY

IPF is a disease of the middle-aged and elderly. Raghu et al.[16,17] estimated an incidence of 58 cases per million per year for ages 18 to 64 and 328 cases per million per year for ages 66 to 69, with a steady increase to 1,439 cases per million per year over age 80 in the United States, but there is considerable country to country variation in incidence numbers. The finding of a UIP picture on a biopsy from someone under age 50 should raise a question of another etiology, particularly an underlying CVD, and we advise noting that point in a diagnosis comment, because the prognosis for UIP in some forms of CVD is much better than that of idiopathic UIP (see Chapter 21).

In most studies, the incidence of IPF is higher in men than in women, and some 70% of cases of IPF occur in current or former cigarette smokers; the characteristic IPF demographic is a male over 60 who is a current or ex-smoker.[4] Lederer and Martinez[18] estimate that IPF accounts for 20% of ILD cases, and chronic HP and CVD-associated ILD for 20% each, but these numbers must be viewed with caution because of the general lack of agreement on the diagnosis of chronic HP (see Chapter 12). Gastroesophageal reflux disease, obstructive sleep apnea, viral infections, and agricultural exposures have also been proposed as causes of IPF, but these putative etiologies are unproven and may simply be associations that reflect the susceptibility of UIP lungs to exogenous insults. We suspect that "IPF" in agricultural workers may actually be chronic HP.

CLINICAL FEATURES

Most cases of UIP present with shortness of breath, sometimes progressing over several years, a restrictive pattern of pulmonary function tests, and a decreased diffusing capacity. Clubbing is very common in UIP, probably more so than in any other forms of ILD. However, these features are not specific and can be seen in many forms of fibrotic ILD. CVD-associated ILD and chronic HP, in particular, can mimic IPF, and thus all patients who might fit the clinical, radiologic, and even pathologic criteria for UIP/IPF need to be evaluated for clinical and serologic evidence of a CVD-associated ILD (Chapter 21) or for potential sensitizing exposures (Chapter 12), as well as for potential occupational exposures.[4]

A small proportion of patients with UIP present for the first time as an acute exacerbation, that is, with the rapid development of hypoxemic respiratory failure and diffuse infiltrates on imaging mimicking acute respiratory distress syndrome (ARDS)/acute interstitial pneumonia (see below and also Chapter 4). In such patients, imaging studies may reveal underlying fibrosis, but sometimes the underlying disease is only demonstrable on biopsy.

IMAGING

The characteristic manifestations of UIP on HRCT are a reticular pattern and honeycombing in a predominantly basal and peripheral distribution[4] (Figs. 6.4 and 6.5). The reticular pattern is commonly associated with traction bronchiectasis and bronchiolectasis. Although ground-glass opacities are commonly seen, they are typically less extensive than the reticular pattern (Figs. 6.6 and 6.7).[19]

A typical UIP pattern on HRCT is highly accurate for the presence of a UIP pattern on surgical lung biopsy, with a positive predictive value (PPV) of 90% to 100%.[20] Therefore, in the appropriate clinical setting, the presence of a characteristic pattern of UIP on HRCT precludes the need for biopsy. A confident diagnosis of UIP on HRCT requires the presence of all of the following four features: reticular pattern, honeycombing, subpleural and basal predominance, and absence of features considered atypical for UIP.[4,20]

It must be emphasized that although a typical HRCT has a high specificity and PPV in the diagnosis of UIP, the characteristic features that allow a confident diagnosis are only present in 50% to 75% of patients.[20] In the remaining 25% to 50% of cases, the HRCT findings are nondiagnostic, atypical, or suggestive of an alternate diagnosis.

It is currently recommended that in patients with clinically suspected IPF, the HRCT findings be classified into four categories: characteristic of UIP (as discussed earlier), probable UIP, indeterminate, or suggestive of an alternate diagnosis.[3,4] Patients with a basal and subpleural predominant reticular pattern with peripheral traction bronchiectasis or bronchiolectasis, no honeycombing, and no features suggestive of an alternative diagnosis are classified

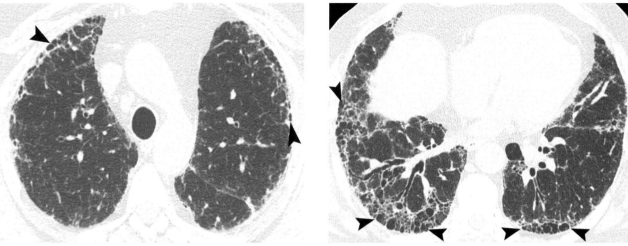

6.4

6.5

FIGURES 6.4 and 6.5. Usual interstitial pneumonia. HRCT at the level of the upper lobes (**Fig. 6.4**) shows mild peripheral reticulation and minimal honeycombing (*arrowheads*). HRCT at the level of the lung bases (**Fig. 6.5**) demonstrates extensive reticulation and honeycombing (*arrowheads*). The patient was a 58-year-old man with IPF.

as having a probable UIP pattern on HRCT (Fig. 6.8). A probable UIP pattern on HRCT has a PPV of 62% to 94% in the diagnosis of UIP depending on the prevalence of UIP. The combination of probable UIP pattern and moderate or extensive traction bronchiectasis in a male patient 60 or more years of age has a specificity of 99% and PPV of 96% in the diagnosis of UIP/IPF.[21]

Patients who do not meet the HRCT criteria for definite UIP or probable UIP and do not have features that suggest an alternative diagnosis are classified as having an indeterminate pattern. Findings considered atypical for UIP on HRCT include upper lobe predominance, peribronchovascular predominance, extensive ground-glass opacities, profuse micronodules, multiple discrete cysts away from honeycombing, diffuse mosaic attenuation/air trapping,

and consolidation.[4,19] The presence of any of these findings should suggest an alternate diagnosis. It must be noted, however, that in patients with clinically suspected IPF, the predictive value of computed tomography (CT) in excluding UIP is low, because up to 60% of patients with CT findings interpreted as suggestive of an alternative diagnosis have histologically proven UIP.[22]

PATHOLOGIC FEATURES

GROSS APPEARANCES

UIP is typically more severe in the lower zones and in the periphery of the lung (Figs. 6.9 to 6.11), but even at presentation, the disease frequently involves the upper zones

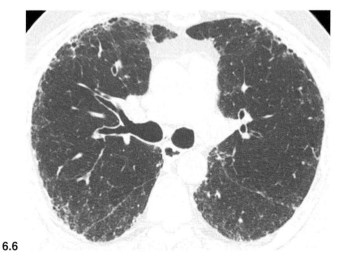

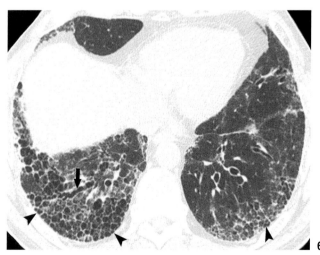

6.6

6.7

FIGURES 6.6 and 6.7. Usual interstitial pneumonia. HRCT at the level of the upper lobes (**Fig. 6.6**) shows mild peripheral reticulation and mild patchy ground-glass opacities. HRCT at the level of the lung bases (**Fig. 6.7**) demonstrates extensive reticulation, honeycombing (*arrowheads*), and patchy ground-glass opacities. Most of the ground-glass opacities are closely associated with areas of reticulation and probably represent fibrosis below the resolution of CT. The patient was a 62-year-old woman with clinical IPF.

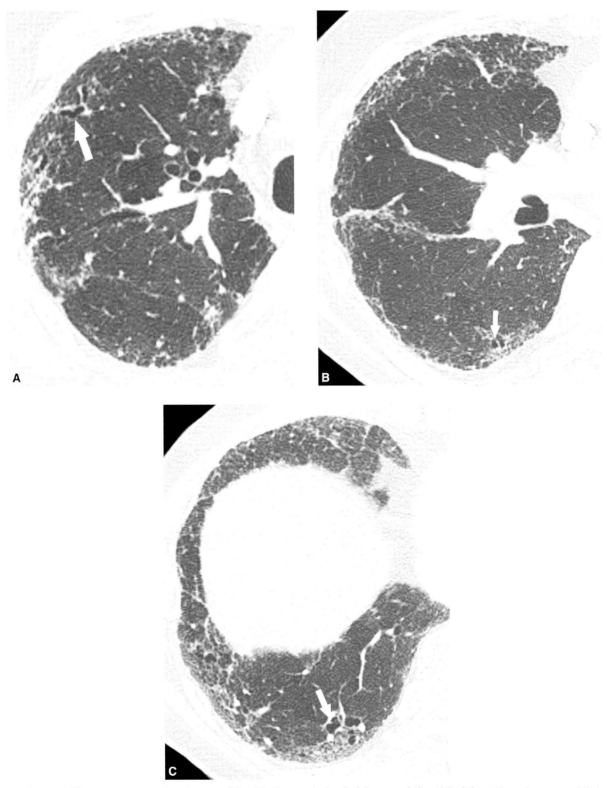

FIGURE 6.8. Probable UIP pattern on HRCT. Images of the right lung at the level of the upper **(A)**, middle **(B)**, and lower lung zones **(C)** demonstrate subpleural reticulation and peripheral traction bronchiectasis (*arrows*) with a slight lower lung predominance and the absence of any atypical features.

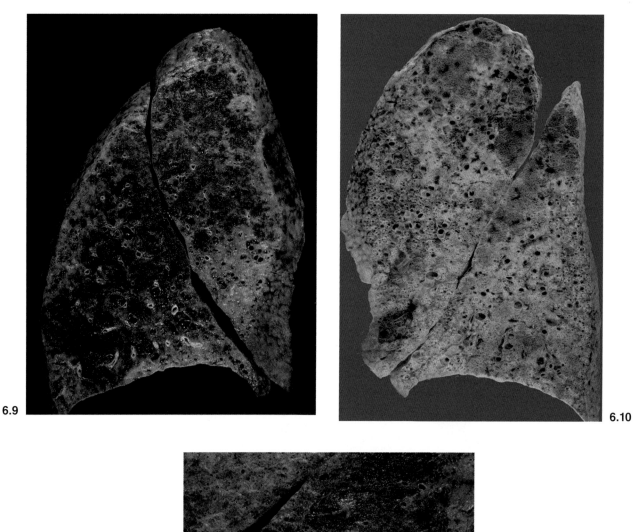

6.9

6.10

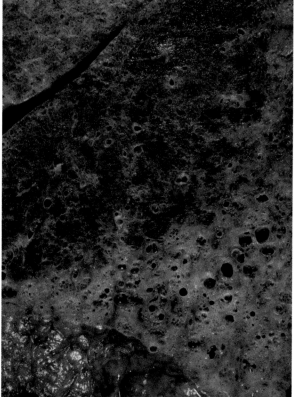

6.11

FIGURES 6.9 to 6.11. Gross images of UIP. The fibrotic process is worse in the periphery compared to the central portions of the lung and tends to be more severe in the lower zones. **Figure 6.11** illustrates an area of fibrosis and honeycombing in the lower portion of the image with irregular extension of fibrous tissue into the more normal lung in the upper portion of the image.

Table 6.2
Fibrosing lung disease that may have an upper zone predominance
Chronic HP (Chapter 12)
Sarcoid (Chapter 13)
Old tuberculosis and fungal infections
Ankylosing spondylitis
Pleuroparenchymal fibroelastosis (Chapter 23)

as well and may show increasing upper zone and central involvement over time. However, fibrosing disease that is predominantly upper zonal is unusual for UIP and suggests the entities shown in Table 6.2.

HONEYCOMBING

Cases of UIP almost always show *honeycombing* (Figs. 6.9 to 6.18) at a gross or microscopic level. Honeycombing is defined as abnormal enlarged airspaces with thick fibrous walls, and for convenience may be broken down into macroscopic honeycombing (visible on imaging and with the naked eye) and microscopic honeycombing, although in reality there is a continuous spectrum of airspace sizes.

Macroscopic honeycombing can be visualized by HRCT and plays an important role in the radiologic diagnosis of UIP (see section Imaging).

There is a mistaken belief that honeycombing is synonymous with UIP, but this is not correct: honeycombing is the end stage of a wide variety of fibrosing lung diseases (Table 6.3). However, most cases of UIP do show honeycombing at a gross or microscopic level or on imaging.

Microscopically, honeycombed spaces may have no lining at all but frequently are lined by metaplastic respiratory epithelium (Figs. 6.16 and 6.17). Honeycombed spaces commonly contain inspissated mucus, inflammatory cells, and sometimes giant cells (Figs. 6.16 to 6.18). These do not indicate any infectious process or any specific disease, but reflect local poor clearance. Interstitial inflammation and lymphoid aggregates can be prominent in honeycombed foci, but the presence of lymphoid aggregates with germinal centers or numerous plasma cells in honeycombed foci should raise a question of underlying CVD.

Unless one has a biopsy with just honeycombing and nothing else, honeycombing is not ordinarily part of a diagnosis; rather, just the underlying entity should be listed (i.e., "UIP" not "UIP with honeycombing"). In our view, a biopsy that only shows honeycombing is not specific (although many such cases turn out to be UIP)

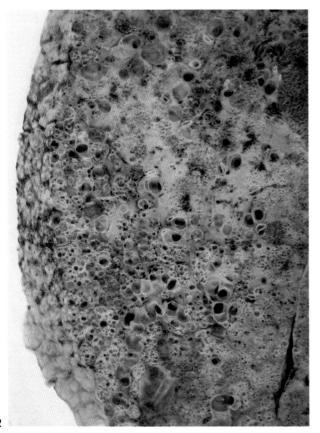

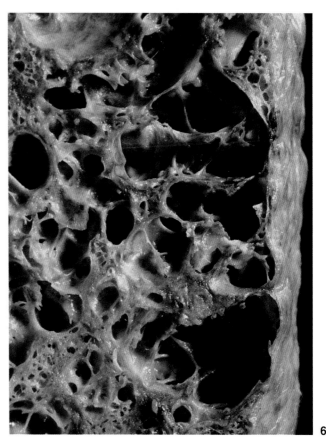

6.12   6.13

FIGURES 6.12 and 6.13. Gross views of macroscopic honeycombing. In **Figure 6.12** there are both honeycombing and extensive sheets of fibrous tissue. The pleura is also cobblestoned in both lungs, a finding that indicates the presence of underlying interstitial fibrosis.

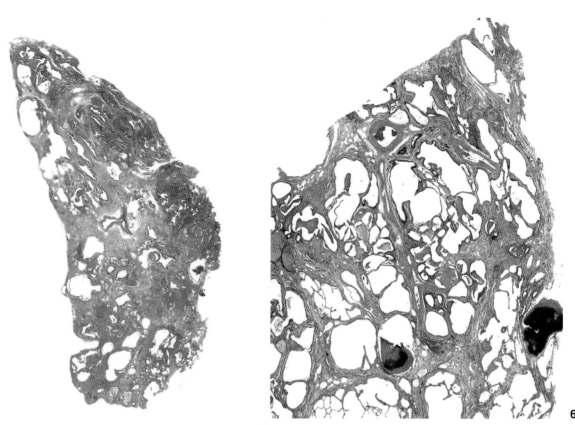

6.14   **6.15**

FIGURES 6.14 and 6.15. Examples of microscopic honeycombing. All of these images are from patients with UIP, but honeycombing is seen in many forms of ILD (see Table 6.3). Many of the airspaces in honeycombed foci are lined by metaplastic bronchiolar epithelium. Although the airspaces of microscopic honeycombing typically have thick fibrous walls, sometimes the walls are relatively thin (**Fig. 6.15**). Note the metaplastic bone in **Figure 6.15**, a frequent but nonspecific occurrence in fibrotic lungs.

and a comment to that effect is appropriate, but the contrary position is discussed in the section Differential Diagnosis and Controversies in the Pathologic Diagnosis of UIP.

PLEURAL COBBLESTONING

In resection specimens and autopsy lungs, the pleura in UIP is usually *cobblestoned* (Figs. 6.12 and 6.13), meaning that it demonstrates irregular bumps surrounded by depressed lines. This effect is caused by underlying scarring causing retraction of the interlobular septa where they insert on the pleura. Like honeycombing it is not specific and can be seen with any process that produces subpleural fibrosis. The pleura may be slightly thickened in UIP, but marked pleural thickening suggests either an underlying CVD, usually rheumatoid arthritis, in which there are repeated effusions, or asbestosis mimicking UIP.

MICROSCOPIC FEATURES OF UIP

The microscopic features of UIP are summarized in Table 6.4. The most characteristic feature of UIP is *patchy interstitial fibrosis* mixed with normal parenchyma. The fibrosis and the patchiness are visible at scanning magnification (Figs. 6.19 to 6.24), and UIP is a disease best diagnosed

at very low power. The fibrosing process typically jumps in a very abrupt fashion from very abnormal to completely normal in the space of less than 1 high-power microscope field (Fig. 6.25). In early disease (Fig. 6.22), the fibrosis may be present only or mostly immediately under the pleura or next to the interlobular septa, so that early UIP sometimes shows a peripheral lobular predominance, but as the disease progresses, more and more of the lobule is occupied by fibrous tissue (Figs. 6.23, 6.24, 6.26, and 6.27). However, fibrosing disease with a centrilobular predominance, meaning fibrosis predominantly around the bronchovascular bundles, is not UIP (see section Differential Diagnosis and Controversies in the Pathologic Diagnosis of UIP).

Two other constant features of UIP are *architectural distortion*, visible as areas of honeycombing or sheets of dense fibrous tissue (Figs. 6.23, 6.26, and 6.27), sometimes with prominent muscular metaplasia of the fibrous tissue (Fig. 6.28), and *fibroblast foci*—tufts of granulation tissue tightly applied to underlying fibrous tissue, with the fibroblasts in the granulation tissue arranged parallel to the underlying lung (Figs. 6.29 to 6.33). Fibroblast foci can be composed of young edematous granulation tissue (Fig. 6.30) or increasingly dense and collagenized granulation tissue (Figs. 6.31 to 6.33) and frequently are covered by cuboidal to flattened epithelial cells (Figs. 6.29 to 6.33).

CHAPTER 6: USUAL INTERSTITIAL PNEUMONIA

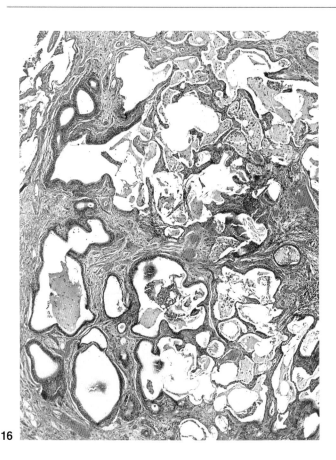

6.16

Table 6.3

Conditions that can have honeycombing

UIP

Desquamative interstitial pneumonia

NSIP (uncommon)

Chronic hypersensitivity pneumonia (sometimes upper zone predominant)

CVD-associated ILD

Pulmonary radiation (localized to radiation port)

Drug reactions

Sarcoidosis (typically upper zone)

Pneumoconioses (asbestosis, hard metal disease, rarely coal worker's pneumoconiosis or silicosis)

Langerhans cell histiocytosis

Healed infections, especially tuberculosis and histoplasmosis (typically upper zone)

Localized nonspecific scars

Fibroblast foci are believed to be the sites of injury in UIP, and repeated (unknown) insults leading to fibroblast foci that turn into dense fibrosis is the process by which UIP is thought to progress.

A myth has grown up that fibroblast foci are specific to UIP. This is not true: fibroblast foci can be seen in any

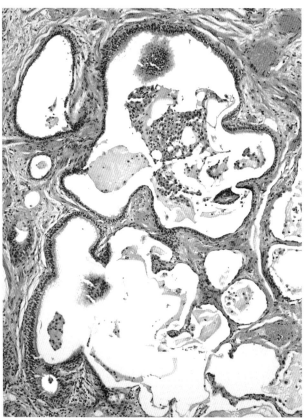

6.17

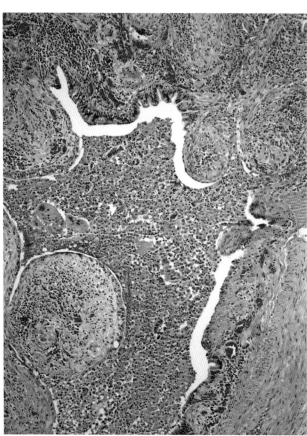

6.18

FIGURES 6.16 to 6.18. Mucus and inflammatory cells in honeycombed airspaces. This is a common finding in areas of honeycombing and is presumed to reflect poor clearance; the presence of inflammatory cells in this setting does not indicate the presence of an infectious process.

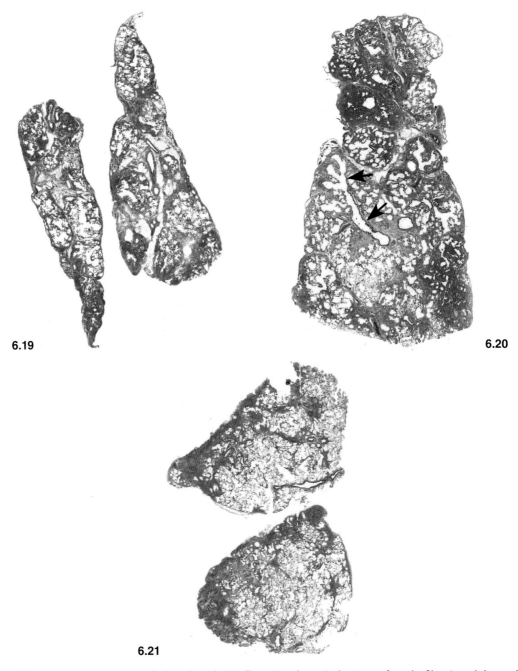

6.19

6.20

6.21

FIGURES 6.19 to 6.21. Scanning power views of relatively early UIP illustrating the typical pattern of patchy fibrosis and the tendency of the fibrosing process to involve the subpleural regions and periphery of the lobules. Note the area of traction bronchiolectasis in **Figure 6.20** (*arrows*). Traction bronchiolectasis is often visible on HRCT and indicates the presence of underlying fibrosis.

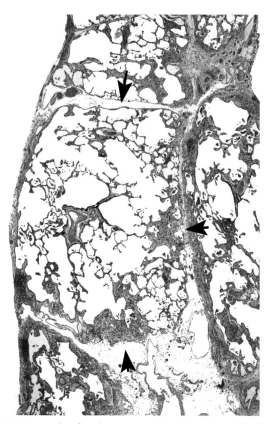

FIGURE 6.22. Example of early or minimal involvement in UIP. The fibrosing process involves the periphery of a lobule with central sparing (*arrows* mark the interlobular septa). This is a characteristic pattern of UIP, but is only occasionally seen.

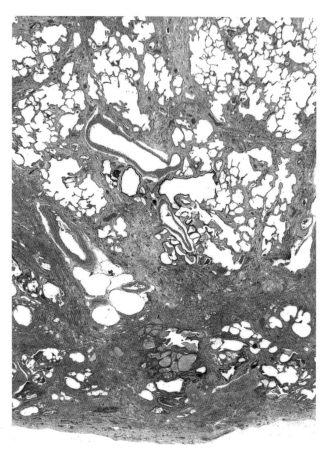

FIGURE 6.23. More advanced UIP. There is marked subpleural fibrosis and honeycombing with extension of fibrosis into the deeper parenchyma in an irregular fashion. The bronchiole in the center of the field shows peribronchiolar metaplasia. An occasional focus of peribronchiolar metaplasia can be seen in any fibrosing interstitial pneumonia, but numerous foci favor chronic HP over UIP (see Chapter 12).

type of fibrosing process in the lung including around nonspecific scars (see below). The separation of fibroblast foci from the granulation tissue plugs of organizing pneumonia (OP) is discussed in Chapter 5 (Table 5.3).

Interstitial inflammation in UIP is composed of lymphocytes and plasma cells and is generally sparse, except in honeycombed foci. Away from honeycombed areas, if there are numerous lymphoid aggregates, especially lymphoid aggregates with germinal centers (Fig. 6.34) or prominent interstitial inflammation (Fig. 6.35), particularly if the plasma cell to lymphocyte ratio away from lymphoid aggregates is greater than 1:1 in a biopsy that otherwise is typical of UIP, one should consider UIP associated with a CVD.[23,24] Chronic HP that mimics UIP (Chapter 12) also may show a fairly marked chronic interstitial inflammatory response, but sometimes is a perfect mimic of UIP/IPF (see Fig. 12.34).

DIFFERENTIAL DIAGNOSIS AND CONTROVERSIES IN THE PATHOLOGIC DIAGNOSIS OF UIP

The morphologic differential diagnosis of UIP is shown in Tables 6.5 and 6.6. Any kind of process that leads to dense fibrosis, including nonspecific scars (Figs. 6.36 and 6.37), can look like UIP at a microscopic level in a local area. If in doubt, consultation with the radiologist is very helpful in showing that a particular process is localized rather than diffuse. Apart from CVD-associated UIP and chronic HP, most of the other processes listed in Table 6.5 may mimic UIP in a given field but don't show a typical UIP picture at low power or on imaging; however, some drug reactions (Fig. 6.38) can produce a UIP picture and in this situation a drug history is crucial for making the correct diagnosis (see Chapter 18).

UIP VERSUS FIBROTIC NONSPECIFIC INTERSTITIAL PNEUMONIA

In general, fibrotic nonspecific interstitial pneumonia (NSIP) shows a fairly homogenous expansion of the alveolar walls with relatively little architectural distortion; the abrupt juxtaposition of normal and very abnormal parenchyma that characterizes UIP is not a part of NSIP (Table 7.3). Fibroblast foci are generally sparse in NSIP,

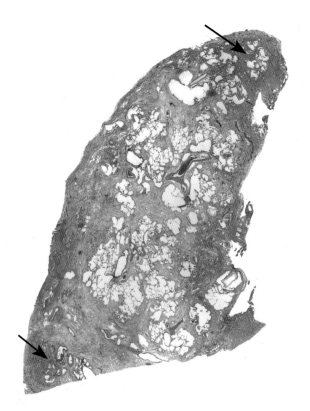

FIGURE 6.24. Whole-mount view of fairly advanced UIP. Even in relatively severe disease, there is still patchy fibrosis with fibrotic foci alternating with normal lung. *Arrows* point out areas of microscopic honeycombing.

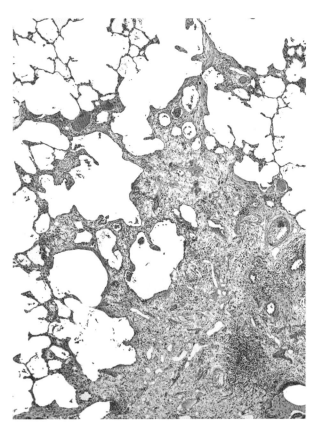

FIGURE 6.25. Characteristic pattern of patchy interstitial fibrosis that abruptly jumps back and forth between very abnormal and perfectly normal alveoli in the space of one high-power field. This kind of patchy fibrosis is sometimes referred to as morphologic heterogeneity and is very typical of UIP.

and if numerous fibroblast foci are present, the possibility of a bad sample of UIP should be considered. However, cases that are true fibrotic NSIP can sometimes show expansion of the alveolar walls to the point of confluence, thus producing relatively large blocks of fibrosis, that is, architectural distortion (Figs. 7.16 and 7.17), and to further add confusion, the confluent foci tend to have incorporated fibroblast foci.[25] However, such biopsies overall still show a relatively homogenous process.

Biopsies of typical UIP can have NSIP-like areas (Fig. 6.39), or if two biopsies are performed, one can show UIP and the other NSIP. When this occurs, the UIP pattern is the one that should be reported, because such cases behave like UIP.[26]

UIP VERSUS CVD-ASSOCIATED UIP

A UIP picture may be seen with any type of CVD (Table 6.6 and see Chapter 21 for more detail), but is particularly common with systemic sclerosis and rheumatoid arthritis and is rare with lupus.[24] UIP in patients with CVD is, pathologically, usually very similar to idiopathic UIP except for increased interstitial cellularity and, particularly, numerous lymphoid nodules or lymphoid nodules with germinal centers (Figs. 6.34 and 6.35). A high ratio of

interstitial plasma cells to lymphocytes (1:1 or greater), measured away from lymphoid aggregates, is strongly suggestive of an underlying CVD.[23] Giant cells and granulomas can be seen in CVD-UIP.[23] However, some cases of CVD-associated UIP are morphologically indistinguishable from UIP/IPF and only serology or clinical history provides a clue to the correct diagnosis. When features suggestive of a CVD are present, this should be noted in the diagnosis line, because the prognosis may be better than idiopathic UIP and treatment is different from UIP/IPF (see section Treatment and Prognosis).

UIP VERSUS CHRONIC HP

The features that allow separation of UIP from chronic HP with a UIP pattern (Table 6.6 and see Chapter 12) are disputed in the literature (reviewed in Churg et al.[6]). Giant cells/granulomas are accepted as features of chronic HP, and also some cases of CVD-associated UIP,[23] and are against a diagnosis of UIP/IPF. Peribronchiolar metaplasia around many bronchioles in a biopsy, certainly when present around more than half the bronchioles, favors chronic HP (Figs. 12.35 and 12.36),[23] but an occasional bronchiole with peribronchiolar metaplasia is not diagnostically

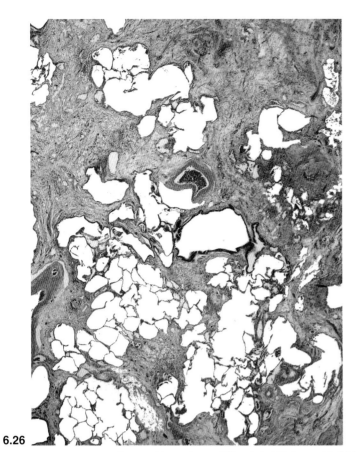

6.26

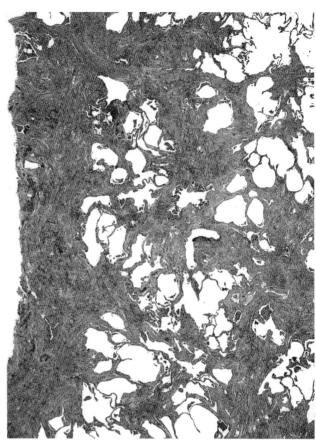

6.27

FIGURES 6.26 and 6.27. More advanced fibrosis in UIP. Even with fairly advanced disease, the characteristic pattern of marked fibrosis abruptly alternating with completely normal alveolar walls is still present. Note the paucicellular nature of the fibrosis; this is typical of idiopathic UIP.

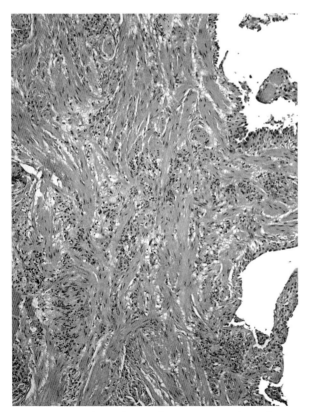

FIGURE 6.28. Smooth muscle metaplasia in UIP. Smooth muscle may replace the fibrous tissue in UIP. This is a common finding that has no diagnostic significance. In the past, muscle metaplasia has sometimes been referred to as "muscular cirrhosis," but this term is archaic and has no diagnostic value.

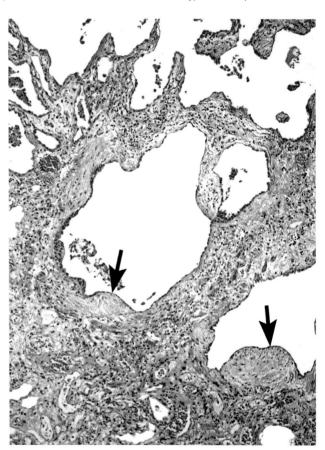

FIGURE 6.29. Fibroblast foci in UIP. Figure 6.29 shows two fibroblast foci (*arrows*) tightly applied to areas of underlying fibrosis.

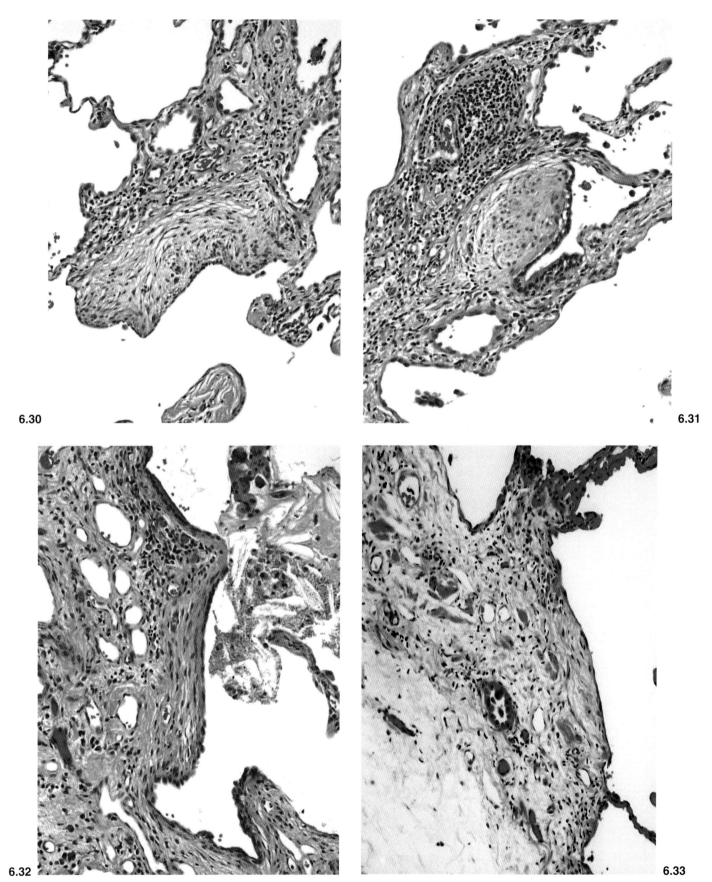

6.30

6.31

6.32

6.33

FIGURES 6.30 to 6.33. Progression of fibroblast foci from early cellular forms (*upper left panel*, **Fig. 6.30**) to (clockwise) progressively more fibrotic forms that eventually become part of the dense fibrosis of UIP. In **Figure 6.32** (*lower left*) the fibroblast focus is almost completely collagenized.

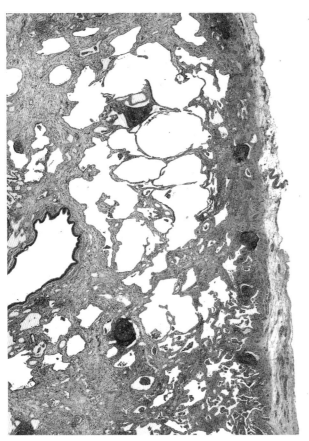

FIGURE 6.34. UIP in a patient with a CVD. Note the numerous lymphoid aggregates, several of which contain germinal centers.

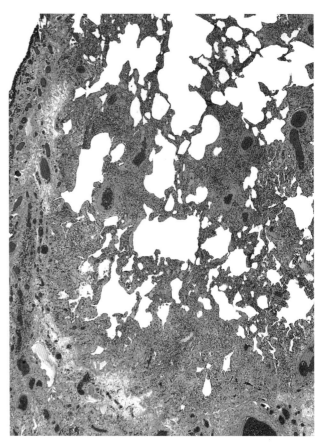

FIGURE 6.35. UIP in a patient with a CVD. There is a fairly marked chronic inflammatory interstitial infiltrate, a finding that takes this out of the idiopathic UIP category.

helpful because it can be seen in many forms of fibrosing interstitial pneumonia (Fig. 6.23).

The major issue of contention is whether any, or how much, peribronchiolar fibrosis (centrilobular fibrosis) can be seen in UIP/IPF or whether peribronchiolar fibrosis automatically removes a case from the UIP/IPF category.[5,6] At present, there is no consensus on this question. In a recent study,[5] 11 pulmonary pathologists reviewed a series of fibrosing interstitial pneumonia cases and were split evenly on the question of whether the type of pattern seen in Figure 6.40 falls within the spectrum of UIP/IPF or is indicative of another diagnosis. The 2018 IPF guideline document[3] illustrated a case similar to Figure 6.40 as an example of "probable UIP," a nebulous term that is itself poorly defined (see later for further comment), but we believe that this morphology somewhat favors chronic HP. This idea was supported in a report from Tanizawa et al.[27] who found that about one-third of UIP cases had centrilobular fibrosis, but centrilobular fibrosis of the sort shown in Figure 6.40 was considerably more common in non-IPF diagnoses (odds ratio for a non-IPF compared to IPF diagnosis of 3.71).

Our view is that isolated foci of peribronchiolar fibrosis with no connection to the pleura or interlobular

Table 6.5

Morphologic differential diagnosis of a UIP pattern on biopsy

Fibrotic forms of HP

Fibrotic forms of CVD-associated ILD

Burnt-out sarcoid (look for granulomas)

Burnt-out Langerhans cell histiocytosis (look for residual active Langerhans cell lesions)

Burnt-out tuberculous or fungal infection (look for granulomas)

Chronic aspiration with scarring (look for foreign body giant cells/lipid droplets)

Organized and honeycombed ARDS (not a good mimic)

Asbestosis and other pneumoconioses such as talcosis (look for asbestos bodies, talc particles)

Old radiation injury (usually localized)

Old drug injury

Old local scars

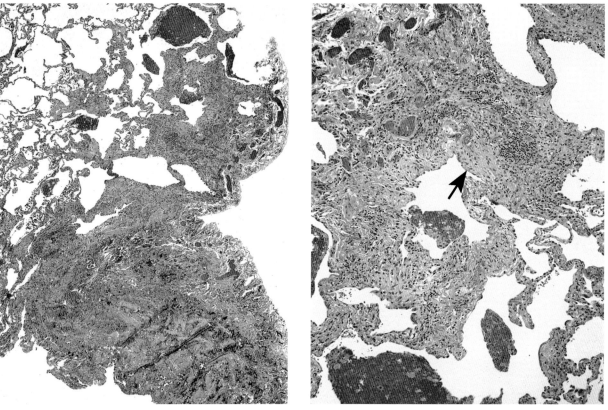

6.36

6.37

FIGURES 6.36 and 6.37. Localized scar mimicking UIP. The patient had had a wedge resection of a lung cancer and then developed a mass lesion at the site of the previous resection. The resulting scar shows patchy fibrosis (**Fig. 6.36**) and even a fibroblast focus (**Fig. 6.37**) (*arrow*). Fibroblast foci are not specific to UIP and can be seen in any kind of fibrosing process. This case illustrates the importance of clinical and radiologic correlation in diagnosing ILD.

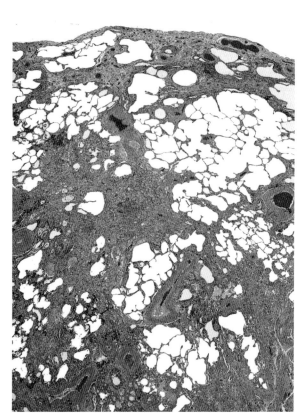

FIGURE 6.38. Drug reaction mimicking UIP. This patient was an elderly woman who received multiple chemotherapeutic drugs for ovarian cancer.

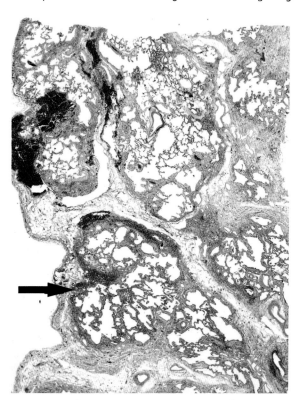

FIGURE 6.39. Fibrotic NSIP-like area in UIP. Most of the biopsy in this case looks like typical UIP with patchy, largely peripheral fibrosis, but one lobule (*arrow*) mimics fibrotic NSIP pattern. In the presence of a typical UIP pattern, the fibrotic NSIP pattern should be ignored, because the presence of a UIP pattern determines prognosis.

Table 6.6			
Pathologic separation of UIP/IPF, chronic HP with a UIP pattern, and CVD-ILD with a UIP pattern			
Feature	**UIP/IPF**	**Chronic HP**	**CVD-ILD**
Extensive peribronchiolar metaplasia (more than half of bronchioles)	Against UIP/IPF	Favors chronic HP	Against CVD-ILD
Giant cells/granulomas	Against UIP/IPF	Can be seen in chronic HP	Can be seen in CVD-ILD
Interstitial cellularity	Paucicellular, few plasma cells or eosinophils	Can be more cellular than UIP/IPF Few plasma cells or eosinophils Can be paucicellular	Often considerable interstitial cellularity, frequently predominance of plasma cells. However, can be paucicellular
Lymphoid aggregates away from honeycombed areas	Can be present in small numbers	Can be present in small numbers	Large numbers favor CVD-ILD
Germinal centers	Rarely present	Rarely present	Support a diagnosis of CVD-ILD particularly if several present
Isolated peribronchiolar fibrosis	Disputed, but probably occurs in UIP/IPF. Many foci of isolated peribronchiolar fibrosis against a diagnosis of UIP/IPF	Often present	Can be present
Bridging fibrosis from peribronchiolar region to subpleural region or interlobular septa	Disputed, but definitely occurs when fibrosis overruns whole lobules	Can be present. Delicate bridges favor CHP	Can be present
Coarse peribronchiolar fibrosis that connects to subpleural fibrosis	Disputed but probably occurs in UIP/IPF; however, favors a non-IPF diagnosis	Can be present	Can be present

septa favor chronic HP over UIP/IPF, particularly when there is minimal or mild subpleural fibrosis/fibrosis adjacent to the interlobular septa, and particularly if there are multiple such peribronchiolar foci (Figs. 12.28 and 12.33). Delicate fibrous bridges between the bronchioles and the pleura or interlobular septa (Figs. 12.37 and 12.38) also favor chronic HP, but coarse fibrotic bridges (Figs. 6.23 and 12.34) are much less specific because as UIP/IPF progresses, it tends to overrun the pulmonary lobule.

GUIDELINE DIAGNOSES OF DEFINITE UIP, PROBABLE UIP, INDETERMINATE FOR UIP, AND ALTERNATIVE DIAGNOSIS

Two recent IPF guidelines[3,4] propose this series of categories for HRCT diagnoses and pathologic diagnoses of suspected UIP/IPF. The imaging categories are discussed earlier and have the advantage that there are a set of positive findings as part of the definitions. The pathology categories of "Definite UIP" and "Alternative Diagnosis" are also clear, but the pathology categories of "Probable UIP" and "Indeterminate for UIP" are nebulous because the definitions essentially say that a given case lacks some or most of the features of definite UIP. In our view, this is so vague as to be unworkable and we don't recommend this usage.

Both position papers also propose that biopsies with pure honeycombing be labeled as "probable UIP." This might not be unreasonable for a case that clinically and radiologically looks like definite UIP/IPF, but the same guidelines make it clear that cases thought to be definite UIP/IPF should not be biopsied. Thus, in practice, pure honeycombing will be seen in biopsies from cases in which the diagnosis of UIP/IPF is in doubt, and, given the numerous possible causes and morphologic nonspecificity of honeycombing (Table 6.3), we suggest that such biopsies should simply be diagnosed as "honeycombing."

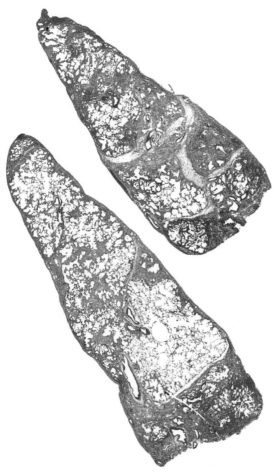

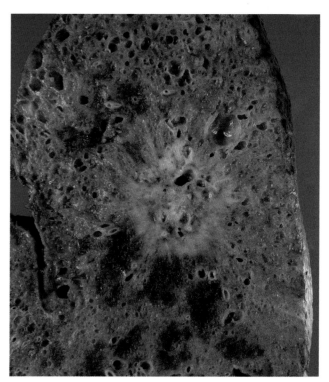

FIGURE 6.41. Lung carcinoma arising in UIP. Note the extensive honeycombing.

FIGURE 6.40. A problem case. The upper section looks like typical UIP/IPF but the lower section has extensive areas with little subpleural fibrosis and greater amounts of centrilobular fibrosis. There is dispute in the literature on the question of whether this pattern is still acceptable as UIP/IPF or is more indicative of another diagnosis, especially chronic HP (see comments in text).

COMPLICATIONS AND CAUSES OF DEATH IN UIP

Table 6.7 lists complications and causes of death in UIP. There is a markedly increased risk of lung cancer (Fig. 6.41), even in nonsmokers, but the overall prognosis of UIP has historically been so poor that the presence of lung cancer seems to have little effect on survival.[28]

Table 6.7

Complications and causes of death in UIP

Carcinoma of lung (~10-fold increased risk)
Pulmonary hypertension/cor pulmonale
Respiratory failure secondary to progressive fibrosis
Pulmonary infections
Acute exacerbation = diffuse alveolar damage or OP
    superimposed on UIP

Pulmonary hypertension is seen in 30% to 80% of UIP patients awaiting transplantation, although the incidence may be lower if all UIP patients are considered,[29] and probably leads to a shortened life expectancy. Microscopically thick-walled pulmonary artery branches are commonly seen in UIP and in virtually all forms of fibrotic ILD; however, most of the time, these changes are nonspecific and it is difficult to reliably predict the presence of pulmonary hypertension from the morphologic findings.

An acute exacerbation is the development of diffuse parenchymal opacities on imaging (Fig. 4.21), usually accompanied by hypoxemia and marked shortness of breath, in a patient with UIP over a time course of 30 days or less and not caused by fluid overload.[30] Acute exacerbations are also seen with other types of fibrosing ILD, but with much lower frequencies (Table 6.8). Many acute exacerbations do not have an identifiable cause, but some are associated with pulmonary infections, aspiration, thoracic surgery or cryobiopsy, and drugs including chemotherapeutic agents and immunosuppressive agents.[30]

The incidence of acute exacerbations in UIP is probably about 5% to 15% of cases per year and increases with increasing disease severity.[30] Acute exacerbations are an important cause of death; in some autopsy series, 50% of UIP deaths have shown morphologic evidence of an acute exacerbation.[31]

Morphologically acute exacerbations look like diffuse alveolar damage, which may be in the acute or organizing phase, or OP, plus an underlying pattern of UIP[32,33]

Table 6.8

Types of fibrosing ILD that are associated with acute exacerbations

Idiopathic UIP (IPF)
UIP Associated with CVD
Fibrotic NSIP
Chronic HP with UIP-like pattern
Desquamative interstitial pneumonia
Asbestosis

(see Figs. 4.21 to 4.25). When the acute injury pattern is spatially separated from the old fibrosis of UIP (Figs. 4.24 and 4.25), the diagnosis is readily made; however, in some instances, the acute injury obscures the underlying disease (Figs. 4.22 and 4.23). A helpful hint is that neither diffuse alveolar damage nor OP should show evidence of old fibrosis; if old fibrosis is present, then the acute injury must be superimposed on some preexisting condition. Sometimes the old fibrosis is much more apparent on imaging studies than on biopsy (Fig. 4.21).

A recent study has looked at the effects of pirfenidone and nintedanib antifibrotic treatment on the morphology of UIP in explanted lungs.[34] For the most part, treatment did not change the microscopic appearances, but there was a decreased incidence of superimposed diffuse alveolar damage, a finding consistent with the observed clinical effects of these agents.

DIAGNOSTIC MODALITIES

As discussed in Chapter 3, UIP cannot be diagnosed on transbronchial or core biopsy. Even if definite fibrosis is present in a transbronchial forceps biopsy, this finding is of no diagnostic utility (see Chapter 3) and we advise not mentioning fibrosis in the diagnosis line in transbronchial biopsies least they be misinterpreted as indicating that UIP or another fibrosing interstitial pneumonia is present.

Whether cryobiopsy is suitable is controversial (see Chapter 3), and in our view cryobiopsies probably do not sample enough tissue to reliably pick up the features that differentiate UIP from chronic HP (see Chapter 12). Current clinical guidelines recommend against using transbronchial forceps or cryobiopsies for a diagnosis of UIP.[3,4] Surgical lung biopsy remains the procedure of choice, and several biopsies of suitably large size (see Chapter 3) should be taken to avoid finding only nonspecific honeycombing.[4]

The use of multidisciplinary discussion (see Chapter 1) greatly increases the accuracy of ILD diagnosis and is particularly valuable in fibrosing interstitial pneumonias such as UIP and its differential diagnoses, because these entities produce the greatest number of problems for clinicians, radiologists, and pathologists.

TREATMENT AND PROGNOSIS

The overall outcome of IPF is poor, with median survival in a recent survey of 24 patient cohorts of 3.2 years.[35] It has been suggested that IPF mortality is increasing in the population, but this is most likely a lead-time and diagnostic bias effect, with improved methods of early radiologic detection and increased numbers of patient diagnosed with IPF, particularly since the introduction of antifibrotic therapy.[35] In fact, a detailed analysis suggests that there is a small but real improvement in survival in more recent cohorts,[35] either because of the use of antifibrotic agents or because of the avoidance of contraindicated drugs (see below).

Until very recently, attempts to treat IPF with drugs have been failures. Steroids, azathioprine, N-acetylcysteine (an antioxidant), interferon-γ, imatinib, endothelin receptor antagonists, and anticoagulants such as warfarin not only are ineffective, but some of these agents alone or in combination (particularly steroids, azathioprine, and N-acetylcysteine) greatly increase mortality.[36]

Starting in 2013, large trials of two antifibrotic therapies for IPF, pirfenidone and nintedanib, were reported and a number of additional trials/analyses of the data have been described (reviewed in Raghu et al.[36] and Richeldi et al.[37]). These are the first drugs that have been shown to slow progression of the disease. Nintedanib is a tyrosine kinase inhibitor that targets multiple growth factor pathways, whereas pirfenidone exerts antifibrogenic effects through uncertain mechanisms that decrease collagen synthesis, fibroblast proliferation, and downregulation of transforming growth factor β signaling. Both agents produced a roughly 50% decrease in forced vital capacity decline and a modest but clear improvement in progression-free survival/decreased mortality at 1 year.[36] Both, but especially nintedanib, also appear to reduce the rate of acute exacerbations. These effects persist with treatment beyond 1 year.[37] A number of other new agents are in clinical trials (reviewed in Lederer and Martinez[18]).

Lung transplantation is an option for younger patients who do not have other significant comorbidities. A recent review[38] reported 3-year survivals of 66% and 5-year survivals of 53% for IPF patients. IPF does not recur in transplanted lungs.

UIP in patients with rheumatoid arthritis appears to have the same poor prognosis as IPF (see Chapter 21), but UIP in other forms of CVD may respond to immunosuppressive agents and/or cyclophosphamide and may have a much better prognosis (see Chapter 21).

The prognosis of acute exacerbations is, overall, very poor, with a short-term mortality of around 50%.[30] Some patients respond to high-dose steroids. Patients with acute exacerbations and a pattern of OP on biopsy seem to do better than those with diffuse alveolar damage.[32]

REFERENCES

1. ATS/ERS international multidisciplinary consensus classification of the idiopathic interstitial pneumonias. *Am J Respir Crit Care Med*. 2002;165:277–304.
2. Travis WD, Costabel U, Hansell DM, et al.; ATS/ERS Committee on Idiopathic Interstitial Pneumonias. An official American Thoracic Society/European Respiratory Society statement: update of the international multidisciplinary classification of the idiopathic interstitial pneumonias. *Am J Respir Crit Care Med*. 2013;188:733–748.
3. Raghu G, Remy-Jardin M, Myers JL, et al.; American Thoracic Society, European Respiratory Society, Japanese Respiratory Society, and Latin American Thoracic Society. Diagnosis of Idiopathic Pulmonary Fibrosis. An Official ATS/ERS/JRS/ALAT Clinical Practice Guideline. *Am J Respir Crit Care Med*. 2018;198:e44–e68.
4. Lynch DA, Sverzellati N, Travis WD, et al. Diagnostic criteria for idiopathic pulmonary fibrosis: a Fleischner Society White Paper. *Lancet Respir Med*. 2018;6:138–153.
5. Hashisako M, Tanaka T, Terasaki Y, et al. Interobserver agreement of usual interstitial pneumonia diagnosis correlated with patient outcome. *Arch Pathol Lab Med*. 2016;140:1375–1382.
6. Churg A, Bilawich A, Wright JL. Pathology of chronic hypersensitivity pneumonitis what is it? What are the diagnostic criteria? Why do we care? *Arch Pathol Lab Med*. 2018;142:109–119.
7. Roggli VL, Gibbs AR, Attanoos R, et al. Pathology of asbestosis—an update of the diagnostic criteria: report of the asbestosis committee of the college of American pathologists and pulmonary pathology society. *Arch Pathol Lab Med*. 2010;134:462–480.
8. Leslie KO, Cool CD, Sporn TA, et al. Familial idiopathic interstitial pneumonia: histopathology and survival in 30 patients. *Arch Pathol Lab Med*. 2012;136(11):1366–1376.
9. Putman RK, Gudmundsson G, Araki T, et al. The MUC5B promoter polymorphism is associated with specific interstitial lung abnormality subtypes. *Eur Respir J*. 2017;50. pii: 1700537.
10. Adegunsoye A, Vij R, Noth I. Integrating genomics into management of fibrotic interstitial lung disease. *Chest*. 2019;155(5):1026–1040.
11. Ley B, Newton CA, Arnould I, et al. The MUC5B promoter polymorphism and telomere length in patients with chronic hypersensitivity pneumonitis: an observational cohort-control study. *Lancet Respir Med*. 2017;5(8):639–647.
12. Juge PA, Lee JS, Ebstein E, et al. MUC5B promoter variant and rheumatoid arthritis with interstitial lung disease. *N Engl J Med*. 2018;379:2209–2219.
13. Yang IV, Fingerlin TE, Evans CM, et al. MUC5B and idiopathic pulmonary fibrosis. *Ann Am Thorac Soc*. 2015;12(suppl 2):S193–S199.
14. Noth I, Zhang Y, Ma SF, et al. Genetic variants associated with idiopathic pulmonary fibrosis susceptibility and mortality: a genome-wide association study. *Lancet Respir Med*. 2013;1:309–317.
15. Hoffman TW, van Moorsel CHM, Borie R, et al. Pulmonary phenotypes associated with genetic variation in telomere-related genes. *Curr Opin Pulm Med*. 2018;24(3):269–280.
16. Raghu G, Chen SY, Yeh WS, et al. Idiopathic pulmonary fibrosis in US Medicare beneficiaries aged 65 years and older: incidence, prevalence, and survival, 2001-2011. *Lancet Respir Med*. 2014;2:566–572.
17. Raghu G, Chen SY, Hou Q, et al. Incidence and prevalence of idiopathic pulmonary fibrosis in US adults 18–64 years old. *Eur Respir J*. 2016;48:179–186.
18. Lederer DJ, Martinez FJ. Idiopathic pulmonary fibrosis. *N Engl J Med*. 2018;378:1811–1823.
19. American Thoracic Society; European Respiratory Society. Idiopathic pulmonary fibrosis: diagnosis and treatment: international consensus statement. *Am J Respir Crit Care Med*. 2000;161:646–664.
20. Song JW, Do KH, Kim MY, et al. Pathologic and radiologic differences between idiopathic and collagen vascular disease-related usual interstitial pneumonia. *Chest*. 2009;136:23–30.
21. Brownell R, Moua T, Henry TS, et al. The use of pretest probability increases the value of high-resolution CT in diagnosing usual interstitial pneumonia. *Thorax*. 2017;72:424–429.
22. Chung JH, Oldham JM, Montner SM, et al. CT-pathologic correlation of major types of pulmonary fibrosis: insights for revisions to current guidelines. *AJR Am J Roentgenol*. 2018;210(5):1034–1041.
23. Churg A, Wright JL, Ryerson CJ. Pathologic separation of chronic hypersensitivity pneumonitis from fibrotic connective tissue disease-associated interstitial lung disease. *Am J Surg Pathol*. 2017;41:1403–1409.
24. Katzenstein AL, Zisman DA, Litzky LA, et al. Usual interstitial pneumonia: histologic study of biopsy and explant specimens. *Am J Surg Pathol*. 2002;26(12):1567–1577.
25. Churg A, Bilawich A. Confluent fibrosis and fibroblast foci in fibrotic non-specific interstitial pneumonia. *Histopathology*. 2016;69:128–135.
26. Monaghan H, Wells AU, Colby TV, et al. Prognostic implications of histologic patterns in multiple surgical lung biopsies from patients with idiopathic interstitial pneumonias. *Chest*. 2004;125:522–526.
27. Tanizawa K, Ley B, Vittinghoff E, et al. Significance of bronchiolocentric fibrosis in patients with histopathologic usual interstitial pneumonia. *Histopathology*. 2019;74(7):1088–1097.
28. Aubry MC, Myers JL, Douglas WW, et al. Primary pulmonary carcinoma in patients with idiopathic pulmonary fibrosis. *Mayo Clin Proc*. 2002;77:763–770.
29. Fell CD. Idiopathic pulmonary fibrosis: phenotypes and comorbidities. *Clin Chest Med*. 2012; 33:51–57.
30. Ryerson CJ, Cottin V, Brown KK, et al. Acute exacerbation of idiopathic pulmonary fibrosis: shifting the paradigm. *Eur Respir J*. 2015;46:512–520.
31. Rice AJ, Wells AU, Bouros D, et al. Terminal diffuse alveolar damage in relation to interstitial pneumonias. An autopsy study. *Am J Clin Pathol*. 2003;119:709–714.
32. Churg A, Wright JL, Tazelaar HD. Acute exacerbations of fibrotic interstitial lung disease. *Histopathology*. 2011;58:525–530.
33. Churg A, Müller NL, Silva CI, et al. Acute exacerbation (acute lung injury of unknown cause) in UIP and other forms of fibrotic interstitial pneumonias. *Am J Surg Pathol*. 2007;31:277–284.
34. Zhang Y, Jones KD, Achtar-Zadeh N, et al. Histopathological and molecular analysis of idiopathic pulmonary fibrosis

lungs from patients treated with pirfenidone or nintedanib. *Histopathology.* 2019;74:341–349.

35. Ryerson CJ, Kolb M. The increasing mortality of idiopathic pulmonary fibrosis: fact or fallacy? *Eur Respir J.* 2018;51. pii: 1702420.

36. Raghu G, Rochwerg B, Zhang Y, et al.; American Thoracic Society; European Respiratory society; Japanese Respiratory Society; Latin American Thoracic Association. An Official ATS/ERS/JRS/ALAT Clinical Practice Guideline: treatment of Idiopathic Pulmonary Fibrosis. An Update of the 2011 Clinical Practice Guideline. *Am J Respir Crit Care Med.* 2015;15;192:e3–e19.

37. Richeldi L, Kreuter M, Selman M, et al. Long-term treatment of patients with idiopathic pulmonary fibrosis with nintedanib: results from the TOMORROW trial and its open-label extension. *Thorax.* 2018;73(6):581–583.

38. Valapour M, Lehr CJ, Skeans MA, et al. OPTN/SRTR 2016 annual data report: lung. *Am J Transplant.* 2018;18(suppl 1):363–433.

Nonspecific Interstitial Pneumonia

NOMENCLATURE ISSUES

Rather like organizing pneumonia (OP), nonspecific interstitial pneumonia (NSIP) is both an idiopathic disease and a pathologic pattern seen in other conditions, most notably collagen vascular diseases and entities with some features of collagen vascular disease (e.g., interstitial pneumonia with autoimmune features [IPAF], see Chapter 21), hypersensitivity pneumonitis, and drug reactions.

There are no universally agreed rules for names to be used in diagnosis, but when the underlying process is clearly not idiopathic NSIP, a qualifying name or a different name may be appropriate. For example, a patient with rheumatoid arthritis and NSIP should be diagnosed with "NSIP associated with rheumatoid arthritis" or "NSIP with features of a collagen vascular disease," assuming such features are present (see below and Chapter 21). A patient with an NSIP pattern on imaging and biopsy, a history of bird exposures, and anti-avian protein antibodies in serum should be diagnosed with hypersensitivity pneumonitis, rather than NSIP.

CLINICAL FEATURES

The clinical features of NSIP depend somewhat on associated conditions, but regardless of etiology, NSIP is usually associated with signs and symptoms of an interstitial lung disease (ILD, Chapter 1).[1] The age range is wide, extending even to children. Symptoms may be present for months to years and can include systemic symptoms such as fever. NSIP is the most common pathologic pattern of ILD in patients with collagen vascular disease,[1] and in such patients, extrapulmonary features of the underlying disease such as arthritis and arthralgias may be evident, but NSIP can also be the first or only manifestation of a collagen vascular disease (see below and Chapter 21).

IMAGING

At initial presentation, NSIP is characterized on high-resolution computed tomography (HRCT) by extensive bilateral ground-glass opacities frequently associated

with mild reticulation but no honeycombing[2] (Figs. 7.1 and 7.2). The parenchymal abnormalities usually

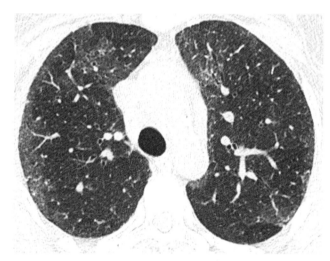

FIGURE 7.1. Nonspecific interstitial pneumonia. HRCT at the level of the upper lobes shows bilateral ground-glass opacities.

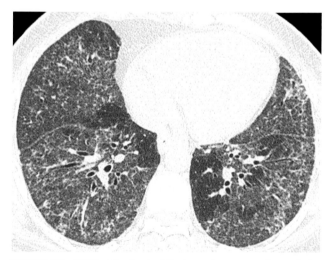

FIGURE 7.2. HRCT at the level of the lower lung zones demonstrates extensive bilateral ground-glass opacities with superimposed mild fine reticulation. Although the upper lobe changes in Figure 7.1 are consistent with cellular NSIP, the reticulation in the lower lobes suggests the presence of some fibrosis. The patient was a 42-year-old woman with NSIP.

involve the lower lung zones predominately and are frequently associated with lower lobe volume loss.[3] A purely ground-glass pattern is seen in cellular NSIP. Reticulation superimposed on ground-glass opacities usually indicates fibrosis and may be seen in mixed cellular and fibrotic NSIP and in fibrotic NSIP. The distribution of the reticulation in the axial plane is variable: It may involve mainly the peripheral regions, have a random distribution, or spare the subpleural parenchyma.[3]

With progression of disease, there is a decrease in the extent of ground-glass attenuation and an increase in reticulation and traction bronchiectasis, and in some cases the development of honeycombing (Figs. 7.3 and 7.4).[2]

Reticulation may become the predominant pattern. Findings that favor NSIP over usual interstitial pneumonia (UIP) in these patients include the presence of extensive traction bronchiectasis with minimal or no honeycombing.

The HRCT manifestations of NSIP at presentation, when there is a predominance of ground-glass opacities, minimal reticulation, and no honeycombing, are easily distinguishable from those of UIP, but are otherwise relatively nonspecific and may mimic a variety of other chronic interstitial diseases, particularly hypersensitivity pneumonitis and desquamative interstitial pneumonia (DIP).[4] When the reticulation becomes extensive, the manifestations of NSIP may mimic those of UIP.[2] Although in certain clinical settings, such as in patients with scleroderma, the HRCT findings may be characteristic enough to strongly suggest NSIP, a definitive diagnosis of NSIP requires surgical lung biopsy.

PATHOLOGIC FEATURES

GROSS APPEARANCE

NSIP typically is deceptively normal on gross examination, even when there is extensive microscopic fibrosis (Fig. 7.5). Honeycombing is uncommon and the presence of extensive honeycombing should raise a question of UIP.

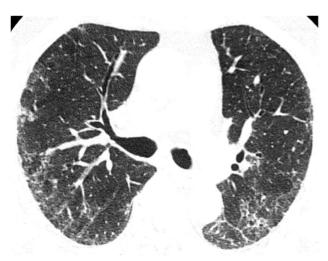

FIGURE 7.3. Nonspecific interstitial pneumonia. HRCT at the level of the upper lobes shows bilateral ground-glass opacities and peripheral reticulation.

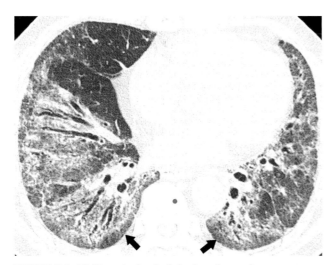

FIGURE 7.4. HRCT at the level of the lung bases demonstrates extensive bilateral ground-glass opacities with superimposed reticulation and traction bronchiectasis. Note lack of reticulation in some of the subpleural lung of the dorsal regions (subpleural sparing) (*arrows*). The patient was a 64-year-old man with fibrotic NSIP.

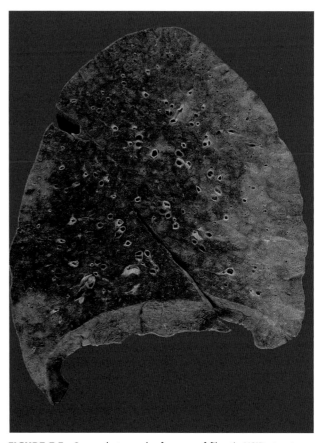

FIGURE 7.5. Gross photograph of a case of fibrotic NSIP at autopsy. Note the absence of honeycombing or obvious architectural distortion.

MICROSCOPIC FEATURES OF NSIP

There is a certain amount of variability in the patterns that different experienced pulmonary pathologists put into the category of NSIP, but the original and prototypical description is that of extremely homogeneous *chronic interstitial inflammation and/or interstitial fibrosis that follows the original alveolar walls* and produces no to minimal architectural distortion (Table 7.1, Figs. 7.6 to 7.8). In most cases, there is neither honeycombing nor sheets of fibrosis. Because of the homogeneity of the process, the scanning power view is that of a lung that is only subtly abnormal (Fig. 7.6).

The term "NSIP" is also often applied to processes where the interstitial inflammation or fibrosis is not completely homogeneous, but rather the lung is abnormal and then the interstitial process becomes less severe, only to reappear again a short distance away (Fig. 7.9). Although this description may sound like UIP at first glance, the important point is that there is still no architectural distortion; rather, the abnormality fades in and out of the parenchyma (Fig. 7.9), whereas in UIP there are abrupt transitions between markedly abnormal fibrotic parenchyma and normal or relatively normal parenchyma (see Figs. 6.22 to 6.27).

In the original description of NSIP by Katzenstein and Fiorelli,[5] cases were divided into purely cellular (Figs. 7.10 and 7.11), purely fibrotic (Figs. 7.9, 7.12, and 7.13), and mixed cellular and fibrotic forms. There has been a tendency over the ensuing years to try to use only cellular or fibrotic as descriptors, but our experience is that some cases show both features (Figs. 7.6 to 7.8). *The presence or absence of fibrosis should always be noted when diagnosing NSIP* because purely cellular forms can completely disappear with treatment, leaving normal parenchyma, whereas the more fibrosis that is present, the less the reversibility and the worse the prognosis. Biopsies are not always

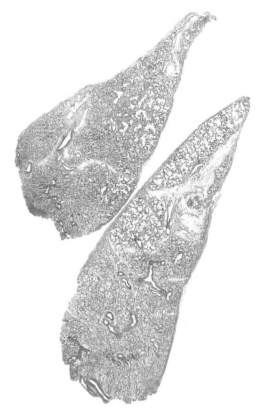

FIGURE 7.6. Scanning power view of a case of mixed cellular and fibrotic NSIP. Although this low-power view does not allow a specific diagnosis, it does show that there is no honeycombing and no architectural distortion.

representative of the amount of fibrosis, and correlation with imaging studies can be helpful.

As is true of UIP, the presence of numerous lymphoid aggregates (Figs. 7.10 to 7.12), and particularly aggregates with germinal centers, suggests an underlying collagen vascular disease or IPAF (see Chapter 21), as does an

Table 7.1
Pathologic features of NSIP
Cellular NSIP: chronic interstitial inflammation following the original alveolar walls
Fibrotic NSIP: old dense interstitial fibrosis following the original alveolar walls
Mixed cellular and fibrotic NSIP: combinations of the above
Tends to be morphologically homogeneous
Small areas of OP may be present
Generally no or only occasional fibroblast foci present, except in areas of confluent fibrosis
Large numbers of lymphoid aggregates suggest underlying collagen vascular disease or related conditions, particularly if germinal centers are present (see Chapter 21)
A high proportion of plasma cells in the interstitial inflammatory infiltrate suggests underlying collagen vascular disease
Usually absence of architectural distortion/honeycombing

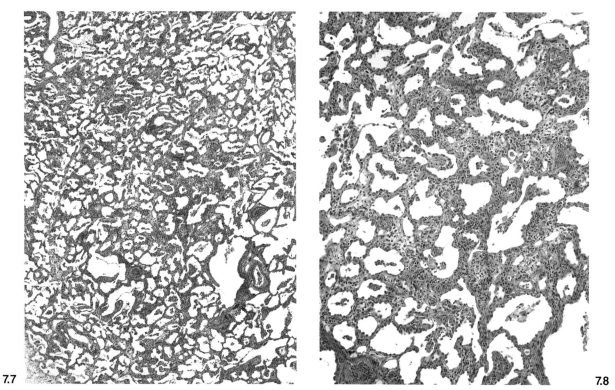

7.7   **7.8**

FIGURES 7.7 and 7.8. Progressively higher power views of the same case. The fibrotic and inflammatory process follows the original alveolar walls; this is the characteristic finding in NSIP.

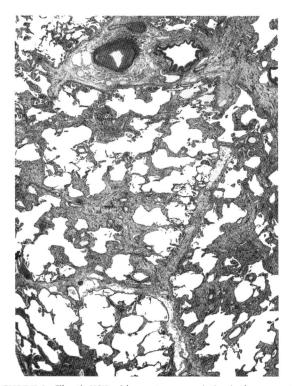

FIGURE 7.9. Fibrotic NSIP with area to area variation in the amount of interstitial fibrous tissue. Even though there is a mild amount of architectural distortion in this biopsy, the fibrosing process fades in and out gradually, as opposed to the abrupt jumps between very fibrotic and completely normal lung that is characteristic of UIP.

interstitial infiltrate with a high proportion of plasma cells. Ignoring lymphoid aggregates, a 1:1 or greater plasma cell to lymphocyte ratio favors a collagen vascular disease or IPAF,[6] and this should be noted in the diagnosis line. It has also been suggested that a thickened pleura is a manifestation of a collagen vascular disease,[7] although it is not clear that this claim has been formally examined. Increased alveolar macrophages may be present (Fig. 7.13), but large numbers of macrophages filling airspaces should raise a question of DIP (see Chapter 8).

MORPHOLOGIC VARIANTS OF NSIP

As noted, honeycombing is unusual in NSIP, but in our experience it is sometimes found in cases of fibrotic NSIP where there is marked expansion of the alveolar walls, such that they tend to become confluent (Figs. 7.14 and 7.15). Sometimes only sheets of fibrosis without honeycombing are seen in such cases (Figs. 7.16 and 7.17). These processes are exceptions to the rule that NSIP does not produce architectural distortion.

Fibroblast foci are occasionally seen in NSIP (Figs. 7.18 and 7.19), but tend to be particularly prominent in areas of confluent fibrosis.[8] However, large numbers of fibroblast foci should raise a question of whether the biopsy is a bad sample of UIP.

Tiny widely spaced foci of OP are fairly common in NSIP of any cause (Figs. 7.20 and 7.21). How much OP

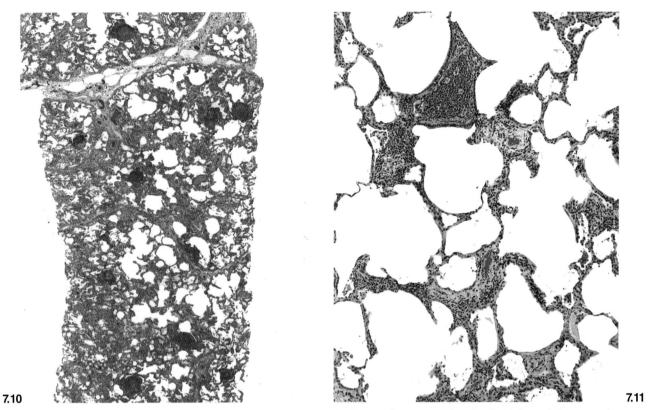

7.10

7.11

FIGURES 7.10 and 7.11. Cellular NSIP in a patient with a collagen vascular disease. The numerous lymphoid nodules and the germinal centers are a hint that the patient has an underlying collagen vascular disease, and this should be noted in the diagnosis line.

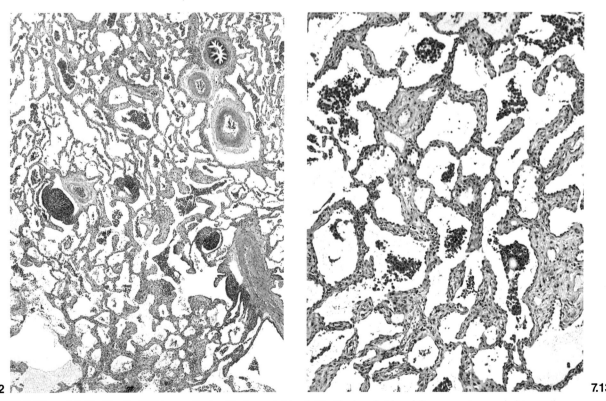

7.12

7.13

FIGURES 7.12 and 7.13. Fibrotic NSIP in a patient with rheumatoid arthritis. The lymphoid nodules suggest an underlying collagen vascular disease. Note the airspace collections lof alveolar macrophages; these are sometimes prominent in NSIP.

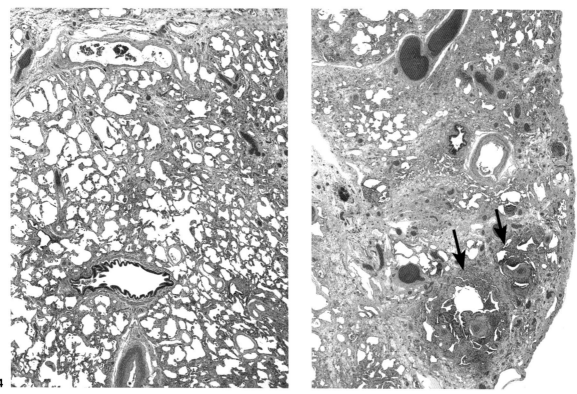

FIGURES 7.14 and 7.15. Fibrotic NSIP with an area of honeycombing (*arrows*). Honeycombing is relatively uncommon in NSIP but does occasionally occur.

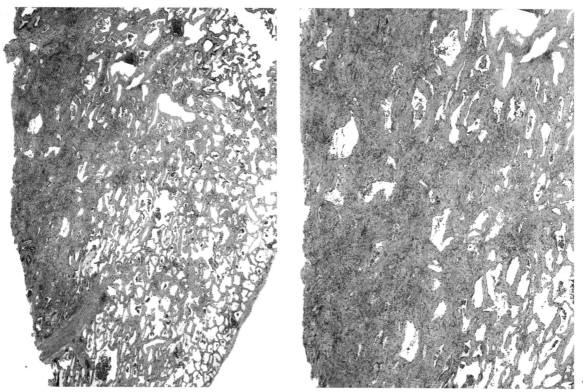

FIGURES 7.16 and 7.17. Fibrotic NSIP with an area of confluence. Confluent foci are formed by progressive expansion of alveolar walls (**Fig. 7.17**) and represent architectural distortion, a relatively uncommon finding in NSIP. Fibroblast foci may be found in increased numbers in confluent areas.

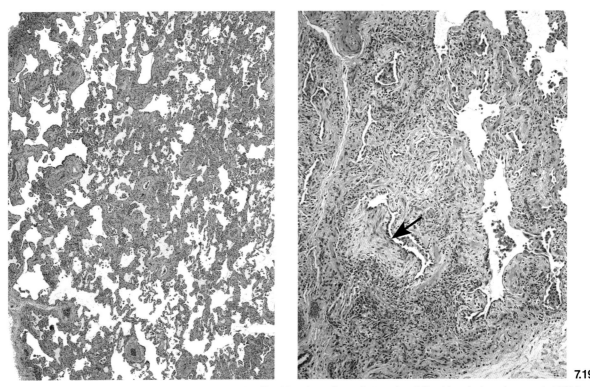

7.18

7.19

FIGURES 7.18 and 7.19. Mixed cellular and fibrotic NSIP with a fibroblast focus (*arrow*). Occasional fibroblast foci can be seen in NSIP but the presence of numerous fibroblast foci raises a question of a bad sample of UIP.

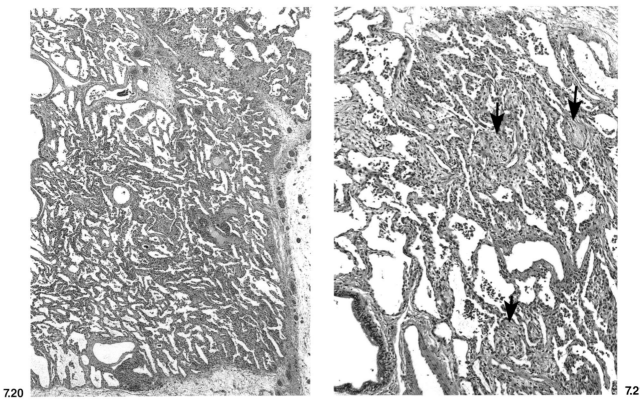

7.20

7.21

FIGURES 7.20 and 7.21. Cellular NSIP with an area of OP visible in **Figure 7.21** (*arrows*). Occasional small foci of OP are not uncommon in NSIP, but if there are numerous foci of OP on a background that is clearly NSIP, the possibility of an underlying collagen vascular disease or IPAF (see Chapter 21) should be raised.

still allows a diagnosis of NSIP is controversial; a review paper on idiopathic NSIP suggested that up to 20% of the parenchyma could show OP.[3] However, extensive areas of OP on a background of NSIP suggests either an underlying collagen vascular disease (and this combination may be apparent on imaging as well) or a bad sample of a case that really is OP and not NSIP, but with the biopsy taken from the edge of the OP lesion (see Chapter 5, Fig. 5.12). Interstitial inflammation is always part of OP and the edge of an OP lesion may have mostly interstitial inflammation and little granulation tissue (Chapter 5, Fig. 5.12). Imaging studies are often very helpful in sorting out these possibilities.

The original description of NSIP included cases with interstitial giant cells or granulomas, but the consensus from more recent studies is that giant cells and granulomas (and Schaumann bodies, which mark the sites of previous granulomas) are not part of NSIP and when present suggest that the correct diagnosis is most likely hypersensitivity pneumonitis (Figs. 7.22 and 7.23)[9] or sometimes a collagen vascular disease (see Chapter 21) or a drug reaction; for example, caused by methotrexate or anti–tumor necrosis factor agents.

Occasionally the fibrosis of NSIP tends to be more subpleural or aligned along interlobular septa, and separation of such cases from UIP can be difficult. Kambouchner et al.[10] suggest that gradual fading of fibrosis into the parenchyma rather than sharp demarcations and a lack/paucity of fibroblast foci favor NSIP.

MOLECULAR AND GENETIC ABNORMALITIES

Little is known about genetic abnormalities associated with NSIP, and the question is confounded by the fact that most cases of NSIP have a defined etiology (collagen vascular disease or other autoimmune disease, hypersensitivity pneumonitis, drug reaction). If one accepts the definition of two or more closely related family members with an interstitial pneumonia as "familial," roughly 85% of such patients have UIP and 10% NSIP.[10] NSIP patients apparently do not have the MUC5B promoter single nucleotide polymorphism or the telomerase mutations that are frequent in idiopathic UIP (idiopathic pulmonary fibrosis), but some have mutations in surfactant protein genes, specifically *SFTPC*.[10]

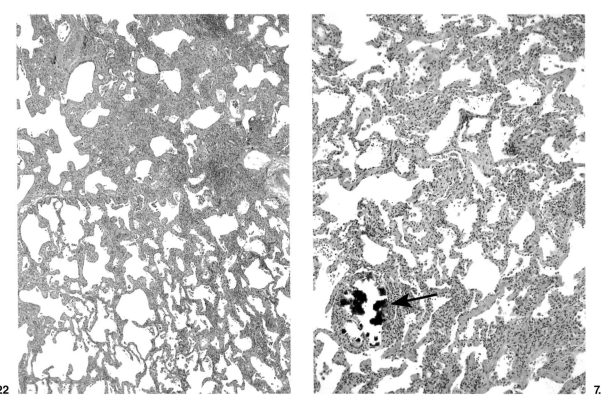

7.22   **7.23**

FIGURES 7.22 and 7.23. Chronic (fibrotic) hypersensitivity pneumonitis mimicking fibrotic NSIP. Most of the biopsy is indistinguishable from idiopathic NSIP, but the Schaumann body (*arrow*) in **Figure 7.23** marks the site of an old granuloma and indicates the correct diagnosis. The patient had known bird exposure.

DIFFERENTIAL DIAGNOSIS/ASSOCIATIONS

NSIP morphology is a frequent finding in lung biopsies from patients with ILD and has a wide differential/etiologic diagnosis (Table 7.2). Hypersensitivity pneumonitis (Figs. 7.22 and 7.23), drug reactions (Figs. 7.24 to 7.26 and see Chapter 18), and collagen vascular diseases, as well as idiopathic pneumonias with autoimmune features[11] are the most common causes of an NSIP pattern (Figs. 7.10 to 7.12), and *we recommend including these entities as important differential diagnoses in a comment when a diagnosis of NSIP is made.*

As noted earlier, NSIP is the most common form of ILD in patients with defined collagen vascular diseases. Some patients with NSIP have clinical or serologic evidence of an underlying collagen vascular disease but do not meet the rheumatologic criteria for a defined collagen vascular disease. This scenario has been described in the literature under a variety of overlapping terms including "lung-dominant connective tissue disease,"[12] "autoimmune-featured ILD,"[13] "IPAF,"[7,14] and "undifferentiated connective disease."[15] If a video-assisted thoracoscopic surgery (VATS) biopsy shows a picture of NSIP with morphologic features suggestive of a collagen vascular disease (many lymphoid aggregates, germinal centers, high proportion of plasma

cells), but there is no clinical evidence of a collagen vascular disease, then the diagnosis line should read: "Surgical lung biopsy showing NSIP with features suggestive of underlying collagen vascular disease/interstitial pneumonia with autoimmune features." This topic is discussed in more detail in Chapter 21.

Cases of idiopathic NSIP are actually relatively uncommon,[3] and some believe that they actually represent undifferentiated connective tissue disease.[15]

DIP (Chapter 8) can progress to fibrosis and when that happens the characteristic airspace alveolar macrophages may persist, but in some cases they disappear, leaving a picture morphologically indistinguishable from fibrotic NSIP (Chapter 8, Figs. 8.22 and 8.23).

Chronic pulmonary hemorrhage can lead to interstitial fibrosis and produce a picture that very much mimics fibrotic NSIP. Clues to the diagnosis are the presence of interstitial hemosiderin or hemosiderin-laden macrophages (Chapter 24, Figs. 24.3 and 24.4) and iron encrustation of the elastic layers of small vessels (Chapter 24, Fig. 24.4). Many such cases reflect underlying vasculitis (capillaritis), typically microscopic polyangiitis.[16]

An identical phenomenon occurs in pulmonary veno-occlusive disease because of chronic alveolar hemorrhage (Chapter 24, Figs. 24.6 and 24.7); such patients have clinical evidence of pulmonary hypertension and thrombosed small intrapulmonary veins (Chapter 24, Fig. 24.8). In veno-occlusive disease, the fibrosing process is limited to the subpleural regions, as opposed to diffuse hemorrhage from capillaritis where the fibrosis is quite widespread.

Other types of fibrosing processes can produce linear fibrosis somewhat mimicking NSIP; these include old Langerhans cell histiocytosis (Chapter 10, Figs. 10.25 and 10.26) and burnt-out sarcoid (Chapter 13, Fig. 13.28). In sarcoid and Langerhans cell histiocytosis, the fibrosis is usually much patchier than in fibrotic NSIP and typical granulomas or stellate nodules may be present. Imaging studies often make the diagnosis clear.

Respiratory bronchiolitis with fibrosis (RBF),[17] also called smoking-related interstitial fibrosis and airspace enlargement with fibrosis (see Chapter 8), may produce a pattern of fibrosis following alveolar walls that mimics fibrotic NSIP (Figs. 8.9 to 8.12); indeed, the original description of RBF[18] was derived from a set of cases initially diagnosed as fibrotic NSIP. Clues to the diagnosis of RBF are that the fibrosing process is sharply localized to an area under the pleura rather than being diffuse, the fibrosis is mixed with enlarged emphysematous airspaces, the process is sometimes wedge shaped with a respiratory bronchiole at the apex of the wedge, and pigmented smoker's macrophages (see Chapter 8) are present in the airspaces. Typically, the fibrosis of RBF is quite hyalinized, as opposed to the fibrosis of NSIP.

Cellular NSIP needs to be separated from lymphocytic interstitial pneumonia (LIP). In LIP, the interstitial

---

Table 7.2

Differential diagnosis and associations of an NSIP pattern

Idiopathic NSIP (exclusionary diagnosis)

Some cases of hypersensitivity pneumonitis (look for giant cells/granulomas)

Drug reactions

Collagen vascular disease (all types, including antisynthetase syndromes) and related conditions (IPAF)

Primary biliary cholangitis

Inflammatory bowel disease

Long-standing and largely burnt-out DIP

Some cases of chronic eosinophilic pneumonia

Old fibrotic DAD/acute respiratory distress syndrome

Some areas of burnt-out Langerhans cell histiocytosis

Edge of OP lesions

Chronic pulmonary hemorrhage (look for interstitial hemosiderin or iron-encrusted vessel elastica)

Pulmonary veno-occlusive disease (look for interstitial hemosiderin or iron-encrusted vessel elastica immediately under the pleura and thrombosed veins)

LIP

RBF (smoking-related interstitial fibrosis, see Chapter 8)

Restrictive allograft syndrome after lung or bone marrow transplantation

Focally in UIP (diagnosis remains UIP)

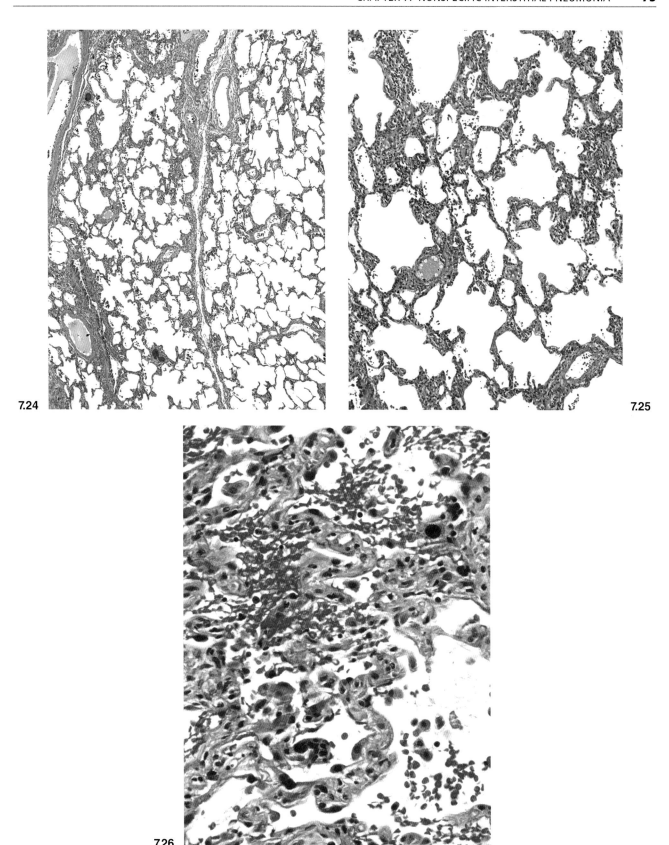

7.24

7.25

7.26

FIGURES 7.24 to 7.26. Busulfan toxicity appearing as cellular NSIP. Note the enlarged hyperchromatic nuclei typical of busulfan in **Figure 7.26**. NSIP is a common drug reaction pattern.

chronic inflammatory infiltrate is much more marked than in cellular NSIP so that the alveolar walls are considerably widened by inflammatory cells and sometimes become confluent (Chapter 19, Figs. 19.10 to 19.16). LIP may also be associated with cysts on computed tomographic imaging and occasionally on biopsy (Chapter 19, Fig. 19.19). Small interstitial granulomas or individual giant cells are common in LIP. Most important, for a diagnosis of LIP, the intensity of the lymphoid infiltrate should be marked enough to make one worry about a lymphoma.

Separation of NSIP from organizing diffuse alveolar damage (DAD) can sometimes be a problem when the organization follows alveolar walls.[9] Apparently interstitial granulation tissue or lightly staining connective tissue in an NSIP pattern favors organizing DAD (Figs. 7.27 and 7.28), whereas the fibrosis of NSIP is generally fairly dense. This distinction is important because the prognosis for such cases is that of DAD and is much worse than that of NSIP.[9] It is possible that such cases end up looking like NSIP if the patient survives.

NSIP-like morphology can also be seen as a local reaction pattern in completely unrelated conditions (Figs. 7.29 and 7.30); it should be remembered that true NSIP is both pathologically and radiologically a diffuse process.

SEPARATION OF UIP AND NSIP

The differential diagnosis that appears to cause the most difficulty is the separation of UIP and some cases of fibrotic NSIP.[19] Part of the problem arises from the fact that fibrotic NSIP-like areas can be present in otherwise perfectly ordinary UIP (Chapter 6, Fig. 6.39), and occasionally such areas occupy most of the biopsy, or if two biopsies are performed, one looks like fibrotic NSIP and one like UIP. However, follow-up data have shown that the presence of a UIP pattern is what determines prognosis,[20,21] so that if unequivocal UIP is present, UIP should be diagnosed and the NSIP component ignored.

Features that suggest one disease or the other are shown in Table 7.3. Architectural distortion (sheets of fibrosis and honeycombing) and patchiness of the process are the most important findings and strongly favor UIP. Sharp transitions between fibrotic and nonfibrotic parenchyma are also much more typical of UIP than NSIP.[9] In most cases, the distinction is easily made at scanning magnification (see Chapter 6, Figs. 6.19 to 6.22). A trick that can be helpful is to ask what happens if one mentally removes the inflammation and/or fibrosis: in NSIP one generally ends up with normal lung parenchyma, whereas in UIP no amount of mental contortion can restore the distorted parenchyma to its normal state.

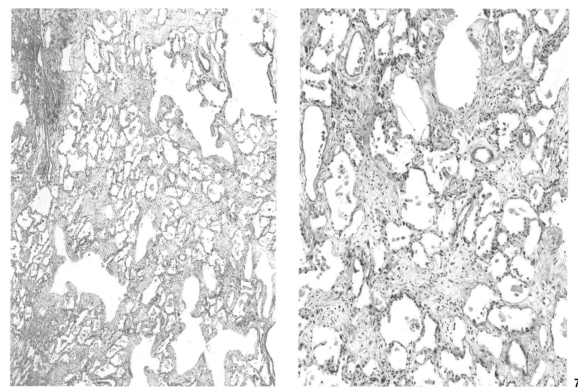

7.27

7.28

FIGURES 7.27 and 7.28. Low- and high-power views of organizing DAD mimicking NSIP. The loose connective tissue that makes up the apparent "interstitial" process is a clue to the correct diagnosis.

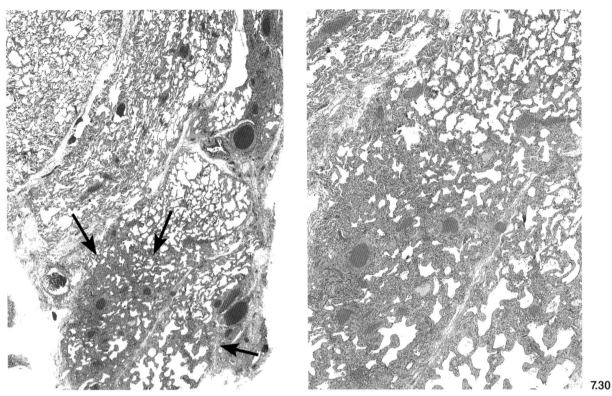

7.29   **7.30**

FIGURES 7.29 and 7.30. A local reaction mimicking NSIP. Images are from a case of spontaneous pneumothorax. The photographed region is immediately under the inflamed pleura. The area bounded by arrows in Fig. 7.29 mimics cellular NSIP (higher power of this area shown in Fig. 7.30), but the rest of the parenchyma is normal. True NSIP is always a diffuse process. This is a localized reaction of no consequence.

Table 7.3

Separation of fibrotic NSIP and UIP

Fibrotic NSIP	UIP
Lack of architectural distortion	Architectural distortion always present
Honeycombing uncommon	Honeycombing seen in most biopsies
Fibrosis evenly spread throughout lobule	Fibrosis most severe under pleura or along interlobular septa
Fibrosing process very homogeneous	Fibrosing process patchy, alternates abruptly with normal or near-normal lung
Fibroblast foci sparse to nonexistent	Fibroblast foci common
Transitions between normal and abnormal parenchyma are gradual	Focal NSIP-like areas may be present but do not change the diagnosis

One report[22] based on biopsies and subsequent explanted lungs has suggested that NSIP can progress to UIP. This is the only morphologic study to have made such a claim, and at present, most pathologists regard the two conditions as completely separate entities.

DIAGNOSTIC MODALITIES

NSIP is a diagnosis that requires evaluation of low-power architecture over a large area. At present only VATS or open biopsies are suitable for this purpose. NSIP cannot be diagnosed on transbronchial biopsy, and in fact, such biopsies are often extremely misleading because many conditions can produce a local area of chronic interstitial inflammation (Figs. 7.29 and 7.30 and Chapter 3, Figs. 3.2 and 3.8). There is no information yet on whether cryobiopsies are useful for diagnosing NSIP.

TREATMENT AND PROGNOSIS

Regardless of etiology, the prognosis of NSIP depends very much on the presence or absence of fibrosis. NSIP is generally treated with immunosuppressive agents (see Chapter 1). NSIP with a purely cellular pattern typically responds to steroids and can completely resolve, whereas with fibrosis, the prognosis is considerably worse, albeit not as poor as the prognosis of idiopathic UIP.[23] For this reason, it is important to always mention the presence or absence of fibrosis when making a diagnosis of NSIP. The presence of OP does not change the prognosis.[24]

There may be differences in NSIP outcome by underlying etiology. Nunes et al.[25] reported that patients with collagen vascular disease–associated NSIP had a better prognosis than cases of idiopathic NSIP, and patients with an NSIP pattern of chronic (fibrotic) hypersensitivity pneumonitis fared worst. However, this report is somewhat hard to interpret because it does not indicate whether all of the NSIP cases were fibrotic or whether some were purely cellular.

REFERENCES

1. Kinder BW. Nonspecific interstitial pneumonia. *Clin Chest Med.* 2012;33:111–121.
2. Silva CI, Müller NL, Hansell DM, et al. Nonspecific interstitial pneumonia and idiopathic pulmonary fibrosis: changes in pattern and distribution of disease over time. *Radiology.* 2008;247:251–259.
3. Travis WD, Hunninghake G, King TE Jr, et al. Idiopathic nonspecific interstitial pneumonia: report of an American Thoracic Society project. *Am J Respir Crit Care Med.* 2008;177:1338–1347.
4. Silva CI, Müller NL, Lynch DA, et al. Chronic hypersensitivity pneumonitis: differentiation from idiopathic pulmonary fibrosis and nonspecific interstitial pneumonia by using thin-section CT. *Radiology.* 2008;246:288–297.
5. Katzenstein AL, Fiorelli RF. Nonspecific interstitial pneumonia/fibrosis. Histologic features and clinical significance. *Am J Surg Pathol.* 1994;18:136–147.
6. Churg A, Wright JL, Ryerson CJ. pathologic separation of chronic hypersensitivity pneumonitis from fibrotic connective tissue disease-associated interstitial lung disease. *Am J Surg Pathol.* 2017;41:1403–1409.
7. Fischer A, Antoniou KM, Brown KK, et al.; "ERS/ATS Task Force on Undifferentiated Forms of CTD-ILD." An official European Respiratory Society/American Thoracic Society research statement: interstitial pneumonia with autoimmune features. *Eur Respir J.* 2015;46:976–987.
8. Churg A, Bilawich A. Confluent fibrosis and fibroblast foci in fibrotic non-specific interstitial pneumonia. *Histopathology.* 2016;69:128–135.
9. Borie R, Kannengiesser C, Crestani B. Familial forms of nonspecific interstitial pneumonia/idiopathic pulmonary fibrosis: clinical course and genetic background. *Curr Opin Pulm Med.* 2012;18:455–461.
10. Kambouchner M, Levy P, Nicholson AG, et al. Prognostic relevance of histological variants in nonspecific interstitial pneumonia. *Histopathology.* 2014;65:549–560.
11. Nascimento ECTD, Baldi BG, Sawamura MVY, et al. Morphologic aspects of interstitial pneumonia with autoimmune features. *Arch Pathol Lab Med.* 2018;142:1080–1089.
12. Fischer A, West SG, Swigris JJ, et al. Connective tissue disease-associated interstitial lung disease: a call for clarification. *Chest.* 2010;138:251–256.
13. Vij R, Noth I, Strek ME. Autoimmune-featured interstitial lung disease: a distinct entity. *Chest.* 2011;140:1292–1299.
14. Suzuki A, Kondoh Y, Fischer A. Recent advances in connective tissue disease related interstitial lung disease. *Expert Rev Respir Med.* 2017;11:591–603.
15. Kinder BW, Collard HR, Koth L, et al. Idiopathic nonspecific interstitial pneumonia: lung manifestation of undifferentiated connective tissue disease? *Am J Respir Crit Care Med.* 2007;176:691–697.
16. Comarmond C, Crestani B, Tazi A, et al. Pulmonary fibrosis in antineutrophil cytoplasmic antibodies (ANCA)-associated vasculitis: a series of 49 patients and review of the literature. *Medicine (Baltimore).* 2014;93:340–349.
17. Churg A, Hall R, Bilawich A. Respiratory bronchiolitis with fibrosis-interstitial lung disease: a new form of smoking-induced interstitial lung disease. *Arch Pathol Lab Med.* 2015;139:437–440.
18. Yousem SA. Respiratory bronchiolitis-associated interstitial lung disease with fibrosis is a lesion distinct from fibrotic nonspecific interstitial pneumonia: a proposal. *Mod Pathol.* 2006;19:1474–1479.
19. Nicholson AG, Addis BJ, Bharucha H, et al. Inter-observer variation between pathologists in diffuse parenchymal lung disease. *Thorax.* 2004;59:500–505.
20. Monaghan H, Wells AU, Colby TV, et al. Prognostic implications of histologic patterns in multiple surgical lung biopsies from patients with idiopathic interstitial pneumonias. *Chest.* 2004;125:522–526.
21. Flaherty KR, Travis WD, Colby TV, et al. Histopathologic variability in usual and nonspecific interstitial pneumonias. *Am J Respir Crit Care Med.* 2001;164:1722–1727.
22. Schneider F, Hwang DM, Gibson K, et al. Nonspecific interstitial pneumonia: a study of 6 patients with progressive disease. *Am J Surg Pathol.* 2012;36:89–93.
23. Nicholson AG, Colby TV, du Bois RM, et al. The prognostic significance of the histologic pattern of interstitial pneumonia in patients presenting with the clinical entity of cryptogenic fibrosing alveolitis. *Am J Respir Crit Care Med.* 2000;162:2213–2217.
24. Huo Z, Li J, Li S, Zhang H, et al. Organizing pneumonia components in non-specific interstitial pneumonia (NSIP): a clinicopathological study of 33 NSIP cases. *Histopathology.* 2016;68:347–355.
25. Nunes H, Schubel K, Piver D, et al. Nonspecific interstitial pneumonia: survival is influenced by the underlying cause. *Eur Respir J.* 2015;45:746–755.

Respiratory Bronchiolitis with Interstitial Lung Disease, Respiratory Bronchiolitis with Fibrosis, and Desquamative Interstitial Pneumonia

NOMENCLATURE AND CONCEPTUAL/ DIAGNOSTIC ISSUES

Respiratory bronchiolitis with interstitial lung disease (RBILD), respiratory bronchiolitis with fibrosis (RBF), and desquamative interstitial pneumonia (DIP) are diseases that occur almost entirely in cigarette smokers, even though RBILD and DIP are frequently included in the idiopathic interstitial pneumonias[1] (see Chapter 1). The relationship of these lesions is not entirely clear. We have proposed[2] that smoker's respiratory bronchiolitis (RB) is

the "baseline" abnormality from which RBILD, RBF, and DIP are derived via two different morphologic pathways as shown in Figure 8.1.

For the pathologist, the diagnosis of RBILD presents an unusual conceptual problem, because *the morphology of RBILD, a disease with clinical features of an interstitial lung disease (ILD; see later), is identical to that of smoker's RB*, a process found incidentally in virtually every cigarette smoker (as can be readily identified by examining any lobe resected for lung cancer in a smoker) and one that is associated with very mild abnormalities of airflow or with

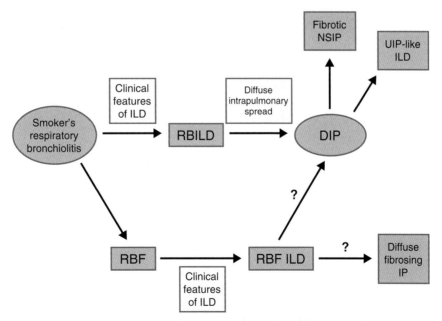

FIGURE 8.1. A conceptual scheme showing the relationships of the entities discussed in this chapter. (Reprinted from Churg A, Hall R, Bilawich A. Respiratory bronchiolitis with fibrosis-interstitial lung disease: a new form of smoking-induced interstitial lunge disease. *Arch Pathol Lab Med.* 2015;139(4):437–440 with permission from Archives of Pathology & Laboratory Medicine. Copyright 2015 College of American Pathologists.)

no detectable functional abnormality. It was originally believed that the presence of interstitial fibrosis associated with RB automatically turned it into RBILD, but more recent studies have shown that this is not true because fibrosis can be seen in both conditions.[3] Pathologic separation of RB and RBILD depends on the clinical and imaging context and cannot be determined from the biopsy alone.

An additional rule is that *a diagnosis of RBILD requires clinical and radiologic evidence of an ILD with no other cause for an ILD evident in the biopsy*; if there is another ILD present, that disease is considered the cause of the clinical interstitial process and smoking-related changes in the respiratory bronchioles are ignored.[3]

The consensus at present is that RBILD and DIP are related processes, with RBILD the earlier and more localized lesion that evolves, with continued smoking, into the more widespread DIP[4] (Fig. 8.1). As one might expect under this scenario, there are cases that are morphologically intermediate between the two.[5]

A further complication is that DIP-like areas can also be found around the lesions of Langerhans cell histiocytosis (Chapter 10), around tumors, and occasionally in other conditions if the patient is a cigarette smoker.[6] DIP, by definition, is a diffuse disease that is not accompanied by other types of ILD, and focal collections of smoker's macrophages in airspaces are not sufficient for a diagnosis of DIP.

RBF[7,8] appears in the literature under a variety of other names including RB-associated ILD with fibrosis,[9] airspace enlargement with fibrosis,[10] smoking-related idiopathic interstitial pneumonia,[11] and smoking-related interstitial fibrosis.[12] The latter term is in theory the best, but because "smoking-related ILD" gets used informally in various contexts, we believe that "RBF" avoids ambiguity.

As is true of RB, RBF is usually an incidental and inconsequential finding in the lungs of cigarette smokers, typically heavy smokers[9,10]; Katzenstein et al.[12] described RBF in 45% of extensively sampled lung resection specimens from cigarette smokers, and Kawabata et al.[10] reported similar lesions in the lungs of 21% of heavy smokers. However, in our experience, such lesions are much less frequent even in resection specimens. On high-resolution computed tomography (HRCT), we observed the distinctive imaging appearance of RBF (see later) in only 7% of a series of 200 smokers with greater than 30 pack-years[8]; similarly, Flaherty et al.[11] found RBF lesions on HRCT in 8% of heavy smokers. These figures should, however, be interpreted in light of the fact that small pathologic lesions are often not visible on HRCT.

In a small minority of cases, the patient has clinical and radiologic evidence of an ILD with RBF as the only pathologic finding on biopsy, and no other findings to account for an ILD. In that setting, the process could be termed respiratory bronchiolitis with fibrosis–interstitial lung disease (RBFILD) by analogy with RBILD.[2] Review of the literature shows that some proportion of cases labeled RBILD in the past, particularly those with considerable fibrosis, are really RBF or RBFILD[13,14] (see Pathologic Features, later).

ETIOLOGIES

Table 8.1 shows etiologies of RBILD, RBF, and DIP. All of the published cases of RBILD and RBF have occurred in cigarette smokers, whereas a minority of DIP cases have occurred in nonsmokers (of tobacco). A list of other putative associations is shown in Table 8.1, although in some of these reports, the patients are also heavy cigarette smokers (for a detailed review, see Godbert et al.[15]), and in some instances the published illustrations raise doubts as to whether the process really is DIP rather than just a localized accumulation of airspace macrophages. However, we have seen unequivocal DIP in heavy marijuana smokers (see later).

CLINICAL FEATURES

Patients with RBILD typically present with shortness of breath, whereas most cigarette smokers with RB are asymptomatic; however, some smokers are short of breath because they have chronic obstructive pulmonary disease (COPD), so shortness of breath does not reliably separate RB and RBILD. Physiologically, patients with RB may have airflow obstruction or no abnormality, but RBILD is characterized by a pure restrictive abnormality, or a combination of a restrictive and obstructive abnormality, or a markedly decreased diffusing capacity.[3] Patients with DIP are usually short of breath and always have a restrictive abnormality and/or a decreased diffusing capacity. Clubbing is seen in some patients with DIP.[15]

RBF/RBFILD is a disease of heavy smokers, typically greater than 30 pack-years, with an average in some series over 50 pack-years.[2] Many cases appear to be incidental findings with no physiologic consequences that can specifically be attributed to RBF. However, a minority of patients have either evidence of an ILD on imaging or a clinical diagnosis of ILD based on a disproportionately decreased diffusing capacity beyond that expected from the degree of cigarette smoke–induced COPD.[7]

Table 8.1
Etiologies of RBILD, RBF, and DIP
Cigarette smoking history: 100% of patients with RBILD and RBF
Cigarette smoking history: 60%–90% of patients with DIP
Other putative causes of DIP
Fumes
Dust
Drugs
Marijuana smoke
Collagen vascular diseases

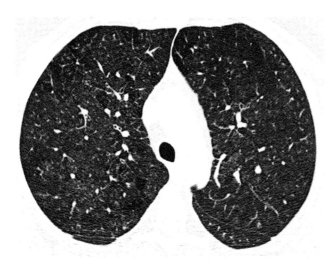

FIGURE 8.2. Respiratory bronchiolitis with interstitial lung disease. HRCT at the level of the upper lobes shows bilateral ground-glass opacities and poorly defined centrilobular nodules. The patient was a 44-year-old woman.

IMAGING

The HRCT manifestations of RBILD consist of centrilobular ground-glass nodules and/or patchy or confluent ground-glass opacities[4,5] (Fig. 8.2). These abnormalities tend to involve mainly the upper lobes but may be diffuse. Upper lobe centrilobular emphysema is seen in almost all cases. A small percentage of patients have mild reticulation mainly in the lower lung zones.[5]

The HRCT findings of RBF may be subtle and easily missed. They typically consist of mild patchy reticulation

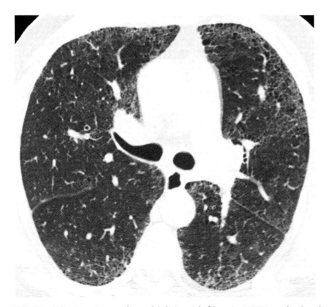

FIGURE 8.3. Respiratory bronchiolitis with fibrosis. HRCT at the level of the right upper lobe bronchus in a patient with extensive RBF shows mild emphysema with adjacent reticulation and ground-glass opacities involving mainly the peripheral regions of the lungs.

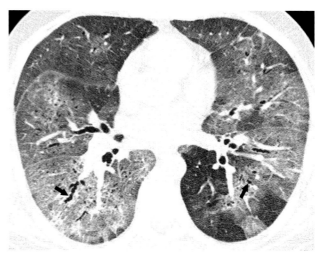

FIGURE 8.4. Desquamative interstitial pneumonia. HRCT at the level of the lower lung zones demonstrates extensive bilateral ground-glass opacities and small focal areas of reticulation. Also noted are mild dilatation and a beaded appearance of some of the lower lobe bronchi (traction bronchiectasis) (*arrows*) consistent with fibrosis. The patient was a 59-year-old man with DIP secondary to marijuana smoke.

adjacent to centrilobular and paraseptal emphysema mainly in the peripheral regions of the upper and middle lung zones with minimal or no reticulation at the lung bases (Fig. 8.3).[7] Almost all patients also have patchy or extensive ground-glass opacities, which may be diffuse or involve predominately the upper or lower lung zones.

The main HRCT feature of DIP is extensive bilateral ground-glass opacification and is present in all cases[5] (Fig. 8.4). It may be diffuse but tends to involve mainly the lower lobes. A reticular pattern may be present in up to 60% of patients but is usually mild and confined to the peripheral regions of the lower lung zones. Honeycombing is uncommon, but numerous small well-defined cysts may occur within the areas of ground-glass attenuation.[5] The computed tomographic findings of RBILD, RBF, and DIP overlap with those of several other ILDs, particularly hypersensitivity pneumonitis and nonspecific interstitial pneumonia (NSIP).

PATHOLOGIC FEATURES

Smoker's RB and RBILD show two features (Table 8.2). First, there is accumulation of smoker's macrophages, that is, macrophages with a light golden or light brown color (Figs. 8.5 to 8.8), in the lumens of respiratory bronchioles and/or in the more distal alveolar ducts or alveoli. The pigment in smoker's macrophages reflects aluminum silicates derived from the smoke and ferruginated by macrophages; it generally appears smooth or finely granular on hematoxylin and eosin stains (Fig. 8.7) and may give a blush of blue color on iron stains (Fig. 8.8). Smoker's pigment needs to be separated from hemosiderin, which is typically coarsely granular (Chapter 24, Figs. 24.3 and 24.4) and which usually stains intensely on iron stains.

Table 8.2

Morphologic criteria for the diagnosis of RB/RBILD and RBF/RBFILD

RB/RBILD	RBF/RBFILD
Smoker's macrophages in lumens of respiratory bronchioles and surrounding alveoli	Morphologic RB usually present
Variable but usually mild interstitial fibrosis confined to the walls of respiratory bronchioles and surrounding alveoli. Interstitial fibrosis may be completely absent.	Distinct but localized patches of interstitial fibrosis present, either immediately under the pleura or extending from a respiratory bronchioles to the pleura
	Fibrosis typically hyalinized and very paucicellular
	Fibrosis usually surrounds emphysematous spaces that contain smoker's macrophages

Second, RB and RBILD are characterized by a variable degree of fibrosis in the walls of the respiratory bronchioles. Fibrosis may be almost nonexistent (Fig. 8.5) or present but confined to the walls of affected respiratory bronchioles and a few surrounding alveoli (Fig. 8.6).

In RBF and RBFILD (Table 8.2), by definition, there is easily visible *but distinctly localized* interstitial fibrosis, which at high power is paucicellular and frequently hyaline[2,8] (Figs. 8.9 to 8.13). The fibrosis usually surrounds emphysematous spaces (Figs. 8.9 to 8.13). Fibrosis may be localized to a fairly shallow area immediately under

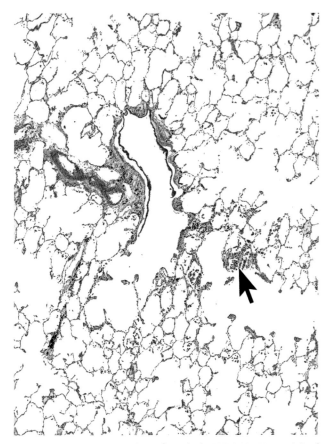

FIGURE 8.5. Low-power view of smoker's RB/RBILD. Note minimal fibrosis of the walls of the bronchiole in this example and collections of pigmented macrophages in alveolar ducts and alveoli (*arrow*). The process in this figure and Figures 8.5 to 8.9 represents RBILD if there is clinical evidence of an ILD and no other cause for an ILD in the biopsy; otherwise, it is simply RB.

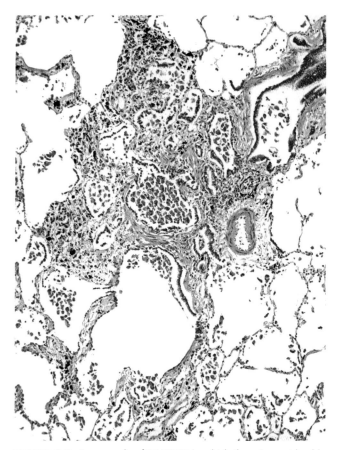

FIGURE 8.6. An example of RB/RBILD in which there is considerable fibrosis in the walls of the respiratory bronchioles. Despite the fibrosis, this is not RBILD unless there is clinical evidence of an ILD and no other cause for such a disease.

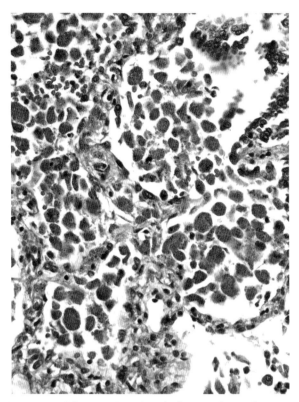

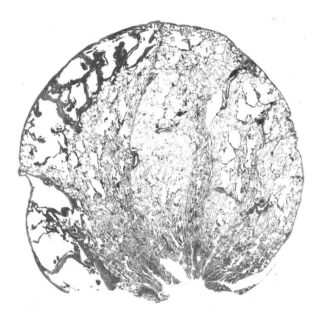

FIGURE 8.9. Low power view of RBF. Note the sharply circumscribed but fairly dramatic subpleural fibrosis mixed with emphysematous airspaces.

FIGURE 8.7. High power view of smoker's macrophages showing typical golden-brown, faintly granular, pigmentation.

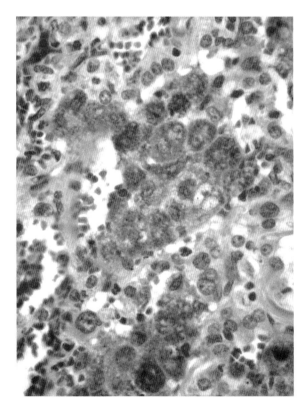

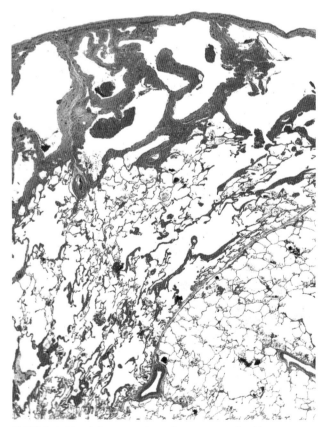

FIGURE 8.8. Iron stain of smoker's macrophage showing a faint blush of blue color. This is the most typical staining reaction. Hemosiderin, which is also golden brown, is distinctly coarser and stains intensely with Perl's iron stain.

FIGURE 8.10. High-power view of Figure 8.9. The fibrosis is very paucicellular, the typical finding in RBF.

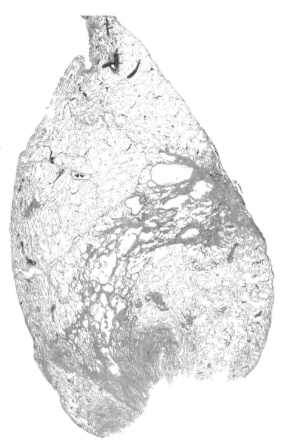

FIGURE 8.11. A case of RBF in which the fibrotic area forms a sharply circumscribed wedge extending to the pleura; note the typical pattern of admixed emphysema. (Reproduced by permission from Reddy TL, Mayo J, Churg A. Respiratory bronchiolitis with fibrosis. High-resolution computed tomography findings and correlation with pathology. *Ann Am Thorac Soc.* 2013;10:590–601.)

the pleura (Figs. 8.9 and 8.10) or may extend in a wedge shape from a respiratory bronchiole to the subpleural region (Fig. 8.11); however, by definition, the fibrosing process spares most of the parenchyma. The airspaces within the areas of fibrosis always contain smoker's macrophages (Figs. 8.12 and 8.13). Fibroblast foci are nonexistent to rare, and the presence of numerous fibroblast foci raises a question of a bad sample of usual interstitial pneumonia (UIP).

In contrast to the distinctly localized abnormalities of RB/RBILD and RBF/RBFILD, in DIP (Table 8.3), there is widespread filling of alveolar spaces by smoker's macrophages, and there is always accompanying widespread chronic interstitial inflammation and/or interstitial fibrosis (Figs. 8.14 to 8.21). The interstitial fibrosis of DIP is, structurally, similar to that of fibrotic NSIP because there is usually no architectural distortion; however, long-standing DIP cases may develop honeycombing, at least on imaging.[16] In some cases of DIP, the alveolar macrophages persist, but in others they disappear over time, leaving a picture that is essentially

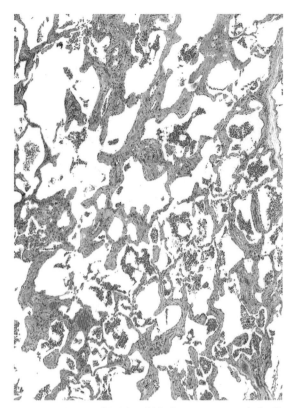

FIGURE 8.12. A case of RBF in which the appearance mimics fibrotic NSIP. However, it is much more paucicellular and hyalinized than NSIP. Collections of smoker's macrophages are present in the emphysematous airspaces. In this case, the fibrosing process was confined to a band immediately under the pleura.

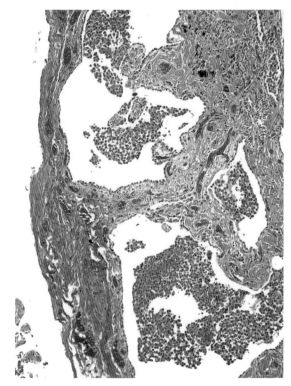

FIGURE 8.13. High-power view of a case of RBF to show the paucicellular hyaline fibrosis and large numbers of airspace macrophages.

Table 8.3
Pathologic features of DIP

Homogeneous process over large areas

Airspaces filled by variably pigmented macrophages that may have the appearance of smoker's macrophages

Lymphoid nodules common

Small numbers of eosinophils common

Interstitial inflammation/fibrosis always present, usually follows original alveolar walls without architectural distortion

Individual microscopic fields indistinguishable from individual fields of RB/RBILD

Long-standing cases may look like fibrotic NSIP or may develop honeycombing

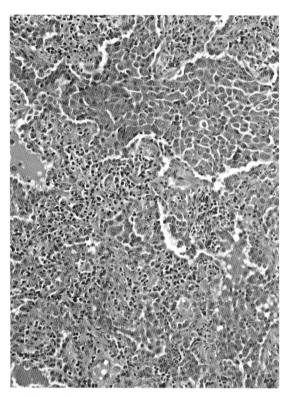

FIGURE 8.16. High-power view of the case shown in Figures 8.14 and 8.15. At this magnification, the interstitial inflammatory infiltrate is clearly visible. DIP always has an interstitial inflammatory infiltrate and/or interstitial fibrosis.

indistinguishable from fibrotic NSIP (Figs. 8.1, 8.22, and 8.23).

Small numbers of eosinophils are also commonly found in DIP, either in the airspaces or in the interstitium (Fig. 8.17), but large numbers of eosinophils should raise a question of chronic eosinophilic pneumonia (Chapter 15). Imaging will almost always sort out

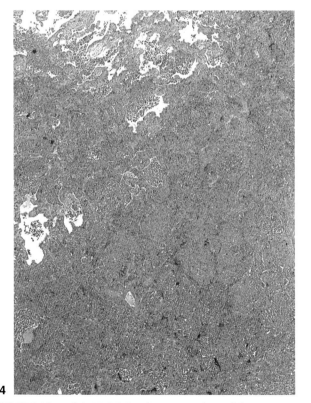

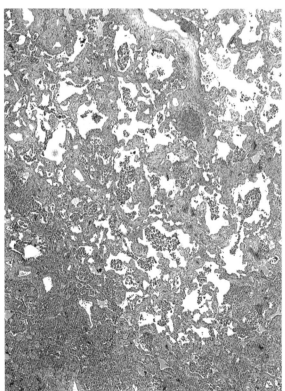

8.14

8.15

FIGURES 8.14 and 8.15. DIP. Two low-power views of the same case. In **Figure 8.14** the process appears almost solid, whereas in **Figure 8.15** collections of airspace macrophages separated from the underlying lung are visible.

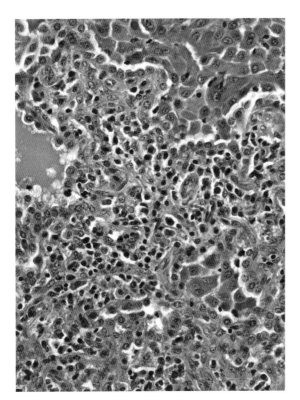

FIGURE 8.17. High-power view of the case shown in Figures 8.14 to 8.16. Scattered eosinophils are present in the interstitial inflammatory infiltrate. Small numbers of eosinophils in the interstitium or airspaces are common in DIP.

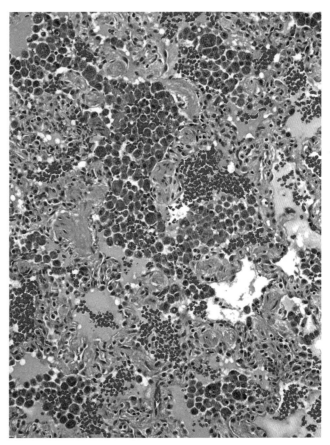

FIGURE 8.19. An example of DIP in which all of the alveolar macrophages are heavily pigmented smoker's macrophages. This occurs in a minority of cases; most cases show only scattered or sometimes no pigmented macrophages.

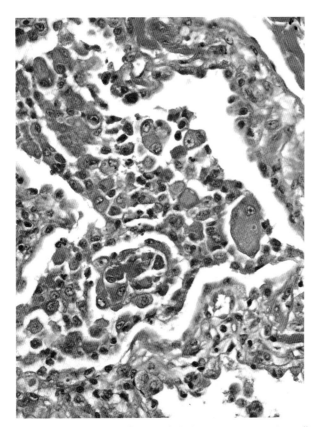

FIGURE 8.18. An example of DIP in which there is an airspace giant cell.

these two possibilities because DIP typically shows diffuse ground-glass opacities with or without reticulation, whereas chronic eosinophilic pneumonia shows localized areas of consolidation that are usually peripheral and may be migratory. Other common microscopic features in DIP include lymphoid nodules (Figs. 8.14 and 8.15) and scattered giant cells (Fig. 8.18).

The alveolar macrophages in DIP have a variable appearance. In most cases, there are relatively few pigmented smoker's macrophages and larger numbers of nonpigmented macrophages, but occasionally the alveoli are completely filled by smoker's macrophages (Fig. 8.19).

Occasional cases fall somewhere between RB/RBILD and DIP because the abnormalities are more widespread than typical RB/RBILD but less widespread than DIP. We suggest that such cases be diagnosed as DIP because the inflammatory/fibrotic process is extending and presumably would end up as DIP, given sufficient time.

DIP has been reported to recur in transplanted lungs[17] (Fig. 8.24). It is not clear if this phenomenon is only seen in patients who continue to smoke.

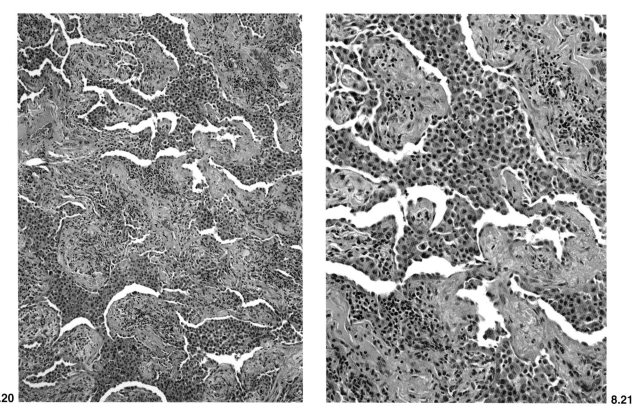

FIGURES 8.20 and 8.21. Low- and high-power views of DIP in a heavy marijuana smoker. There is distinct interstitial fibrosis.

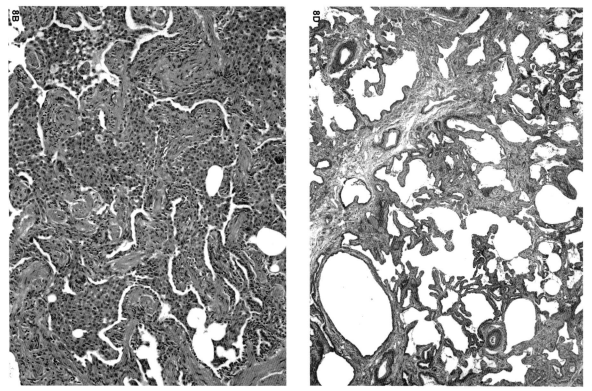

FIGURES 8.22 and 8.23. Transformation of DIP into a picture of fibrotic NSIP. This patient had a biopsy showing DIP 3 years before undergoing lung transplantation. These images are from the explanted lung. In **Figure 8.22** the appearance is still that of DIP, but most of the explanted lung looked like fibrotic NSIP (**Fig. 8.23**). (Reproduced by permission from Tazelaar HD, Wright JL, Churg A. Desquamative interstitial pneumonia. *Histopathology.* 2011;58:509–516.)

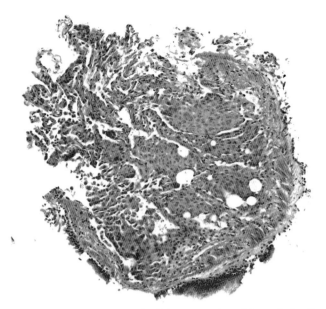

FIGURE 8.24. Recurrence of DIP in a transplanted lung. Ordinarily transbronchial biopsies are not suitable for the diagnosis of DIP, but they are sometimes useful for assessing recurrent disease in lung transplants.

DIAGNOSTIC MODALITIES

RBILD, RBF/RBFILD, and DIP require evaluation of low-power architecture over a large area. As such, transbronchial biopsy cannot be used and video-assisted thoracoscopic surgery biopsy is required. Whether cryobiopsy could be utilized for these diagnoses has not been established.

DIFFERENTIAL DIAGNOSIS

RB/RBILD is distinctive and there is a very limited differential diagnosis. One never sees the metaplastic bronchiolar epithelium of peribronchiolar metaplasia (Chapter 23, Figs. 23.16 to 23.18) in RB/RBILD, nor the narrowed or obliterated lumen of constrictive bronchiolitis (bronchiolitis obliterans, Chapter 20, Figs. 20.23 to 20.27), nor is there marked inflammation in the walls of the respiratory bronchioles such as is present with infectious bronchiolitis (Chapter 20, Figs. 20.7 to 20.10). RB/RBILD is commonly associated with centrilobular emphysema, and centrilobular emphysematous spaces may themselves have smoker's macrophages as well as fibrosis in the walls of the spaces, but the airspaces are markedly dilated (Chapter 9, Figs. 9.11 and 9.12).

The major differential diagnosis of RBF/RBFILD is a diffuse fibrosing interstitial pneumonia, and in fact the original report of RBF by Yousem[9] described cases extracted from a series of lesions initially thought to be fibrotic NSIP. Over a localized area, RBF certainly can mimic fibrotic NSIP (Fig. 8.12), although NSIP typically does not have the enlarged airspaces of RBF. But no true fibrosing

interstitial pneumonia (UIP, NSIP, DIP, chronic hypersensitivity pneumonitis, connective tissue disease–associated ILD) is localized to small patches in the fashion of RBF/RB-FILD. As well, true fibrosing interstitial pneumonias may be paucicellular, but the fibrosis is never hyaline. In an equivocal case, imaging will usually sort out the problem.

On the chest radiograph, RBF can also be mistaken for asbestosis. Bledsoe et al.[18] described 24 cases with ILO readings of 1/0 or greater and histories of asbestos exposure in whom the clinical/radiologic diagnosis was asbestosis, but on pathologic review 18/24 were thought to actually be RBF. This topic is considered further in Chapter 22.

The differential diagnosis of DIP is shown in Table 8.4. Smoker's macrophages can be seen focally around any lesion in cigarette smokers, for example, in Langerhans cell histiocytosis, or around tumors, and in that setting the macrophages should be ignored. Alveolar macrophages can accumulate around any kind of inflammatory mass lesion (Figs. 8.25 and 8.26), but DIP is always a diffuse disease and does not form masses. Smoker's macrophages may also be seen in airspaces in otherwise unremarkable lungs (Fig. 8.27), but airspace macrophages by themselves do not qualify for a diagnosis of DIP. DIP is always a diffuse disease with interstitial inflammation/fibrosis as well as airspace macrophages.

Any cause of airway obstruction, for example, a tumor, will lead to collections of macrophages behind the obstructing lesion (so-called golden pneumonia, visible as a gold color on gross examination). In contrast to DIP, obstructing lesions typically are segmental or subsegmental and not diffusely present throughout the lung. The macrophages that accumulate behind obstructions are finely foamy and do not have smoker's pigment, and in general obstructing lesions don't lead to interstitial inflammation/fibrosis, something that is always present in DIP.

Widespread filling of alveoli by coarsely foamy macrophages without pigment can also be seen in patients treated with amiodarone (Figs. 8.28 and 8.29) or statins, and sometimes in patients inhaling lipids. In immunocompromised hosts, slightly foamy macrophages containing large numbers of *Mycobacterium avium intracellulare*

Table 8.4
Differential diagnosis of DIP
Smoker's macrophage collections around lesions of Langerhans cell histiocytosis and sometimes around tumors and other lesions
Drug reactions, especially to amiodarone, statins
Obstructive pneumonias with collections of foamy macrophages
Rhodococcus and *Mycobacterium avium* infections in immunocompromised hosts
Chronic eosinophilic pneumonia

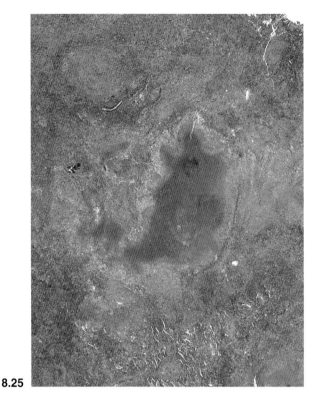

8.25

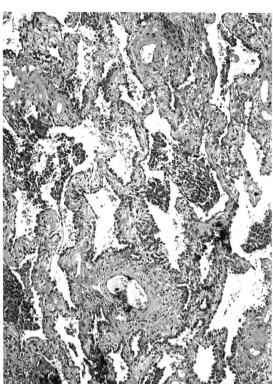

8.26

FIGURES 8.25 and 8.26. Mimics of DIP. Localized reaction around a tuberculous granuloma (**Fig. 8.25**) mimicking DIP (**Fig. 8.26**). DIP is always diffuse and should not be associated with mass lesions.

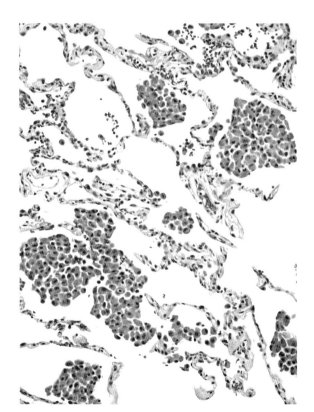

FIGURE 8.27. Mimics of DIP. In this example, there are collections of smoker's macrophages in the airspaces, but no interstitial inflammatory infiltrate or interstitial fibrosis, features that are required for the diagnosis of DIP.

or *Rhodococcus* organisms can fill alveolar spaces, but again these macrophages are distinctly different from the macrophages of DIP, and there is generally no interstitial reaction.

Chronic eosinophilic pneumonia (Chapter 15, Figs. 15.12 and 15.13) may have large numbers of macrophages in the airspaces and an interstitial inflammatory reaction, but also has large numbers of eosinophils in the airspaces, much greater numbers than are found in DIP. On imaging, chronic eosinophilic pneumonia typically forms discrete areas of consolidation that are frequently subpleural.

Hard metal disease (giant cell interstitial pneumonia, tungsten carbide pneumoconiosis) usually is characterized by fibrosis and inflammation limited to the walls of small airways with an associated giant cell and macrophage response; however, occasionally hard metal disease spreads through the parenchyma and can mimic DIP (see Chapter 22).

PROGNOSIS

The prognosis of RBILD is good, with all cases except one in the literature at least stabilizing in response to smoking cessation/steroids.[3] There is limited information about the prognosis of RBF/RBFILD, but on imaging most such cases are either stable or a small proportion show minimal localized progression,[11] and RBF/RBFILD appears to be morphologic dead end that does not progress to a diffuse

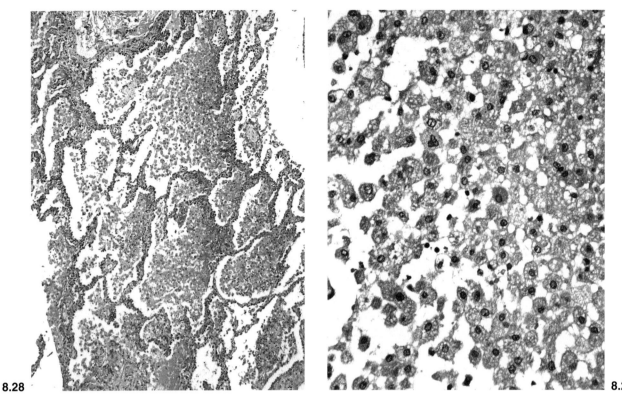

8.28   8.29

FIGURES 8.28 and 8.29. Amiodarone toxicity mimicking DIP. The airspaces are filled by macrophages, but they are coarsely foamy, the typical pattern seen with amiodarone. Obstructive pneumonia behind mass lesions can produce a similar pattern, but with generally more finely foamy macrophages.

fibrosing interstitial pneumonia. RBF/RBFILD is always seen in heavy smokers, and progressive disease in such patients is much more likely to be a manifestation of underlying COPD.

The prognosis for DIP is, overall, remarkably good, especially considering how much such cases resemble fibrotic NSIP, with long-term survivals of about 70% to 95% in various series. Steroids and smoking cessation are the usual approach to therapy; macrolides have been successfully used in some patients. Smoking cessation by itself has led to improvements in a few patients. Spontaneous remissions have been reported, although it is unclear whether these patients also stopped smoking.[15] In some patients, the alveolar macrophages disappear and the disease becomes indistinguishable from fibrotic NSIP (Figs. 8.22 and 8.23).[19] Other patients develop radiologic honeycombing and end-stage fibrosis,[16] but the pathologic findings in such lungs are not known.

REFERENCES

1. Travis WD, Costabel U, Hansell DM, et al.; ATS/ERS Committee on Idiopathic Interstitial Pneumonias. An official American Thoracic Society/European Respiratory Society statement: update of the international multidisciplinary classification of the idiopathic interstitial pneumonias. *Am J Respir Crit Care Med.* 2013;188:733–748.

2. Churg A, Hall R, Bilawich A. Respiratory bronchiolitis with fibrosis-interstitial lung disease: a new form of smoking-induced interstitial lung disease. *Arch Pathol Lab Med.* 2015;139:437–440.

3. Churg A, Müller NL, Wright JL. Respiratory bronchiolitis/interstitial lung disease: fibrosis, pulmonary function, and evolving concepts. *Arch Pathol Lab Med.* 2010;134:27–32.

4. Heyneman LE, Ward S, Lynch DA, et al. Respiratory bronchiolitis, respiratory bronchiolitis-associated interstitial lung disease, and desquamative interstitial pneumonia: different entities or part of the spectrum of the same disease process? *AJR Am J Roentgenol.* 1999;173:1617–1622.

5. Sverzellati N, Lynch DA, Hansell DM, et al. American Thoracic Society-European Respiratory Society classification of the idiopathic interstitial pneumonias: advances in knowledge since 2002. *Radiographics.* 2015;35:1849–1871.

6. Vassallo R, Jensen EA, Colby TV, et al. The overlap between respiratory bronchiolitis and desquamative interstitial pneumonia in pulmonary Langerhans cell histiocytosis: high-resolution CT, histologic, and functional correlations. *Chest.* 2003;124:1199–1205.

7. Reddy TL, Mayo J, Churg A. Respiratory bronchiolitis with fibrosis: high resolution computed tomography findings and correlation with pathology. *Ann Am Thorac Soc.* 2013;10:590–601.

8. English C, Churg A, Lam S, et al. Respiratory bronchiolitis with fibrosis: prevalence and progression. *Ann Am Thorac Soc.* 2014;11:1665–1666.

9. Yousem SA. Respiratory bronchiolitis-associated interstitial lung disease with fibrosis is a lesion distinct from fibrotic

nonspecific interstitial pneumonia: a proposal. *Mod Pathol.* 2006;19:1474–1479.

10. Kawabata Y, Takemura T, Hebisawa A, et al. Eosinophilia in bronchoalveolar lavage fluid and architectural destruction are features of desquamative interstitial pneumonia. *Histopathology.* 2008;52:194–202.

11. Flaherty KR, Fell C, Aubry MC, et al. Smoking-related idiopathic interstitial pneumonia. *Eur Respir J.* 2014;44:594–602.

12. Katzenstein AL, Mukhopadhyay S, Zanardi C, et al. Clinically occult interstitial fibrosis in smokers: classification and significance of a surprisingly common finding in lobectomy specimens. *Hum Pathol.* 2010;41:316–325.

13. Myers JL, Veal CF Jr, Shin MS, et al. Respiratory bronchiolitis causing interstitial lung disease: a clinicopathologic study of six cases. *Am Rev Respir Dis.* 1987;135:880–884.

14. Yousem SA, Colby TV, Gaensler EA. Respiratory bronchiolitis-associated interstitial lung disease and its relationship to desquamative interstitial pneumonia. *Mayo Clin Proc.* 1989;64:1373–1380.

15. Godbert B, Wissler MP, Vignaud JM. Desquamative interstitial pneumonia: an analytic review with an emphasis on aetiology. *Eur Respir Rev.* 2013;22:117–123.

16. Kawabata Y, Takemura T, Hebisawa A, et al.; Desquamative Interstitial Pneumonia Study Group. Desquamative interstitial pneumonia may progress to lung fibrosis as characterized radiologically. *Respirology.* 2012;17:1214–1221.

17. King MB, Jessurun J, Hertz MI. Recurrence of desquamative interstitial pneumonia after lung transplantation. *Am J Respir Crit Care Med.* 1997;156:2003–2005.

18. Bledsoe JR, Christiani DC, Kradin RL. Smoking-associated fibrosis and pulmonary asbestosis. *Int J Chron Obstruct Pulmon Dis.* 2014;19;10:31–37.

19. Tazelaar HD, Wright JL, Churg A. Desquamative interstitial pneumonia. *Histopathology.* 2011;58:509–516.

Combined Pulmonary Fibrosis with Emphysema

NOMENCLATURE AND CONCEPTUAL ISSUES

A mixture of emphysema and interstitial fibrosis in theory can be seen in the lungs of any patient with an interstitial lung disease (ILD) who smokes, and, in general, we advise not reporting the presence of emphysema in a video-assisted thoracoscopic (VATS) biopsy because such biopsies are never performed to diagnose emphysema. However, in practice there are three different scenarios in which this combination is of interest and/or can cause diagnostic confusion when reviewing pathologic material: combined pulmonary fibrosis and emphysema (CPFE), centrilobular emphysema with bands of fibrosis across the enlarged airspaces, and respiratory bronchiolitis with fibrosis (RBF, and see Chapter 8).

CLINICAL FEATURES

The clinical disease known as "combined pulmonary fibrosis with emphysema" is typically seen in heavy smokers who have underlying chronic obstructive lung disease as well as an ILD that is most commonly usual interstitial pneumonia (UIP), either idiopathic pulmonary fibrosis (IPF) or UIP associated with a collagen vascular disease, particularly rheumatoid arthritis or systemic sclerosis.[1-3] Less frequently other types of fibrosing interstitial pneumonias have been reported in CPFE, although the descriptions in the literature are very poorly detailed. As UIP/IPF, rheumatoid arthritis, and emphysema are all diseases of cigarette smokers, the existence of this combination is not surprising, but occasional cases are also seen in never or light smokers with connective tissue disease.[3]

There is disagreement in the literature about how much emphysema is required for the diagnosis. Jacob et al.[4] made a diagnosis of CPFE, using any amount of emphysema on high-resolution computed tomography (HRCT) as the criterion, in 39% of a consecutive series of 272 IPF patients, but others have found a much smaller proportion when using a higher emphysema cutoff.[5]

CPFE has attracted considerable clinical attention because it presents a confusing pulmonary function picture with apparently preserved lung volumes and a markedly decreased diffusing capacity in the face of signs, symptoms, and imaging of an ILD.[1] For the pathologist it often presents a very unusual morphologic appearance as well (see below).

Pulmonary hypertension is common in CPFE patients,[1,2,6] and there has been considerable debate about whether the combination is associated with disproportionate elevations of pulmonary artery pressure; however, in two large series of CPFE patients, pulmonary artery pressures were found to be about that expected from adding the contributions of emphysema and pulmonary fibrosis, both diseases that by themselves are associated with pulmonary hypertension, and there was no evidence of a multiplicative interaction.[7]

IMAGING

The HRCT findings of CPFE consist of upper lobe emphysema and predominantly lower lobe ILD (Figs. 9.1 and 9.2). In the majority of patients, the ILD manifests

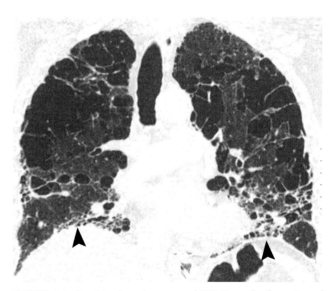

FIGURE 9.1. Combined emphysema and UIP. Coronal reformation of a volumetric HRCT demonstrates extensive upper lobe bullous emphysema and basal ILD (*arrowheads*).

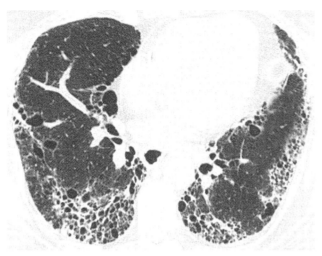

FIGURE 9.2. HRCT at the level of the lung bases in the same patient shows subpleural reticulation and honeycombing characteristic of UIP. The patient was a 67-year-old man who had a 100-pack-year smoking history.

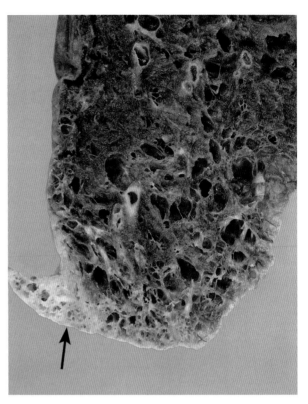

FIGURE 9.3. CPFE. This patient has underlying UIP, which is largely hidden by the emphysema. However, the inferior portion of the lobe shows obvious fibrosis (*arrow*).

as reticulation and honeycombing, involving mainly the subpleural regions and lung bases, a pattern characteristic of UIP.[1,8] Ground-glass opacities are present in approximately two-thirds of the patients but they are usually mild and admixed with reticular opacities and honeycombing.[1] In some patients, however, the ILD results in predominately ground-glass opacities with or without associated reticulation and traction bronchiectasis, a pattern that is suggestive of nonspecific interstitial pneumonia (NSIP) or desquamative interstitial pneumonia (DIP).[8,9]

PATHOLOGIC FEATURES

Most of the cases of CPFE that have been described in the literature have been called UIP with emphysema or NSIP with emphysema, largely on the basis of imaging, and very few have had biopsy confirmation of these diagnoses.[1,2] Some patients by description probably have underlying DIP[1,2] or respiratory bronchiolitis-associated interstitial lung disease (RBILD).[2] There is only one reasonably large (22 cases) series of CPFE patients with pathologic descriptions, and in all of them the underlying fibrosing interstitial pneumonia was UIP.[10]

On morphologic examination, CPFE shows a very variable combination of a fibrosing interstitial pneumonia and emphysema (Figs. 9.3 to 9.10). The pathologic findings can be confusing, particularly because on gross examination of lobectomy or large wedge resections, the emphysema can hide the presence of interstitial fibrosis (Figs. 9.3 and 9.7). In such specimens, there is usually enough tissue available to find areas typical of the fibrotic lung disease, either grossly (Figs. 9.3 and 9.7) or microscopically (Fig. 9.10).

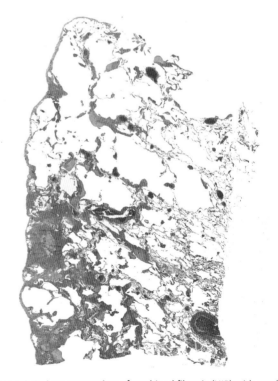

FIGURE 9.4. Low-power view of combined fibrosis (UIP) with emphysema (same case as Fig. 9.3). Because of the emphysema, the fibrosing process has much larger airspaces than are typical of UIP and the process does not look like UIP.

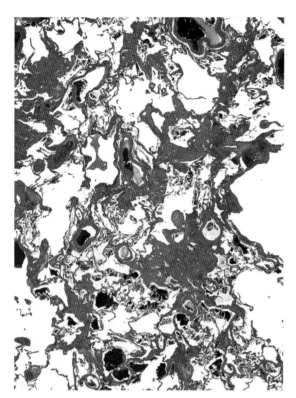

FIGURE 9.5. Another area of the same case. The process is clearly a fibrosing interstitial pneumonia, but because of the emphysema, the fibrosis is much more irregular than is typical of UIP. When presented with this type of odd morphology, review of the CT imaging can be very helpful in pointing to the correct diagnosis.

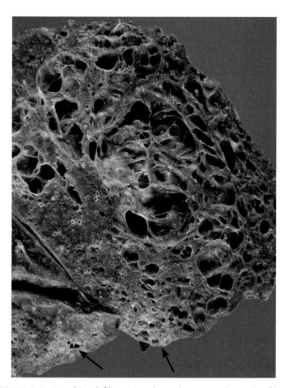

FIGURE 9.7. Combined fibrosis and emphysema where the fibrotic component is chronic hypersensitivity pneumonitis. As in Figure 9.3, the emphysema hides the diffuse fibrosis, but fibrosis is grossly visible away from the emphysematous areas (*arrows*).

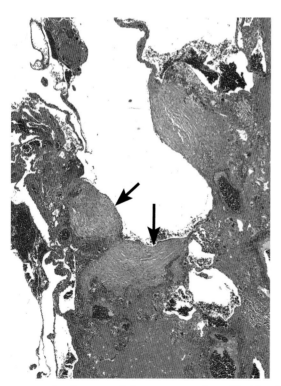

FIGURE 9.6. Another area of the same case shows fibroblast foci (*arrows*) around greatly enlarged airspaces.

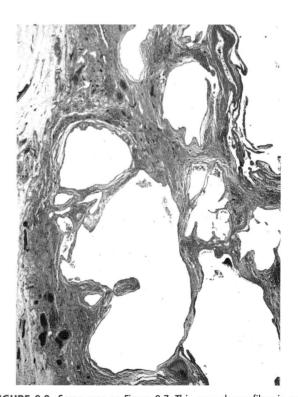

FIGURE 9.8. Same case as Figure 9.7. This area shows fibrosis surrounding emphysematous spaces and mimicking honeycombing. However, the metaplastic bronchiolar epithelium usually seen in honeycombed spaces is absent and there are no inspissated secretions.

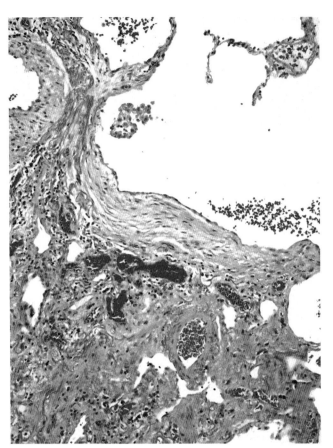

FIGURE 9.9. A fibroblast focus surrounding an emphysematous space in the same case.

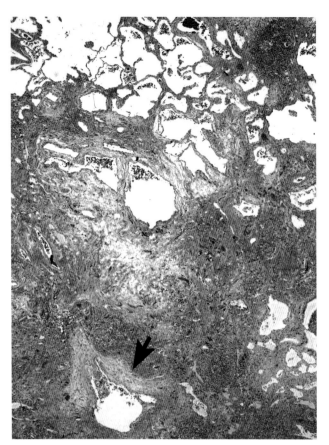

FIGURE 9.10. Another area of this case without emphysema shows a pattern more like that of UIP (some cases of chronic hypersensitivity pneumonitis look like UIP, see Chapter 12). A fibroblast focus is present at the *arrow*.

However, in surgical lung biopsies there may only be an admixture, sometimes producing an unusual pattern of enlarged airspaces with fibrous walls (Figs. 9.4 to 9.6), which occasionally mimics honeycombing (Fig. 9.8). But unlike honeycombing, there is no metaplastic bronchiolar epithelium in the enlarged spaces and usually no inspissated secretions (Fig. 9.8). Inomata et al.[10] point out that these airspaces are frequently over 10 mm in diameter, something that is not typical of honeycombing; rather, these enlarged airspaces appear to represent emphysematous foci with fibrosis that has developed around them. Fibroblast foci may also be present in the enlarged airspaces (Figs. 9.6 and 9.9), and fibroblast foci are never a feature of pure emphysema.

Even where the airspaces are not very large, the interstitial fibrosis is often distorted by emphysema (e.g., Figs. 9.4 and 9.5), and it may not be possible to readily classify the type of fibrosing interstitial pneumonia from a biopsy. The presence of easily identifiable fibroblast foci (Figs. 9.6, 9.9, and 9.10) suggests that the underlying process is probably UIP, but reference to the HRCT imaging may provide a better guide.

CENTRILOBULAR EMPHYSEMA WITH FIBROSIS

The second setting is a combination of fibrosis and emphysema in which the patient does not have a diffuse ILD at all, but rather has ordinary centrilobular emphysema with fibrous bands in the enlarged airspaces (Figs. 9.11 and 9.12). Fibrosis associated with centrilobular (Figs. 9.11 and 9.12) or paraseptal emphysema is actually quite common,[11] but does not change the underlying diagnosis of emphysema, and in fact we avoid mentioning fibrosis in a diagnosis of centrilobular emphysema, because it has no prognostic or management significance and is likely to confuse clinicians.

RESPIRATORY BRONCHIOLITIS WITH FIBROSIS

RBF, also known as smoking-related interstitial fibrosis, airspace enlargement with fibrosis, and RBILD with fibrosis (see Chapter 8), consists of distinctly localized,

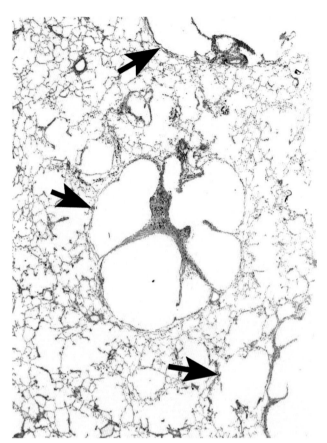

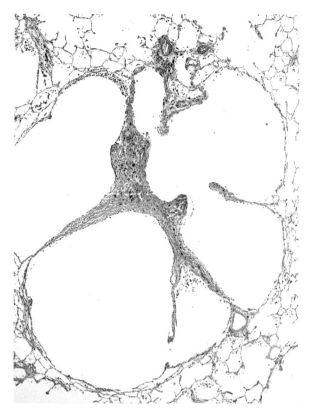

FIGURE 9.12. A higher-power view of the central lesion in Figure 9.11.

FIGURE 9.11. Centrilobular emphysema with fibrosis. Three separate foci of centrilobular emphysema (*arrows*) show varying degrees of fibrosis as bands crossing the enlarged airspace. This is a common finding in centrilobular emphysema; the proper diagnosis is "centrilobular emphysema" and not "centrilobular emphysema with fibrosis" because the latter term can be mistaken for CPFE, and fibrosis of this type in emphysema has no known functional consequences.

typically subpleural, regions of paucicellular and often hyaline-appearing interstitial fibrosis mixed with emphysema (Figs. 9.13 and 9.14, and see Chapter 8). Smoker's macrophages are present in the enlarged airspaces. In a given medium-power field, RBF can mimic some form of CPFE (Fig. 9.14), but in contradistinction to CPFE, which by definition must have an underlying *diffuse* fibrosing interstitial pneumonia, in RBF the process forms patches spacially restricted to the immediate subpleural region (Fig. 9.13), or sometimes with extension from a respiratory bronchiole to the pleura (see Fig. 8.11 in Chapter 8), and this type of circumscription is never present in UIP, NSIP, chronic hypersensitivity pneumonitis, or DIP. When RBF is visible on HRCT, it manifests as subpleural patches of reticulation mixed with emphysema and usually associated with bilateral ground-glass opacities (see Fig. 8.3 in Chapter 8). RBF is discussed in more detail in Chapter 8.

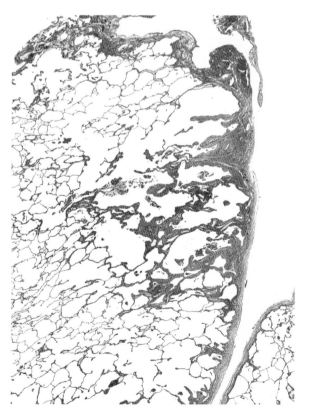

FIGURE 9.13. RBF for comparison to CPFE. Note the distinct circumscription of the fibrosing process, a finding characteristic of RBF as opposed to the diffuse fibrosis typical of CPFE.

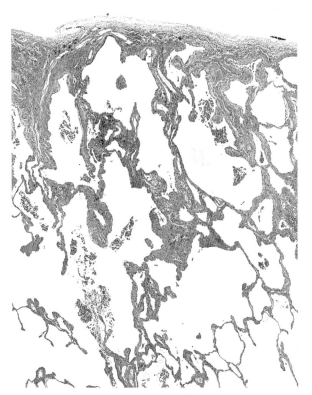

FIGURE 9.14. Higher-power view of the fibrotic area in Figure 9.13. If one had this field alone, it would be impossible to determine whether the fibrosing process is localized or diffuse, but reference to CT imaging usually resolves the problem. Additional illustrations of RBF are shown in Chapter 8.

DIAGNOSTIC MODALITIES

CPFE is usually diagnosed on imaging alone, but if tissue is required, then a VATS biopsy must be performed. Transbronchial biopsy produces no useful information in this setting. The possible utility of cryobiopsy in this setting is not known.

PROGNOSIS

The prognosis of CPFE has been the subject of considerable debate and has been variably reported as equal to, or better than, or worse than that of UIP alone.[12–16] However, more recent data derived from a large cohort of UIP patients showed that for a given amount of radiologic fibrosis, CPFE patients had worse survival compared with those with UIP and no emphysema.[4] The presence of significant

pulmonary hypertension is a major determinant of mortality, with 1-year survival of about 60%.[7,13,14]

REFERENCES

1. Cottin V, Nunes H, Brillet PY, et al. Combined pulmonary fibrosis and emphysema: a distinct underrecognised entity. *Eur Respir J.* 2005;26:586–593.
2. Cottin V, Cordier JF. Combined pulmonary fibrosis and emphysema in connective tissue disease. *Curr Opin Pulm Med.* 2012;18:418–427.
3. Papaioannou AI, Kostikas K, Manali ED, et al. Combined pulmonary fibrosis and emphysema: the many aspects of a cohabitation contract. *Respir Med.* 2016;117:14–26.
4. Jacob J, Bartholmai BJ, Rajagopalan S, et al. Functional and prognostic effects when emphysema complicates idiopathic pulmonary fibrosis. *Eur Respir J.* 2017;50(1). pii: 1700379.
5. Ryerson CJ, Hartman T, Elicker BM, et al. Clinical features and outcomes in combined pulmonary fibrosis and emphysema in idiopathic pulmonary fibrosis. *Chest.* 2013;144:234–240.
6. Fell CD. Idiopathic pulmonary fibrosis: phenotypes and comorbidities. *Clin Chest Med.* 2012;33:51–57.
7. Jacob J, Bartholmai BJ, Rajagopalan S, et al. Likelihood of pulmonary hypertension in patients with idiopathic pulmonary fibrosis and emphysema. *Respirology.* 2017;23:593–599.
8. Attili AK, Kazerooni EA, Gross BH, et al. Smoking-related interstitial lung disease: radiologic-clinical-pathologic correlation. *Radiographics.* 2008;28:1383–1396.
9. Jankowich MD, Rounds SI. Combined pulmonary fibrosis and emphysema syndrome: a review. *Chest.* 2012;141:222–231.
10. Inomata M, Ikushima S, Awano N, et al. An autopsy study of combined pulmonary fibrosis and emphysema: correlations among clinical, radiological, and pathological features. *BMC Pulm Med.* 2014;14:104.
11. Wright JL, Tazelaar HD, Churg A. Fibrosis with emphysema. *Histopathology.* 2011;58:517–524.
12. Jankowich MD, Rounds S. Combined pulmonary fibrosis and emphysema alters physiology but has similar mortality to pulmonary fibrosis without emphysema. *Lung.* 2010;188:365–373.
13. Kurashima K, Takayanagi N, Tsuchiya N, et al. The effect of emphysema on lung function and survival in patients with idiopathic pulmonary fibrosis. *Respirology.* 2010;15:843–848.
14. King TE Jr, Pardo A, Selman M. Idiopathic pulmonary fibrosis. *Lancet.* 2011;378:1949–1961.
15. Mejía M, Carrillo G, Rojas-Serrano J, et al. Idiopathic pulmonary fibrosis and emphysema: decreased survival associated with severe pulmonary arterial hypertension. *Chest.* 2009;136:10–15.
16. Cottin V, Le Pavec J, Prévot G, et al. Pulmonary hypertension in patients with combined pulmonary fibrosis and emphysema syndrome. *Eur Respir J.* 2010;35:105–111.

Langerhans Cell Histiocytosis (Eosinophilic Granuloma of Lung)

NOMENCLATURE AND CONCEPTUAL ISSUES

Langerhans cell histiocytosis (LCH) is a proliferation of Langerhans cells, which are a form of dendritic cell. The older term "eosinophilic granuloma of lung" is sometimes also applied to these lesions, but is misleading because there are no granulomas in eosinophilic granuloma and eosinophils may be abundant, scarce, or completely absent. The even older name, "histiocytosis X" is best avoided, because it includes a number of quite disparate entities: LCH (with the term sometimes used for disseminated disease), Letterer–Siwe disease, and Hand–Schiller–Christian disease, the latter two disseminated and sometimes aggressive conditions usually seen in infants and children. The disseminated forms seen in children are now more frequently referred to as systemic LCH.[1]

The current belief is that LCH is a myeloid neoplasm with the neoplastic cell being a clonal dendritic cell at various stages of differentiation,[2] and therefore some cases have been treated with inhibitors directed at specific molecular abnormalities[3] (see section Etiology and Molecular Pathogenesis, and Treatment and Prognosis). However, although this idea may be conceptually correct, most cases of pulmonary LCH remain localized to the lung and behave as an inflammatory process that may resolve or may cause parenchymal scarring (see section Treatment and Prognosis), rather than "metastasizing" in the fashion of a neoplasm.

ETIOLOGY AND MOLECULAR PATHOGENESIS

LCH in adults is usually a disease of current or ex-cigarette smokers, but in France, 20% of cases of LCH are associated with marijuana smoking.[1] In humans, and in experimental animal models, cigarette smoke functions as a dendritic cell attractant.[4] Smoking promotes survival of dendritic cells via antiapoptotic mechanisms, and increased numbers of CD1A-positive Langerhans cells can be found even in the lungs of healthy smokers. Cigarette smoke is also believed

to induce senescence, but not cell death, in many cell types including Langerhans cells, and senescent cells are typically associated with a proinflammatory state.[5] LCH cells in the lung express differentiation markers similar to those seen after exposure to pathogens or activating cytokines.

Considerable information is now available on the molecular changes in LCH and it has been suggested[1,2] that all cases have mutations that affect the mitogen-activated protein kinase pathway, a pathway that transduces external cell membrane signals to the nucleus, leading to a variety of effects, most notably cell proliferation. Durham[2] has proposed that when mutations arise in a population of self-renewing dendritic cell precursors, the result is a systemic LCH disease, whereas mutations that arise in differentiated dendritic cell populations lead to localized LCH disease.

Roughly 35% to 50% of cases of pulmonary LCH and more than 50% of cases of systemic LCH have *BRAF* V600E mutations[2] (Table 10.1). This is the same mutation that is seen in a variety of other neoplasms, including melanomas, colon carcinomas, and thyroid

Table 10.1

Mutations and translocations reported in LCH

Common
  BRAF V600E
  MAP2K1
Uncommon
  KRAS
  NRAS
  ARAF
  BRAF not V600E
  ERRB3
  BRAF indels
ETV3-NCOA2 translocation

From Durham BH. Molecular characterization of the histiocytoses: neoplasia of dendritic cells and macrophages. *Semin Cell Dev Biol.* 2019;86:62–76.

carcinomas, and leads to constitutive activation of *BRAF* and subsequent activation of the downstream MAP kinases extracellular signal-regulated kinase (ERK) and ERK kinase (also called MEK).[3] *BRAF* V600E mutations can often be detected in LCH by immunohistochemistry; for example, Roden et al.[6] found positive BRAF V600E staining in 25/43 (28%) cases of pulmonary LCH and 19/54 (35%) cases of extrapulmonary LCH (see section Immunohistochemistry).

In LCH, the second most common mutation (around 20% of cases) is in *MAP2K1* (also called *MEK1*), and a variety of other mutations and occasional translocations are found in a small proportion of cases[2] (Table 10.1); these are all mutually exclusive with *BRAF* V600E. At present, detection of these mutations requires direct sequencing. However, all of these mutations, including those in *BRAF*, activate ERK and sustained ERK activity leads to accumulation of cyclin D1, which can be detected in LCH lesions by immunochemistry[7] (see section Immunohistochemistry).

CLINICAL FEATURES

LCH patients are typically young adults, most of whom are short of breath, but about 20% are asymptomatic[1,8,9] and the lesions are picked up on routine chest radiographs. Another 15% present with spontaneous pneumothorax, which may be recurrent.[10] Systemic complaints, particularly fever and weight loss, are seen in 15% to 20%. Pulmonary function tests may demonstrate a restrictive or an obstructive defect (the latter reflecting the fact that LCH lesions obliterate small airways), or sometimes just an isolated reduction in diffusing capacity.[1]

IMAGING

The characteristic high-resolution computed tomography (HRCT) manifestations of LCH consist of nodules and cysts in the upper and middle lung zones with relative sparing of the lung bases (Figs. 10.1 to 10.3). The nodules predominate in the early stages and the cysts in the later stages.[11] The nodules can have smooth or irregular margins, usually measure less than 10 mm in diameter, and have a centrilobular distribution. The cysts may have thin or thick walls. In the early stages, the cysts usually measure less than 1 cm in diameter and are round or ovoid. In the later stages, the cysts become confluent, larger than 2 cm in diameter and often have bizarre configurations.[12] HRCT shows no consistent central or peripheral predominance of lesions, but in nearly all cases, the lung bases are relatively spared.

In the majority of patients, the manifestations of LCH are characteristic enough to allow a confident diagnosis on HRCT.[13] Centrilobular emphysema can

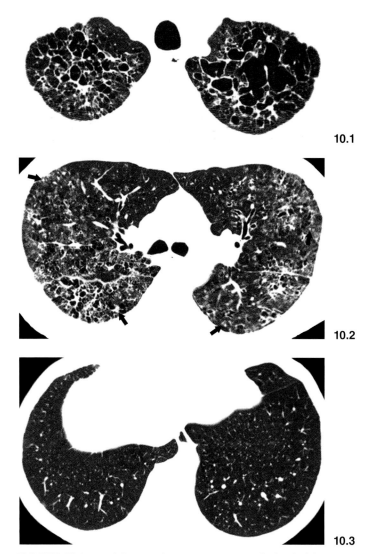

FIGURES 10.1 to 10.3. LCH. Figure 10.1: HRCT at the level of the lung apices demonstrates multiple thin- and thick-walled cysts of various sizes and shapes and a few small nodules. **Figure 10.2:** HRCT at the level of the main bronchi shows multiple cysts and small nodules of various sizes and shapes (*arrows*). Also noted are ground-glass opacities presumably due to respiratory bronchiolitis. **Figure 10.3:** HRCT at the level of the lung bases shows normal parenchyma.

usually be readily distinguished by the lack of visible walls and the presence of small vessels within the focal areas of lung destruction. The cysts in lymphangioleiomyomatosis are typically diffused throughout the lungs without any zonal predominance and are seldom associated with nodules. It should be noted, however, that in patients with mild LCH, the abnormalities may be missed or misinterpreted as being due to respiratory bronchiolitis or other causes of multiple small nodules or cysts (Figs. 10.4 and 10.5). Many LCH lesions are positive on PET scans.[1]

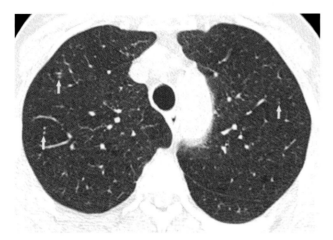

FIGURE 10.4. HRCT at presentation shows mild emphysema and a few poorly defined nodular opacities (*straight arrows*) in the upper lobes. This CT was interpreted as showing only emphysema and a few indeterminate small nodules.

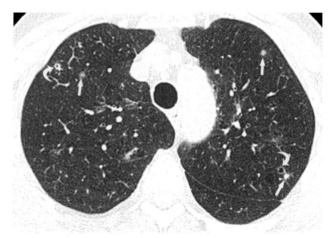

FIGURE 10.5. HRCT 10 months later demonstrates several nodular opacities (*straight arrows*) and two cystic lesions (*curved arrows*). The diagnosis of pulmonary Langerhans was suggested and confirmed at surgical biopsy.

PATHOLOGIC FEATURES

As a mnemonic tool, LCH lesions can be divided into early or cellular phase (Table 10.2) and the late or scarred phase (Table 10.2), but it is common to find mixtures of the two in a biopsy.

The early phase consists of nodules that are grossly rounded to stellate (Fig. 10.6) and microscopically appear quite cellular at low power (Figs. 10.7 to 10.9). The lesions are centered on respiratory bronchioles and frequently obliterate the bronchiolar lumens. At high power, they consist of a mixture of Langerhans cells, which resemble macrophages but have grooved nuclei, eosinophils, and often some numbers of smoker's macrophages (Figs. 10.10 to 10.12). The number of eosinophils is extremely variable and some cases have almost none (compare Figs. 10.10 and 10.11); an apparent absence of eosinophils does not invalidate the diagnosis of LCH, because it is the Langerhans cell that is really the diagnostic feature.

Table 10.2

Pathologic findings in LCH

Early lesions

Cellular rounded to stellate nodules centered on respiratory bronchioles

Occasionally areas with an interstitial pattern

Cellular lesions contain a variable mixture of eosinophils, Langerhans cells, chronic inflammatory cells, and smoker's macrophages

Cysts may be present

Aggregates of S-100, CD1a, Langerin, or cyclin D1-positive cells

Eosinophils may be scarce

Late lesions

Irregular paucicellular scars that may be nodular or stellate or sometimes linear

Scars centered on respiratory bronchioles

No subpleural predominance

Fibrous walled cysts associated with scars may be present

Usually few or no S-100/CD1a/Langerin positive cells

Respiratory bronchioles and/or accompanying pulmonary artery branches may be obliterated

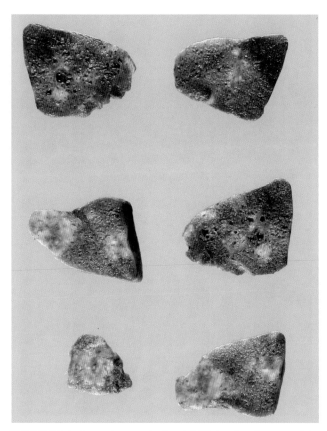

FIGURE 10.6. Gross photograph of early LCH showing discrete nodules that, grossly, cannot be distinguished from a neoplasm. (Case Courtesy Dr. Julia Flint.)

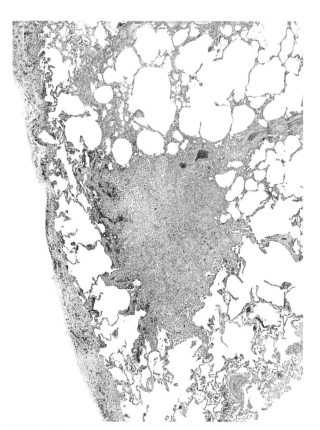

FIGURE 10.8. Low-power view of a nodule of early LCH. Note the stellate shape, which is very common in LCH nodules.

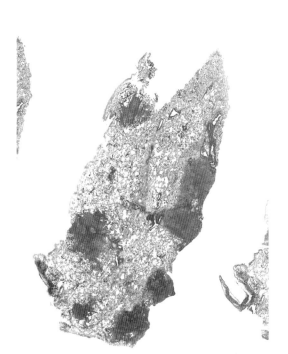

FIGURE 10.7. Whole-mount view of early LCH showing cellular, stellate to irregular, nodules.

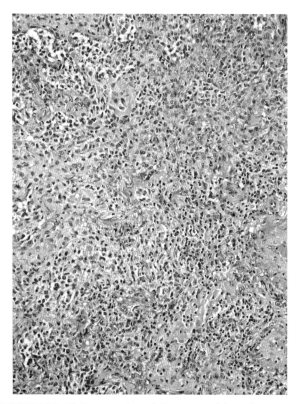

FIGURE 10.9. High-power view of the same nodule. Early LCH nodules are densely cellular.

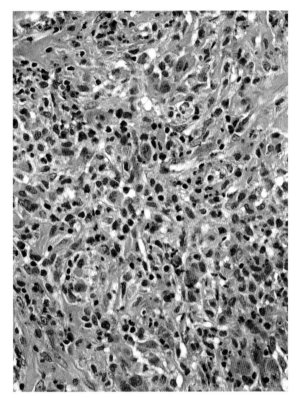

FIGURE 10.10. Early LCH nodule comprising Langerhans cells and fairly numerous eosinophils.

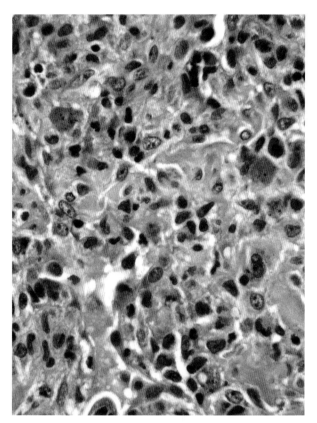

FIGURE 10.12. High-power view showing the bland and sometimes convoluted nuclei of Langerhans cells and a few smoker's macrophages.

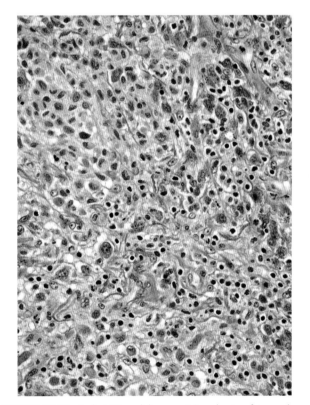

FIGURE 10.11. Early LCH nodule comprising sheets of Langerhans cells with only rare eosinophils. Eosinophils can be completely absent in LCH. Note the numerous smoker's macrophages, a common finding in and around LCH nodules.

Occasionally Langerhans cells proliferate in the interstitium rather than forming distinct nodules (Figs. 10.13 to 10.17) and mimic an interstitial pneumonia, although, as opposed to true interstitial pneumonias, such LCH lesions are always quite localized. Areas of organizing pneumonia (OP) may also be present with the lesions of early LCH (Fig. 10.18). Vascular obliteration is sometimes seen in early lesions (Fig. 10.19).

Early-phase LCH nodules frequently become cystic (Fig. 10.20), perhaps because narrowing of bronchiolar lumens leads to a ball valve effect. If the cysts are immediately subpleural, they can rupture into the pleural space producing a pneumothorax. The cysts often have strange shapes, and recent imaging data suggest that the peculiar shapes arise from fusion of cysts.[13]

Late lesions of LCH are composed of fibrous scars that may be rounded or stellate or more or less linear and grossly can produce a form of honeycombing (Fig. 10.21), although unlike the honeycombing of usual interstitial pneumonia (UIP), old LCH tends to have cystic spaces but no sheets of fibrous tissue, nor does it have the metaplastic bronchiolar epithelium, mucus collections, and inflammatory cells found in true honeycombing (see Figs. 6.16 to 6.18). Rather the lesions of old LCH consist of paucicellular fibrous scars that sometimes can be seen to be centered around respiratory bronchioles or are at least centrilobular

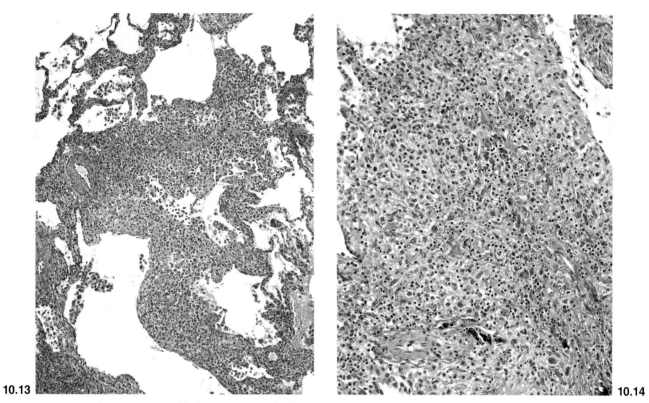

FIGURES 10.13 and 10.14. Low- and high-power views of early LCH with an interstitial pattern. Early LCH lesions are not always nodules, but even when apparently interstitial, the process is circumscribed.

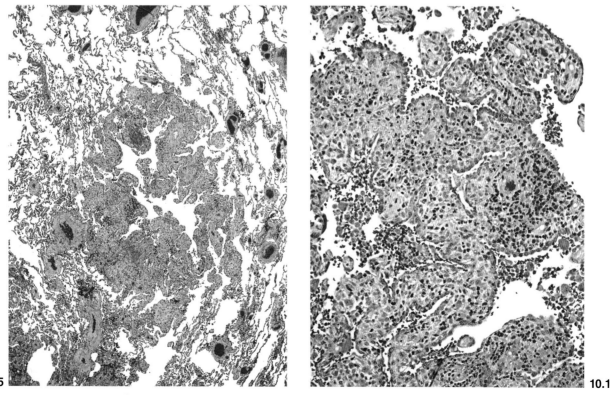

FIGURES 10.15 to 10.17. See figure legend 10.17.

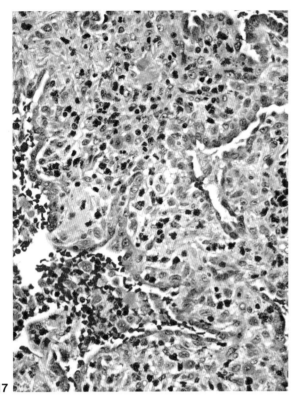

10.17

FIGURES 10.15 to 10.17. Another example of early LCH with an interstitial pattern of growth.

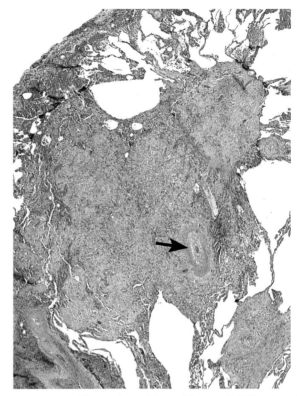

FIGURE 10.19. Obliterated vessel (*arrow*) in an early LCH nodule. Because LCH nodules typically form around respiratory bronchioles, they tend to engulf and obliterate pulmonary artery branches, eventually leading to pulmonary hypertension.

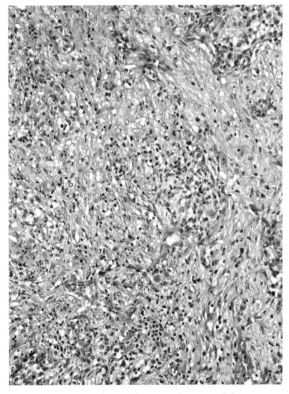

FIGURE 10.18. Areas of OP within an early LCH nodule.

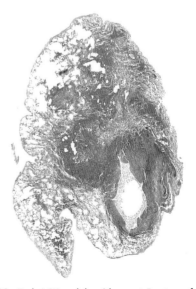

FIGURE 10.20. Early LCH nodule with a cyst. Rupture of cysts into the pleural space accounts for the high incidence of pneumothorax in LCH.

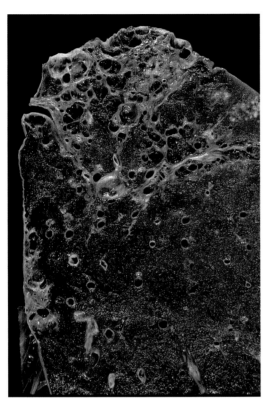

FIGURE 10.21. Gross view of late stage fibrotic LCH in the apex of the lung. LCH typically involves the upper lung zones and spares the lung bases.

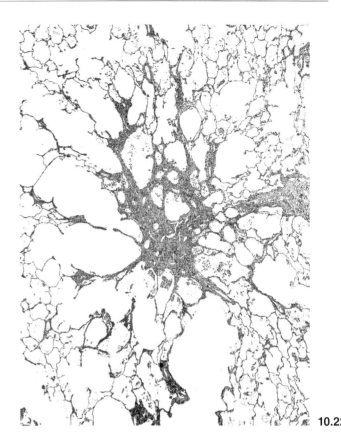

10.22

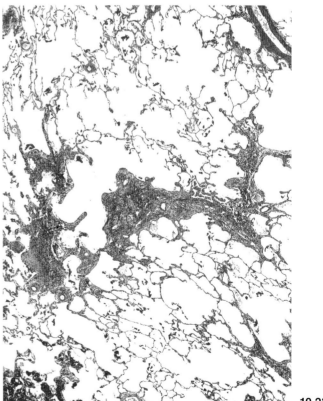

10.23

in distribution (Figs. 10.22 to 10.26). Old scarred LCH never shows the subpleural distribution of UIP nor the homogenous scarring of fibrotic nonspecific interstitial pneumonia (NSIP) and typically spares the lung bases.

Depending on the age of the lesion, small numbers of Langerhans cells and/or eosinophils may be present in late lesions (Figs. 10.27 and 10.28), but the older the lesion, the fewer such cells are found, and very old lesions are almost completely acellular. LCH scars can obliterate respiratory bronchioles and also the accompanying small pulmonary artery branches; if enough arterial branches are destroyed, pulmonary hypertension develops.

Because LCH is a disease of smokers, LCH biopsies may also have focal desquamative interstitial pneumonia (DIP)-like areas and smoker's respiratory bronchiolitis, but the convention is that these lesions are ignored, unless there is true widespread DIP (see Chapter 8) and not just collections of smoker's macrophages in alveoli.

IMMUNOHISTOCHEMISTRY

Langerhans cells are strongly S-100 and CD1a positive (Figs. 10.29 and 10.30), and this is a useful test when the identity of a cellular lesion is uncertain. Langerhans cells are also positive for Langerin (CD207), but few

FIGURES 10.22 to 10.24. Examples of different patterns of localized scarring in late stage LCH. Irregular or stellate centrilobular scars should suggest a diagnosis of old burnt out LCH; however, they can also be seen in old sarcoid.

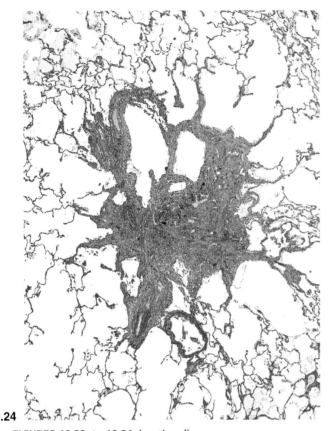

10.24

FIGURES 10.22 to 10.24. (*continued*)

laboratories have Langerin antibodies available and Langerin staining does not offer any advantage over S-100 and CD1a.

Care needs to be taken in interpreting these stains because any kind of inflammatory process in the lung will have a few Langerhans cells.[14] A positive diagnosis requires sheets or nodules of positive staining cells (Figs. 10.29 and 10.30) and not just scattered individual staining cells.[14]

S-100, CD1a, Langerin, and presumably cyclin D1 staining is less useful in older lesions because the Langerhans cells disappear.[14] But occasionally small aggregates of staining cells are still present and this is helpful in determining the etiology of a diffuse scarring process (Figs. 10.31 to 10.33).

As mentioned above, a proportion of pulmonary LCH cases have *BRAF* V600E mutations and will stain with antibodies to BRAF V600E (Figs. 10.34 to 10.36). This finding may be of therapeutic importance (see below) but should not be relied on for diagnosis because many cases do not stain for V600E protein.

Shanmugam et al.[7] have recently reported that all LCH lesions stain for cyclin D1, and this is potentially a very useful marker (Figs. 10.37 to 10.39), as these authors found that non neoplastic Langerhans cells, for example, in lymph nodes in dermatopathic lymphadenopathy, do not stain. LCH lesions also stain for phospho-ERK (pERK).[7] However, in our experience pERK staining can

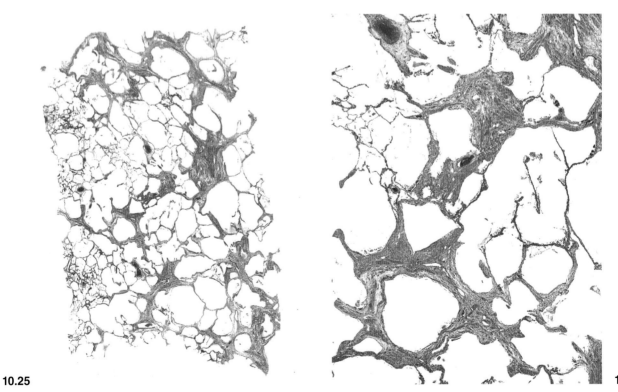

10.25

10.26

FIGURES 10.25 and 10.26. Diffuse scarring in late stage LCH. Although not specific, diffuse scarring of this type with bizarre shapes and a centrilobular distribution should suggest a diagnosis of old burnt out LCH.

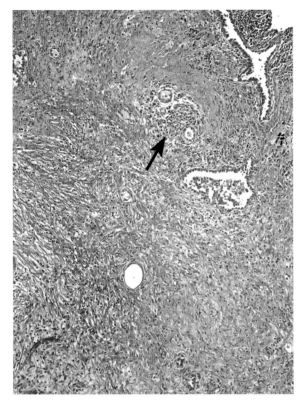

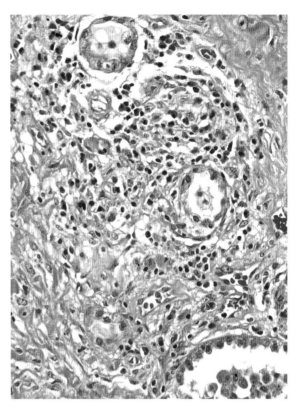

FIGURE 10.27. A largely scarred nodule of LCH in which there is a tiny focus of residual eosinophils and Langerhans cells (*arrow*).

FIGURE 10.28. High-power view of the region at the *arrow* in Figure 10.27. Foci such as this in otherwise scarred nodules allow a definitive diagnosis of LCH.

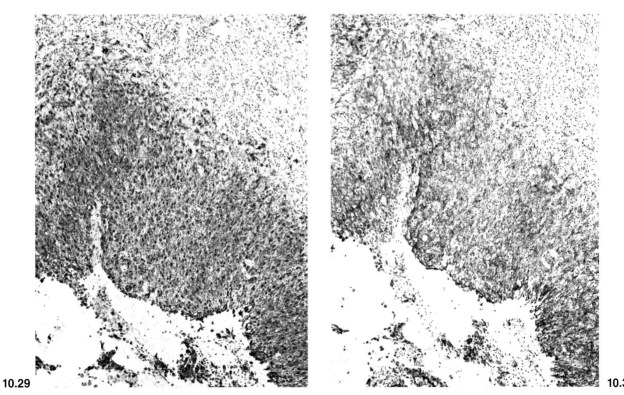

10.29   10.30

FIGURES 10.29 and 10.30. Staining for S-100 (**Fig. 10.29**) and CD1a (**Fig. 10.30**) in a nodule of early LCH. No other lesion produces this pattern of sheets of S100/CD1a-positive cells. However, Langerhans cells disappear as the lesions age, so that negative staining in old fibrotic lesions does not rule out LCH.

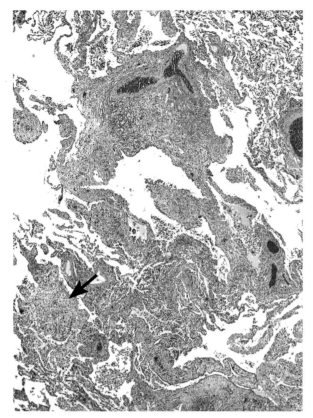

FIGURE 10.31. Low-power view of an LCH lesion that has largely scarred; however, a more cellular area is present at the arrow.

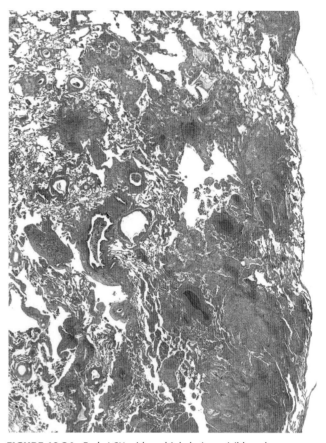

FIGURE 10.34. Early LCH with multiple lesions visible at low power.

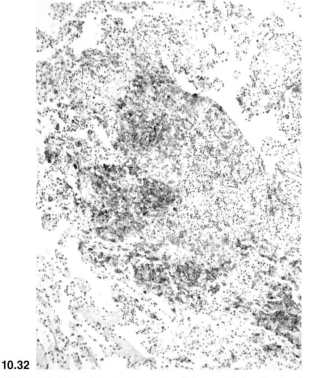

10.32

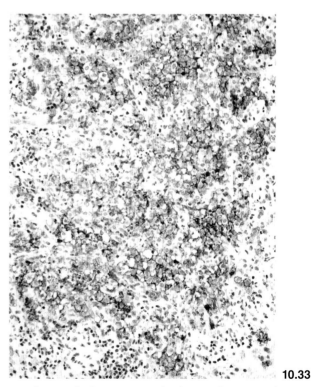

10.33

FIGURES 10.32 and 10.33. CD1a stain of the same lesion showing the area at the *arrow* in Fig. 10.31. Note the absence of staining in the scarred area but intense and concentrated staining in the cellular area. Staining for S-100 or CD1a sometimes is useful for picking out residual diagnostic cellular foci when the morphologic pattern is not specific in late stage LCH, but only positively staining cellular aggregates of the type shown here are diagnostic.

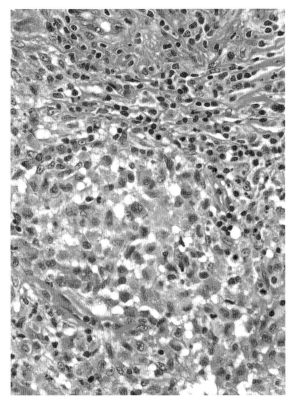

FIGURE 10.35. High-power view of one of the lesions shown in Figure 10.34 demonstrating numerous Langerhans cells and rare eosinophils.

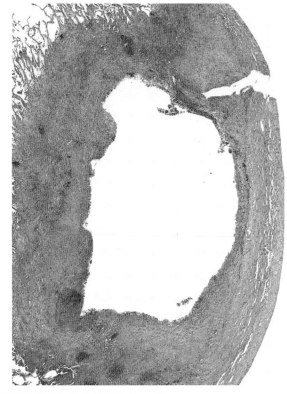

FIGURE 10.37. Early LCH that is cystic.

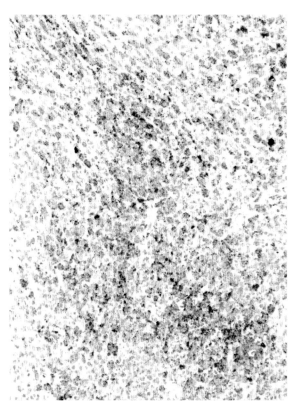

FIGURE 10.36. The lesion shown in Figure 10.35 stains extensively for BRAF V600E.

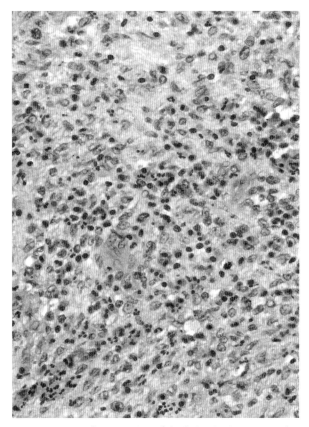

FIGURE 10.38. High-power view of the lesion in Figure 10.37 showing Langerhans cells and numerous eosinophils.

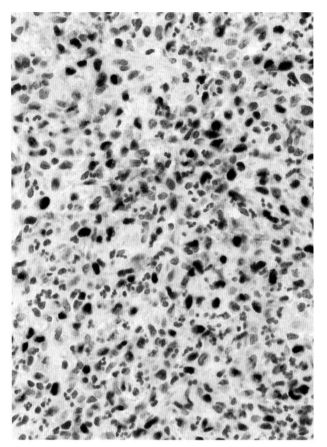

FIGURE 10.39. The lesion is strongly positive for cyclin D1.

be technically difficult, is sensitive to fixation conditions, and offers no advantage over cyclin D1 staining.

DIAGNOSTIC MODALITIES

In many instances, HRCT is diagnostic in LCH and no biopsy is required. Transbronchial biopsy is sometimes diagnostic (see Figs. 3.4 and 3.5), but because the lesions of LCH are scattered, the yield on transbronchial biopsies is fairly low.[15] If the lesions are large enough, they can, occasionally, be picked up on core needle biopsy,[16] and positive results have also been reported with cryobiopsy.[17] However, Video-assisted thoracoscopic surgery biopsy is the usual procedure of choice.

DIFFERENTIAL DIAGNOSIS

Table 10.3 shows the differential diagnosis of LCH. At first glance this appears quite broad, but, in practice, is generally straightforward. At low power, cellular early lesions of LCH mimic neoplasms, but at high power the only neoplasm that might be confused with LCH is classical Hodgkin disease involving the lung, because Hodgkin disease is typically centered around airways and usually has some number of eosinophils. However, Hodgkin disease does

Table 10.3
Differential diagnosis of LCH

Reactive eosinophilic pleuritis
- Common in cases of pneumothorax
- Also seen with drugs, tumors
- Cells are S-100/CD1a negative

Chronic eosinophilic pneumonia
- Eosinophils, no Langerhans cells, usually not nodules

Metastatic tumor (cellular nodules)
Hodgkin disease involving the lung
UIP or NSIP (vs. forms of LCH with extensive scarring)
Old burnt out sarcoid
Erdheim–Chester disease

not have Langerhans cells or smoker's macrophages and Reed–Sternberg cells are not present in LCH.

Reactive eosinophilic pleuritis is a non neoplastic process in which there are large numbers of eosinophils in the pleura, usually as a reaction to an inflammatory process, a tumor, a drug, or a spontaneous pneumothorax[18] (Figs. 10.40 and 10.41). The latter situation can raise a question of underlying LCH, but usually it is clear in bullectomy specimens that LCH is not present. The infiltrating cells in chronic eosinophilic pleuritis are macrophages or mesothelial cells, neither of which are S-100 or CD1a positive. If in doubt, imaging will show an absence of parenchymal nodules/cysts in reactive eosinophilic pleuritis.

Chronic eosinophilic pneumonia (see Chapter 15) can be localized and thus somewhat mimic LCH. However, microscopically eosinophilic pneumonias typically have large numbers of eosinophils, often admixed with OP, and Langerhans cells are sparse to absent. Imaging again will readily sort this out, because chronic eosinophilic pneumonia appears as consolidative lesions that are typically peripheral and are often migratory.

Erdheim–Chester disease (see Chapter 23) is characterized by radiologic sclerosis of the long bones, chronic bone pain, and infiltration of a variety of extra-osseous sites by CD68 and Factor 13a-positive macrophages that may be foamy, and many cases have *BRAF* V600E mutations[2] (see Chapter 23). In the lung, these macrophages are found primarily in the pleura, the interlobular septa, and around the bronchovascular bundles. The macrophages are accompanied by variable degrees of fibrosis (see Figs. 23.11 to 23.15). Collections of Erdheim–Chester cells around bronchovascular bundles (see Fig. 23.13) can somewhat mimic LCH, but Langerhans cells are never foamy, and Erdheim–Chester disease does not have eosinophils and usually does not have smoker's macrophages. Erdheim–Chester cells do not stain for CD1a or Langerin and usually not for S-100. HRCT findings in the chest in

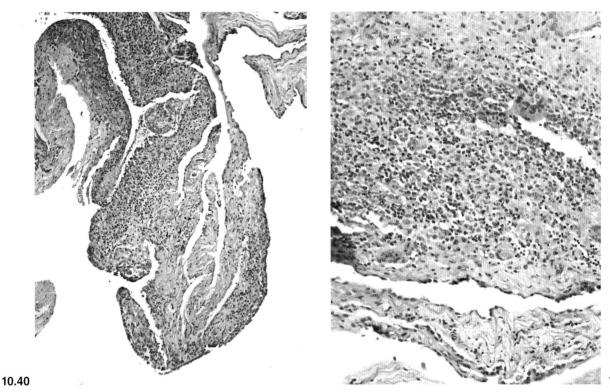

10.40   **10.41**

FIGURES 10.40 and 10.41. Low- and high-power views of reactive eosinophilic pleuritis. The high-power view mimics LCH. Both LCH and reactive eosinophilic pleuritis are associated with pneumothorax, but LCH will have nodules in the lung on imaging, whereas reactive eosinophilic pleuritis will not. The proliferating cells in reactive eosinophilic pleuritis are histiocytes or mesothelial cells and are negative with S-100/CD1a.

Erdheim–Chester disease are also distinct from Langerhans, with marked septal thickening (Fig. 23.10, and see Chapter 23).

In terms of fibrotic mimics, UIP and NSIP do not show stellate scars, and true honeycombing with metaplastic bronchiolar epithelium, such as is seen in UIP (see Chapter 6), is not found in LCH. Sarcoid most commonly scars as nodules, but occasionally sarcoid can scar in a more or less linear fashion with a bronchovascular predominance. When the lesions are not completely scarred and granulomas are still present, separation from LCH is easy, but completely burnt out sarcoid with linear scars is not easily distinguished (see Fig. 13.27).

TREATMENT AND PROGNOSIS

Some cases of LCH remit spontaneously or with smoking cessation,[8,9] but persistent smoking may be associated with progressive disease.[1] Steroids have been used in progressive disease, but the efficacy of steroids remains unproven. Cladribine (2-chlorodeoxyadenosine) has been shown to improve function and shrink cysts in some cases. A small number of patients treated with the BRAF V600E inhibitor, Vemurafenib, have been reported[3] with reversal or at least stabilization of disease. There is also a report of clinical and radiologic improvement in a patient with a

MAP2K1 (MEK1) mutation treated with the MEK1 inhibitor, Trametinib.[19]

In the past, LCH was believed to have an excellent prognosis, but more recent data make it clear that the long-term prognosis is guarded.[8,19] Overall, about one-half of patients stabilize or improve and the remainder progress.[1] Vassallo et al.[8] reported a 15-year survival of about 50% in patients before the days of BRAF inhibitor therapy. Some patients develop significant airflow obstruction.[9,20] Patients may die of respiratory failure secondary to extensive scarring, but pulmonary hypertension is also very common in long-term LCH survivors,[8,20] presumably because the centrilobular lesions pick off pulmonary artery branches when they scar. Patient with pulmonary LCH also have an increased incidence of lymphomas, especially Hodgkins disease, and lung cancers.[21]

Patients that go on to extensive scarring have been treated with lung transplantation. LCH can recur in the transplanted lung, particularly if the patient continues to smoke or resumes smoking.[22]

REFERENCES

1. Vassallo R, Harari S, Tazi A. Current understanding and management of pulmonary Langerhans cell histiocytosis. *Thorax.* 2017;72:937–945.

2. Durham BH. Molecular characterization of the histiocytoses: neoplasia of dendritic cells and macrophages. *Semin Cell Dev Biol.* 2019;86:62–76.

3. Diamond EL, Subbiah V, Lockhart AC, et al. Vemurafenib for BRAF V600-mutant Erdheim-Chester disease and Langerhans cell histiocytosis: analysis of data from the histology-independent, phase 2, open-label VE-BASKET study. *JAMA Oncol.* 2018;4:384–388.

4. Vassallo R, Walters PR, Lamont J, et al. Cigarette smoke promotes dendritic cell accumulation in COPD; a Lung Tissue Research Consortium study. *Respir Res.* 2010;11:45.

5. Wei W, Ji S. Cellular senescence: molecular mechanisms and pathogenicity. *J Cell Physiol.* 2018;233:9121–9135.

6. Roden AC, Hu X, Kip S, et al. BRAF V600E expression in Langerhans cell histiocytosis: clinical and immunohistochemical study on 25 pulmonary and 54 extrapulmonary cases. *Am J Surg Pathol.* 2014;38:548–551.

7. Shanmugam V, Craig JW, Hornick JL, et al. Cyclin D1 is expressed in neoplastic cells of Langerhans cell histiocytosis but not reactive Langerhans cell proliferations. *Am J Surg Pathol.* 2017;41:1390–1396.

8. Vassallo R, Ryu JH, Colby TV, et al. Pulmonary Langerhans'-cell histiocytosis. *N Engl J Med.* 2000;342:1969–1978.

9. Suri HS, Yi ES, Nowakowski GS, et al. Pulmonary Langerhans cell histiocytosis. *Orphanet J Rare Dis.* 2012;7:16.

10. Mendez JL, Nadrous HF, Vassallo R, et al. Pneumothorax in pulmonary Langerhans cell histiocytosis. *Chest.* 2004;125:1028–1032.

11. Brauner MW, Grenier P, Tijani K, et al. Pulmonary Langerhans cell histiocytosis: evolution of lesions on CT scans. *Radiology.* 1997;204:497–502.

12. Kim HJ, Lee KS, Johkoh T, et al. Pulmonary Langerhans cell histiocytosis in adults: high-resolution CT-pathology comparisons and evolutional changes at CT. *Eur Radiol.* 2011;21:1406–1415.

13. Bonelli FS, Hartman TE, Swensen SJ, et al. Accuracy of high-resolution CT in diagnosing lung diseases. *AJR Am J Roentgenol.* 1998;170:1507–1512.

14. Webber D, Tron V, Askin F, et al. S-100 staining in the diagnosis of eosinophilic granuloma of lung. *Am J Clin Pathol.* 1985;84:447–453.

15. Housini I, Tomashefski JF Jr, Cohen A, et al. Transbronchial biopsy in patients with pulmonary eosinophilic granuloma. Comparison with findings on open lung biopsy. *Arch Pathol Lab Med.* 1994;118:523–530.

16. Mukhopadhyay S, Eckardt SM, Scalzetti EM. Diagnosis of pulmonary Langerhans cell histiocytosis by CT-guided core biopsy of lung: a report of three cases. *Thorax.* 2010;65:833–855.

17. Fruchter O, Fridel L, El Raouf BA, et al. Histological diagnosis of interstitial lung diseases by cryo-transbronchial biopsy. *Respirology.* 2014;19:683–688.

18. Askin FB, McCann BG, Kuhn C. Reactive eosinophilic pleuritis: a lesion to be distinguished from pulmonary eosinophilic granuloma. *Arch Pathol Lab Med.* 1977;101:187–191.

19. Lorillon G, Jouenne F, Baroudjian B, et al. Response to trametinib of a pulmonary Langerhans cell Histiocytosis harboring a MAP2K1 deletion. *Am J Respir Crit Care Med.* 2018;198:675–678.

20. Tazi A, Marc K, Dominique S, et al. Serial computed tomography and lung function testing in pulmonary Langerhans' cell histiocytosis. *Eur Respir J.* 2012;40:905–912.

21. Egeler RM, Neglia JP, Aricò M, et al. The relation of Langerhans cell histiocytosis to acute leukemia, lymphomas, and other solid tumors. The LCH-Malignancy Study Group of the Histiocyte Society. *Hematol Oncol Clin North Am.* 1998;12:369–378.

22. Dauriat G, Mal H, Thabut G, et al. Lung transplantation for pulmonary Langerhans' cell histiocytosis: a multicenter analysis. *Transplantation.* 2006;81:746–750.

Introduction to Granulomatous Forms of Interstitial Lung Disease

Table 11.1 summarizes various types of interstitial lung disease (ILD) that are always or sometimes characterized by granulomas. This grouping is useful for the pathologist as a mnemonic because it limits the differential diagnosis, but it is only a mnemonic as most of these entities have no relationship to each other.

This approach also has more limitations than is commonly appreciated. Apart from hot tub lung, none of the diseases listed in Table 11.1 always has granulomas (even sarcoid may lack granulomas when it is burnt out), so that an absence of granulomas is not necessarily evidence against the diagnosis in question. Furthermore, pathologists tend to separate granulomas into nonnecrotizing (frequently, but not always accurately, called, "sarcoidal") and necrotizing, with the implication that the latter are infectious, but this separation is much less clear in actual practice as many of the entities in Table 11.1 can sometimes contain necrotizing granulomas.

There is no ideal way to group all of these entities, so hypersensitivity pneumonitis and sarcoid are considered in separate chapters (see Chapters 12 and 13); granulomatous drug reactions in Chapter 18; and aspiration, which may manifest in the lung as a bronchiolitis but also as organizing pneumonia, primarily in Chapter 20, but also in Chapter 5; and Chapter 14 has been reserved for conditions that are frequently granulomatous and that do not fit comfortably elsewhere (common variable and selective immunoglobulin A deficiency; primary biliary cholangitis; and inflammatory bowel disease).

Table 11.2 lists causes of granulomas in the lung that are not related to ILD, and these should always be kept in mind when a granuloma is encountered, because, apart from sarcoid, granulomatous ILD is relatively uncommon.

Table 11.1

ILD that can be characterized by granulomas

Disease	Granulomas always present?/ ever necrotizing?
Hypersensitivity pneumonitis (see Chapter 12)	No/no
Hot tub lung (see Chapter 12)	Yes/sometimes
Sarcoid (see Chapter 13)	No/sometimes
Drug reactions (see Chapter 18)	No/rare
Common variable immunodeficiency and other genetic causes of immunodeficiency (see Chapter 14)	No/rare
Aspiration (see Chapters 5 and 20) including aspiration-related bronchiolitis	No/sometimes
Lymphocytic interstitial pneumonia (see Chapter 19)	No/no
Primary biliary cholangitis (see Chapter 14)	No/no
Crohn disease (see Chapter 14)	No/sometimes

Table 11.2

Other causes of granulomas in the lung

Disease	Granulomas always present?/always necrotizing?
Infections	
Typical mycobacterias	Yes, except in some immunocompromised hosts/yes
Atypical mycobacteria	Yes, except in some immunocompromised hosts/may or may not be necrotizing
Common fungal infections (*Blastomyces, Coccidioides, Histoplasma, Cryptococcus*[a])	Yes, except in some immunocompromised hosts[a]/yes
Aspergillus sp.	Uncommon/usually necrotizing
Pneumocystis	Uncommon/usually necrotizing
Vasculitis	
Wegener granulomatosis (granulomatosis with polyangiitis)	Usually, but may manifest as only hemorrhage/granulomas always necrotizing when present
Churg-Strauss syndrome (eosinophilic granulomatosis with polyangiitis)	Often absent/granulomas always necrotizing when present
Severe asthma	No/no

[a]Cryptococcal infections may show no host response, even in nonimmunocompromised individuals.

Hypersensitivity Pneumonitis

DEFINITIONS, NOMENCLATURE, AND CONCEPTUAL ISSUES

Hypersensitivity pneumonitis (HP) has been referred to in the past as extrinsic allergic alveolitis, but the latter term has almost entirely disappeared, and we shall only use HP. Because chronic HP (see definition below) can have a usual interstitial pneumonia (UIP) pattern on imaging or biopsy, we explicitly use the term UIP/idiopathic pulmonary fibrosis (IPF) in this chapter to indicate UIP that is the radiologic/pathologic pattern of IPF.

HP is a lung-limited hypersensitivity reaction to an inhaled antigen. Traditionally, HP is divided into acute, subacute, and chronic (meaning fibrotic) forms (Table 12.1) and this convention is followed here. However, there is considerable clinical debate about whether cases can really be separated in this fashion,[1-3] and some authors view "chronic" HP as any case of HP where signs and symptoms have persisted for a long period (generally 6 months or a year), whether there is evidence of fibrosis.[4] We prefer not to use this type of categorization because it produces overlapping patterns on imaging and pathology, and, more important, obliterates clear prognostic differences between traditional subacute and chronic (fibrotic) disease[5,6] (see section Treatment and Prognosis), but the reader needs to be aware of the different ways in which these set of terms are used when reviewing the literature.

An additional problem in regard to chronic HP is a frequent lack of agreement at the clinical, radiologic, and pathologic level on the features that allow this diagnosis and the distinction from other forms of fibrotic interstitial lung disease (ILD). This issue is well illustrated in the study of Walsh et al.[7] in which seven experienced multidisciplinary discussion groups reviewed the same 70 ILD cases. Agreement was good for UIP/IPF (weighted kappa 0.71) and for collagen vascular disease (CVD)-associated ILD (weighted kappa 0.73), but poor for chronic HP (weighted kappa 0.29). In fact, it is likely that some proportion of cases called UIP/IPF are actually chronic HP: Morell et al.[8] reported that 20 of 46 patients who fit the 2011 ATS/ERS clinical and radiologic IPF guidelines could be reclassified as HP after evaluation of inhalation challenge, lavage lymphocytes, serum antibodies, and/or biopsy. In the era in which

Table 12.1

Definition and separation of HP subtypes

Acute form
  Known exposure to an antigen (often very
    high dose)
  Dyspnea, chills, fevers, shortness of breath
    4–6 hours after exposure; resolves by 48 hours
Subacute form
  Known exposure to an antigen
  Insidious onset of shortness of breath over weeks to
    months
  Often inspiratory rales
  Generally mild restrictive pulmonary function/
    decreased diffusing capacity
  Sometimes mild airflow obstruction
  Lymphocytosis in BAL (>20% and especially >40%)
  Specific precipitating serum antibodies or positive
    inhalation challenge
  Specific radiologic and pathologic features (see text)
Chronic form
  Fibrotic ILD with specific radiologic and pathologic
    features
  Known exposure to an antigen
  Insidious onset of shortness of breath
  Restrictive pulmonary function/decreased diffusing
    capacity
  Specific precipitating serum antibodies or positive
    inhalation challenge
  Lymphocytosis in BAL (>20% and especially >40%)

most fibrosing ILD were treated with steroids, this issue was not critical, but since the introduction of antifibrotic therapy for UIP/IPF, the separation of chronic HP from UIP/IPF has assumed considerable importance because chronic HP is treated with immunosuppressive therapy[9] and immunosuppressive therapy is contraindicated in UIP/IPF (see Chapter 6 and section Treatment and Prognosis).

Table 12.1 lists a set of notional defining features for the various types of HP, of which exposure to an offending agent is clinically the most important.[3,10] However, in a substantial proportion of cases, typically around 25% to 30% cases for subacute HP and 50% or more cases for chronic HP,[3,10,11] no antigen can be identified. Broncho-alveolar lavage (BAL) is also a useful test: the finding of a high proportion of lymphocytes, at a minimum 20% and particularly values greater than 40% of cells, supports a diagnosis of HP, but in a significant number of chronic HP cases, particularly those with a UIP pattern, lympho-cytosis is not found.[3] The presence of an elevated titer of antigen-specific IgG antibodies can be used to support a diagnosis of HP, although standardly available tests appear to be very insensitive or do not evaluate the appropriate antigens, and only a few laboratories have the ability to detect more unusual antibodies.[11] Inhalation challenge is similarly available only in a few very specialized centers.[11] Given these constraints, the fundamental diagnosis of HP frequently reduces to that of an ILD with characteristic findings on imaging and biopsy.

ETIOLOGIES

HP is usually caused by inhaled organic antigens, but a small number of cases related to exposure to inorganic chemicals have also been described (Table 12.2). Expo-sures may be occupational or environmental (Table 12.2).

Table 12.2	
Etiologies and names of HP caused by specific types of exposures[a]	
Name	**Etiologic agents**
Bird fancier's lung[b]/pigeon[b] breeder's lung	Avian proteins in droppings, feathers, feather-filled pillows, and duvets
Farmer's lung[b]	Moldy hay and grains
Hot tub lung[b]	Atypical mycobacteria colonizing hot tubs, saunas, and showers
Humidifier lung[b]/airconditioner lung	Humidifiers and forced air heating and cooling systems colonized by various organisms, most commonly *Aureobasidium pullulans* and thermophylic *Actinomycetes* species
Household mold-induced HP[b]	Moldy walls, floors, and ceilings
Bagassosis	Moldy sugar cane
Baker's lung	Contaminated flour
Cheese washer's lung	Moldy cheese
Chemical worker's lung	Isocyanates and trimellitic anhydride
Coffee worker's lung	Coffee bean dust
Detergent lung	Enzyme-containing detergents
Fuel chip HP	Moldy wood fuel chips
Malt worker's lung	Moldy whiskey maltings
Maple bark stripper's disease	Moldy maple bark
Metalworker's/machine operator's	Microorganism-contaminated metalworking fluids HP
Miller's lung	Contaminated grain
Mollusk shell HP	Oyster and sea-snail shells
Mushroom worker's lung	Mushroom compost
Pituitary snuff-taker's disease	Bovine and porcine pituitary snuff
Suberosis	Moldy cork dust
Swimming pool HP	Swimming pools contaminated with endotoxin, *Candida* sp., thermophylic actinomycetes, etc.
Wood pulp and woodworker's	Pine or redwood extracts/moldy wood lung (sequoiosis)
Summer-type HP (Japan)	Homes contaminated by *Trichosporon cutaneum* or *Cryptococcus albidus*
Tobacco worker's lung	Tobacco

[a]For a more extensive list of causes of HP, etiologic agents and specific antigens, see Morell et al.[11]
[b]Common causes of HP in North America.

At first glance, Table 12.2 implies that there are huge numbers of HP cases, but many of the causes listed are confined to very specific industries that employ small numbers of workers at particular locations and are unlikely to be encountered by most physicians. The most common etiologies seen in North America are farming, household birds, hot tub lung, contaminated humidifiers, and household molds.[12,13] In other parts of the world this breakdown is different; for example, in Mexico and Spain many individuals raise pigeons and avian protein-induced HP (often called "pigeon breeder's lung") is very common.[14] In Japan, household mold contamination by *Trichosporon cutaneum* or *Cryptococcus albidus* produces the so-called "summer-type" HP. In India, HP is the most common form of ILD, and, in many cases, is linked to mold contamination of air coolers.[15]

For reference purposes, Table 12.2 follows the common convention of labeling HP of specific etiologies with different names, but this can produce confusion, and it is preferable to specifically use "hypersensitivity pneumonitis" when actually diagnosing HP of any cause; for example, "HP caused by bird exposure" rather than "bird fancier's lung," or "HP caused by maple bark stripping" rather than "maple bark stripper's disease."

MOLECULAR/GENETIC FACTORS AND THEIR POTENTIAL ROLE IN DIAGNOSIS

The development of HP appears to reflect sensitization to an antigen in an individual with a predisposing genetic background, but there is relatively little information on genetic changes in HP. Polymorphisms in TNFα promoters confer differing risks of developing disease, and some forms of HP are associated with specific human leukocyte antigen (HLA) alleles (HLA-DR3 in pigeon breeders, HLA-DQ3 in Japanese summer-type HP, and HLA-A, HLA-B, and HLA-C loci antigens in farmer's lung).[16]

Ley et al.[17] reported that the minor alleles of MUC5B rs35705950 are present in 25% to 30% of patients with chronic HP compared with roughly 10% of healthy controls. Chronic HP patients frequently have short telomeres in peripheral blood leukocytes as well.[17] In the study of Ley et al.,[17] the extent of radiologic fibrosis was associated with the presence of MUC5B rs35705950 minor alleles, and short telomere length was associated with the presence of UIP-like features on biopsy, and reduced survival.

These data primarily provide estimates of risk, but are not diagnostically useful, because an increased frequency of MUC5B rs35705950 minor alleles and short telomeres are also seen in UIP/IPF as well as in rheumatoid arthritis patients with a UIP picture, and probably other forms of fibrotic ILD as well[16,17] (see Chapter 6 for additional discussion).

CLINICAL FEATURES

Table 12.1 also summarizes the clinical features of HP. The acute form is caused by exposure to high levels of the offending antigen and appears as a flu-like illness with the abrupt onset of fever, chills, and shortness of breath a few hours after exposure. If the exposure does not continue, the process resolves spontaneously, typically within 48 hours, but can recur with subsequent exposures.

Subacute HP is the form most commonly encountered and is believed to reflect continuing fairly low-level exposure to the antigen in question. It usually presents with the insidious onset of shortness of breath over weeks to months, occasionally accompanied by fever. Patients typically have Velcro rales at the lung bases and a mild restrictive functional abnormality with a decreased diffusing capacity; however, minor degrees of airflow obstruction may also be found because the process pathologically involves the bronchioles.

The exact sequence of events behind chronic HP is unclear; some authors suggest that it reflects frequent exposure to high levels of antigen, whereas others believe it is caused by long-term low-level exposures. Most cases present in a fashion similar to that of subacute HP, but the pulmonary functional changes are often more marked, patients may be clubbed, and, by definition, there is evidence of fibrosis on biopsy or on imaging.

Although the traditional teaching is that cigarette smoking protects against HP, in our experience, many patients with chronic HP are current or former smokers, and this appears to be particularly true for HP patients with a UIP pattern on imaging or biopsy.[18]

IMAGING

Computed tomography is seldom performed in acute HP because the clinical manifestations are characteristic and the symptoms usually resolve rapidly. The few reported cases demonstrate extensive bilateral ground-glass opacities with or without dependent areas of consolidation and centrilobular nodules (Fig. 12.1).

The vast majority of HP patients who undergo high-resolution computed tomography (HRCT) have subacute HP. The typical finding consists of a heterogeneous appearance of the lung parenchyma (mosaic attenuation) with patchy or confluent ground-glass opacities and scattered lobular areas of decreased attenuation and vascularity[19] (Fig. 12.2). Another common finding is the presence of small centrilobular nodular opacities of ground-glass attenuation. Expiratory HRCT typically shows multifocal lobular air trapping. The abnormalities can be diffuse but tend to have a lower zone predominance. In the proper clinical context, the HRCT findings are often characteristic enough to strongly suggest the diagnosis.[19]

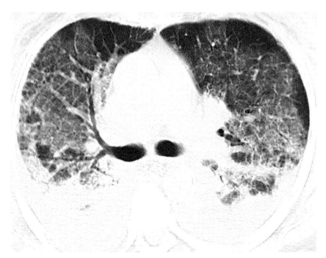

FIGURE 12.1. Acute HP. HRCT at the level of the upper lobes shows extensive bilateral ground-glass opacities and dependent areas of consolidation. The appearance is consistent with diffuse alveolar damage. The patient was a 69-year-old woman with acute HP due to avian antigens (chicken).

The fibrosis in chronic HP is manifested by reticulation, traction bronchiectasis, and, commonly, honeycombing (Figs. 12.3 and 12.4). The distribution of the fibrosis is variable. It may have a random cephalocaudal distribution or predominate in the upper, mid, or lower lung zones, but often spares the extreme lung bases.[20] It may have a random distribution in the transverse plane or show a peribronchial or subpleural predominance. The majority of patients have associated findings of subacute HP, which are helpful in the differential diagnosis of other fibrotic lung diseases (Figs. 12.3 and 12.4). It should be noted, however, that confident distinction of chronic HP from

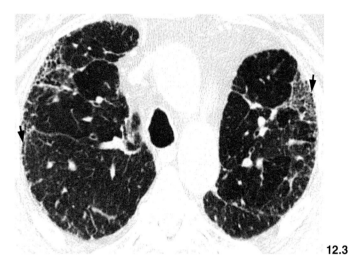

12.3

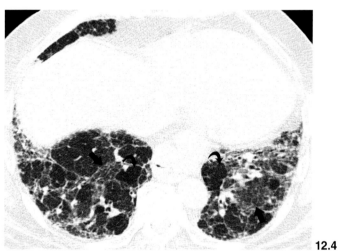

12.4

FIGURES 12.3 and 12.4. Chronic HP. **Figure 12.3:** HRCT at the level of the upper lobes shows peripheral reticulation and minimal honeycombing (*small arrows*). **Figure 12.4:** HRCT at the level of the lung bases demonstrates mild patchy reticulation and marked inhomogeneity of the lung parenchyma with areas of normal attenuation, patchy ground-glass opacities (*straight arrows*), and lobular areas of decreased attenuation and vascularity (*curved arrows*). The patient was a 68-year-old man with chronic HP due to avian antigens.

IPF and from fibrotic nonspecific interstitial pneumonia (NSIP) on HRCT can only be made in approximately 50% of cases.[20] When the extent of mosaic attenuation or air trapping on HRCT is greater than the extent of reticulation and the abnormalities have a diffuse cross-sectional distribution, HP specificity is high and the risk of false-positive diagnosis is low, but this combination of findings is present in only 18% to 55% of patients.[21]

PATHOLOGIC FEATURES

The pathologic features of HP are summarized in Table 3.5. Acute HP (Table 12.3) is rarely biopsied and its pathology is poorly defined. Diffuse alveolar damage, extensive

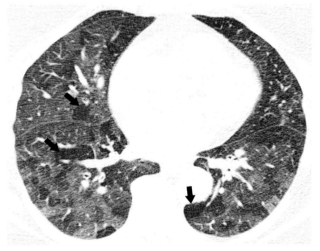

FIGURE 12.2. Subacute HP. HRCT demonstrates extensive bilateral ground-glass opacities and lobular areas of decreased attenuation and vascularity (*arrows*). The patient was an 86-year-old man with subacute HP due to household mold.

Table 12.3

Pathologic features of acute HP

Very poorly defined in the literature because most
   patients with acute HP are not biopsied
Reported reactions include:
   Diffuse alveolar damage/extensive alveolar fibrin
      deposition
   Acute bronchiolitis
   Capillaritis/vasculitis
   Cellular NSIP-like picture
   Subacute HP pattern
Granulomas may be present

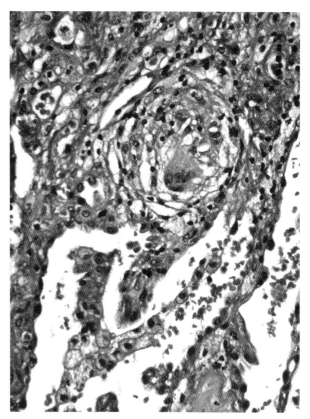

FIGURE 12.6. Acute HP. Another area of the same case showing a loose granuloma.

alveolar fibrin deposition, acute bronchiolitis, a cellular NSIP-like picture, vasculitis/capillaritis, and areas that look like subacute HP have all been described, but only in case reports and small series.[22,23] The few convincing cases that we have seen have had diffuse alveolar damage and granulomas as well (Figs. 12.5 and 12.6).

Subacute HP (Table 12.4) is the form most commonly encountered in biopsies and usually shows a mild chronic interstitial inflammatory infiltrate that is most marked around the bronchovascular bundles in the centers of the lobules and fades off as one gets away from the bronchovascular bundles (Figs. 12.7 to 12.12). Sometimes, there is chronic inflammation in the walls of the bronchioles as well (Fig. 12.13), a process that some authors refer to as a "bronchiolitis." A minority of cases of subacute HP do not show bronchiolocentricity, but have a much more even distribution of interstitial inflammation and produce a cellular NSIP pattern (Figs. 12.14 to 12.16). Small amounts of organizing pneumonia (OP) are occasionally present in cases of subacute HP.

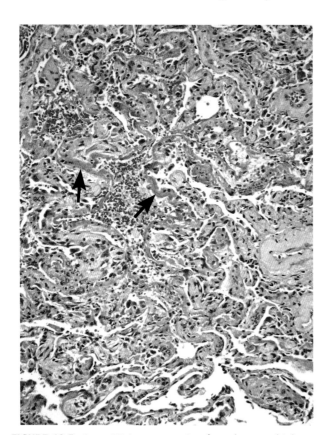

FIGURE 12.5. Acute HP. Low-power view from the same bird exposure case as Figure 12.1 showing hyaline membranes (*arrows*).

Table 12.4

Pathologic features of subacute HP

Interstitial pneumonia with lymphocytes and plasma
   cells most often in a peribronchovascular (centrilobular) distribution
Chronic inflammation may involve walls of bronchioles ("bronchiolitis")
Some cases show a more homogenous cellular NSIP-
   type pattern
Nonnecrotizing granulomas or single giant cells or
   Schaumann bodies, often around bronchioles, in
   about two-thirds of cases.
Granulomas/giant cells may be present in airspaces

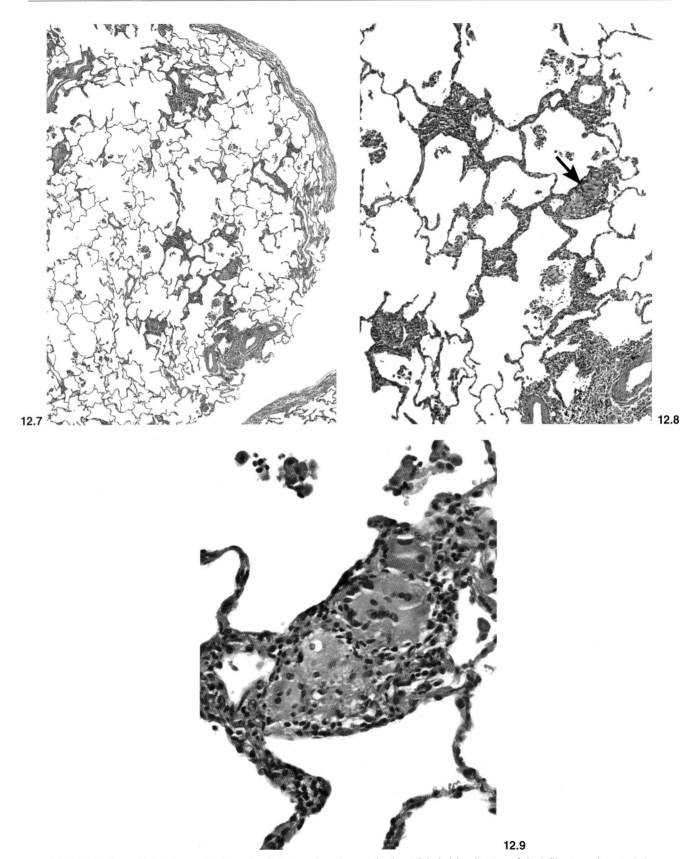

FIGURES 12.7 to 12.9. Subacute HP. Note the distinct peribronchovascular (centrilobular) localization of the infiltrate, a characteristic finding in most cases of subacute HP. A granuloma is present at the *arrow* in **Figure 12.8** and is shown at higher power in **Figure 12.9**. Patient was exposed to birds and had positive serology for avian proteins.

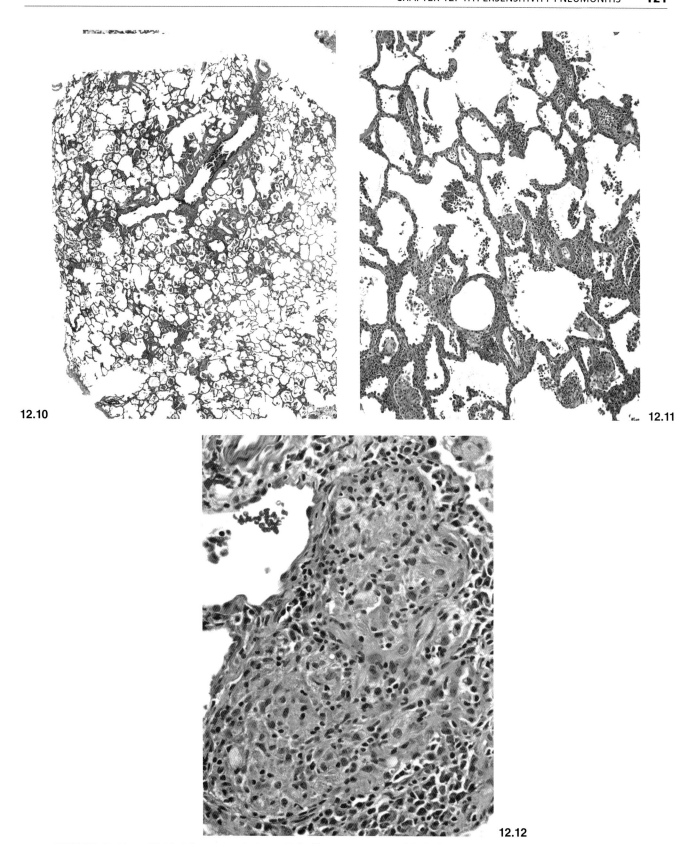

FIGURES 12.10 to 12.12. Subacute HP. The interstitial infiltrate is again centrilobular, but more extensive than the example shown in Figures 12.7 to 12.9. **Figure 12.12** shows a somewhat indistinctly defined granuloma. Patient was exposed to birds.

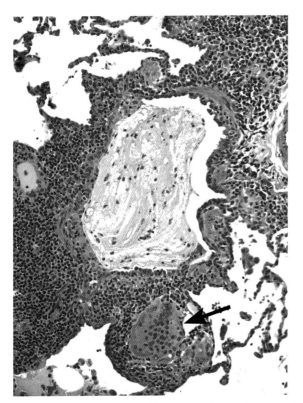

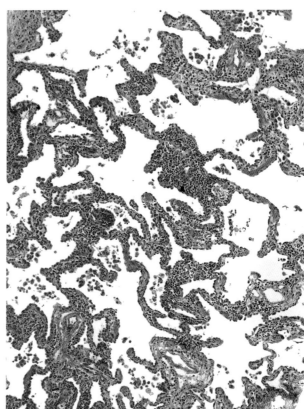

12.15

FIGURE 12.13. So-called "bronchiolitis" in subacute HP. Note the giant cells in the peribronchiolar inflammatory infiltrate (*arrow*). This is a common finding in HP but is not entirely specific because it can occasionally be seen with aspiration.

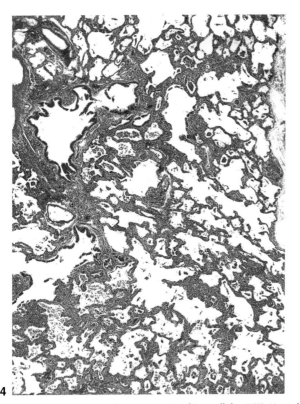

12.14

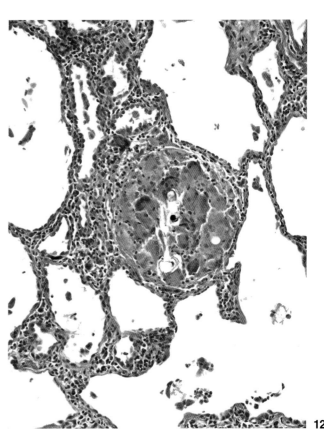

12.16

FIGURES 12.14 to 12.16. Subacute HP mimicking cellular NSIP. Note the absence of peribronchovascular accentuation. On the biopsy, only the presence of granulomas (**Fig. 12.16**) indicates the correct diagnosis. Patient worked on a farm.

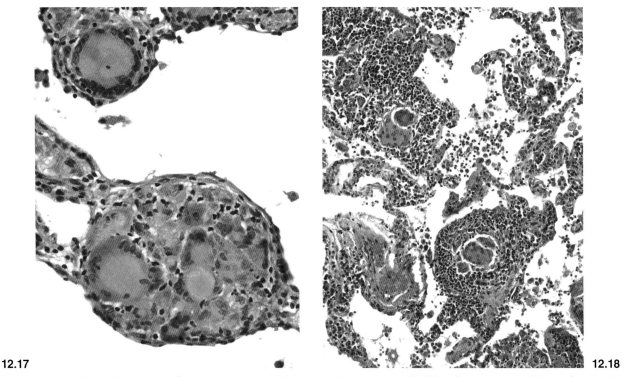

12.17   12.18

FIGURES 12.17 and 12.18. Examples of granulomas and individual giant cells in subacute HP. Although granulomas in HP are often described as poorly formed, in many instances they are quite distinct, but they always lack the peripheral concentric fibrosis often seen in sarcoid (compare Chapter 13, Fig. 13.5).

Noncaseating granulomas or individual giant cells or Schaumann bodies are found in about two out of three cases of subacute HP, but the number of granulomas/giant cells is extremely variable from case to case. Although the traditional teaching is that the giant cells/granulomas of HP are interstitial, they can sometimes be found in the airspaces as well.[24] Giant cells, granulomas, and Schaumann bodies (Figs. 12.17 to 12.20) usually are associated with areas of interstitial inflammation, including in the walls of involved bronchioles (Fig. 12.13); the combination of

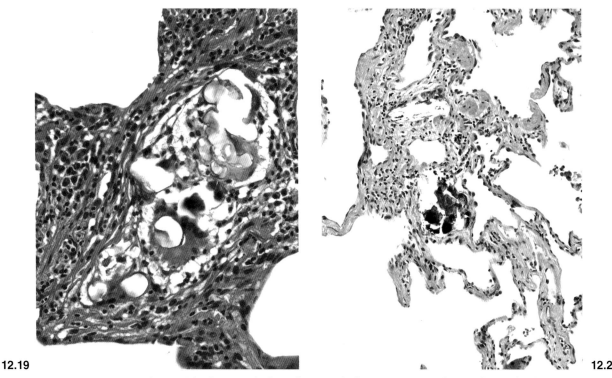

12.19   12.20

FIGURES 12.19 and 12.20. Granulomas with Schaumann bodies. Schaumann bodies are common in the granulomas of HP but can sometimes be seen in sarcoid granulomas. In **Figure 12.20** (chronic HP), all the giant cells have disappeared leaving only the Schaumann bodies.

giant cells or granulomas in the midst of a chronic inflammatory infiltrate in a bronchiolar wall is very suggestive of HP but is not entirely specific because granulomas with inflammation can also be seen in bronchiolar walls after aspiration (see Figs. 20.21 and 20.22) and in mycobacterial infections. Sarcoid granulomas are also commonly found in bronchial walls and around bronchioles but often show concentric lamellar fibrosis (see Figs. 13.15 and 13.16) and typically lack the chronic inflammatory infiltrate.

Granulomas in HP are frequently referred to as "poorly formed" in the literature, but this is not always true: sometimes the granulomas are vague (Fig. 12.12), but more often they are quite distinct (Figs. 12.16 and 12.17). What is never present in HP, however, is the concentric lamellar fibrosis typically seen in sarcoid granulomas (see Fig. 13.5). The granulomas of HP frequently contain Schaumann bodies (Figs. 12.16, 12.19, and 12.20). These structures are not disease-specific and may be seen in persisting granulomas of any cause, but are uncommon in infectious granulomas and in our experience are considerably less frequent in sarcoid than in HP. Schaumann bodies are also useful diagnostically, because, in some cases of HP, all the granulomas have disappeared but Schaumann bodies remain (Figs. 12.20). Giant cells and granulomas in HP may contain cholesterol clefts (Figs. 12.22 and 12.23).

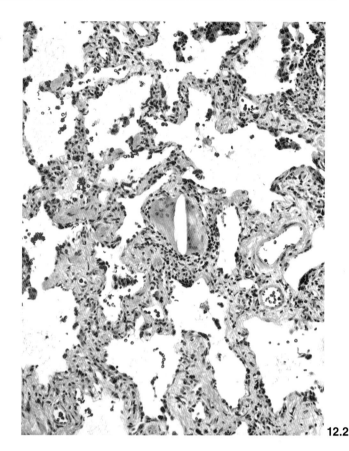
12.22

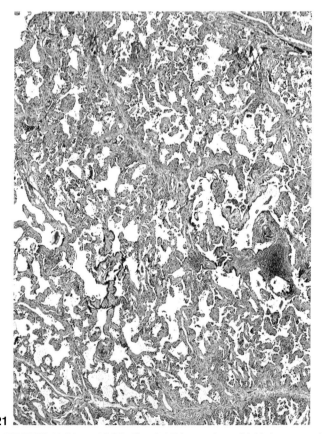
12.21

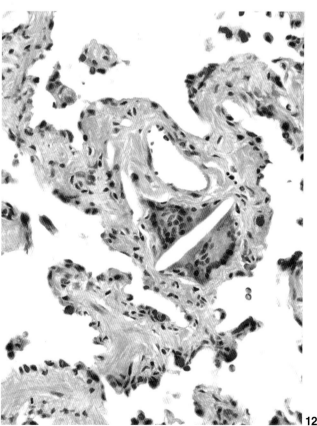
12.23

FIGURES 12.21 to 12.23. Chronic HP in a patient with bird exposure. In this example the disease mimics fibrotic NSIP; however, there are interstitial giant cells as well (**Figs. 12.22** and **12.23**) clues to the correct diagnosis.

Table 12.5

Pathologic features of chronic HP

Old fibrosis present with possible patterns of:
Fibrotic NSIP
UIP
Only peribronchiolar (centrilobular) fibrosis
Combinations of peribronchiolar and UIP-like
fibrosis
Fibrotic bands bridging peribronchiolar and sub-
pleural/paraseptal regions
So-called idiopathic bronchiolocentric interstitial
fibrosis pattern
Interstitial, nonnecrotizing granulomas, giant cells, or
Schaumann bodies in almost 50% of cases
Areas of typical subacute HP may be present
Peribronchiolar metaplasia associated with a large pro-
portion of bronchioles may be present
Fibroblast foci may be present
Relatively low ratio of interstitial plasma cells to
lymphocytes

Chronic HP (Table 12.5) has a much more variable appearance, and there is considerable dispute in the literature about the morphologic features of chronic HP, particularly the features that separate chronic HP from UIP/IPF[25] (reviewed in Churg et al.,[26] and see section Differential Diagnosis), but the essential requirement for a diagnosis of chronic HP of any pattern is old fibrosis. Honeycombing may be present, grossly or microscopically. The fibrosis of chronic HP can be predominantly upper, mid-, or lower zonal, but fibrosis that is milder in the bases than in the upper or mid-zones favors chronic HP over UIP, although this distribution is usually more accurately evaluated on HRCT than biopsy (see below).

Conceptually, the fibrosing process in chronic HP can be divided into a fibrotic NSIP-like form (Figs. 12.21 and 12.22), a UIP-like form (Figs. 12.24 to 12.27), and a centrilobular fibrosis form (Figs. 12.28 to 12.31), with variable combinations of the latter two patterns quite common (Figs. 12.32 to 12.34). In some cases, a biopsy from one lobe looks like UIP, but from another lobe or another area, has predominantly centrilobular fibrosis (Figs. 12.33 and 12.34). As in subacute HP, granulomas, giant cells, or Schaumann bodies may be found (Figs. 12.23 and 12.30); however, as

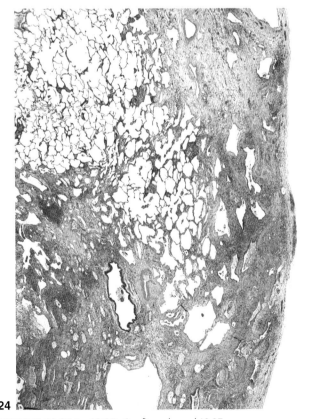

12.24

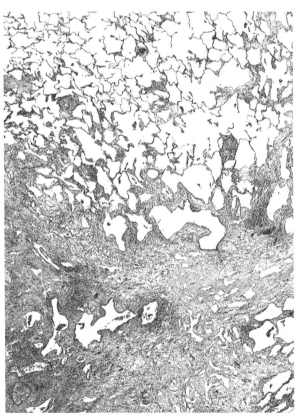

12.25

FIGURES 12.24 to 12.27. See figure legend 12.27

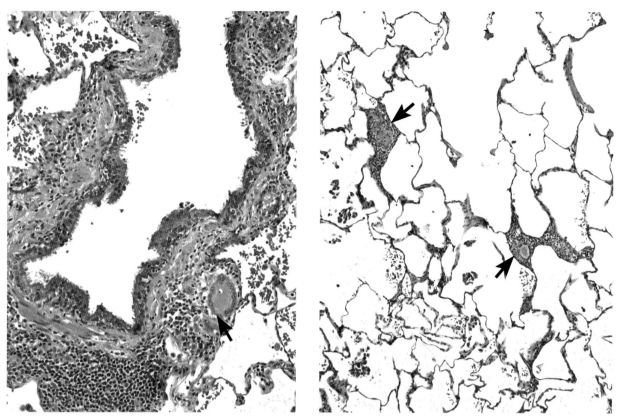

12.26

12.27

FIGURES 12.24 to 12.27. Chronic HP in a patient exposed to household mold. This example resembles UIP with patchy subpleural fibrosis (**Figs. 12.24** and **12.25**). However, there are also areas typical of subacute HP in the form of peribronchiolar (**Fig. 12.26**, *arrow*) and interstitial (**Fig. 12.27**, *arrows*) giant cells and granulomas. Although this case shows patterns clearly identifiable as HP, some cases of chronic HP are indistinguishable from UIP.

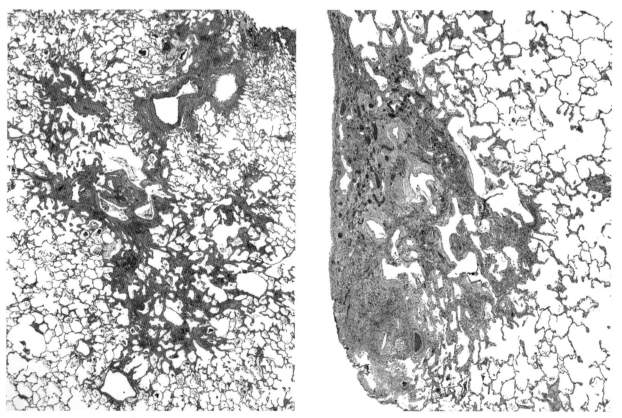

12.28

12.29

FIGURES 12.28 to 12.31. See figure legend 12.31

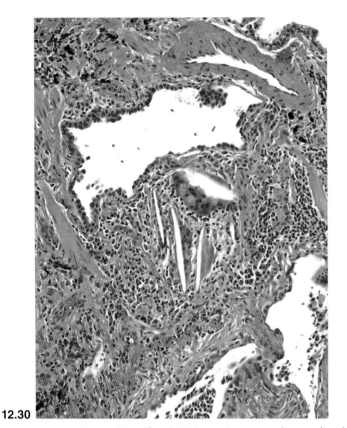
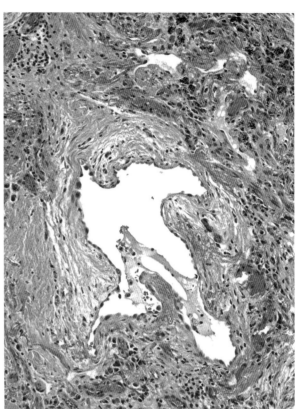

12.30   12.31

FIGURES 12.28 to 12.31. Chronic HP in a patient exposed to metal working fluid. **Figure 12.29** shows localized centrilobular fibrosis, one of the patterns seen in chronic HP. Subpleural fibrosis somewhat resembling UIP is also present (**Fig. 12.29**). At high-power view, giant cells with cholesterol clefts are present (**Fig. 12.30**) as well as fibroblast foci (**Fig. 12.31**).

noted above, at least 50% of chronic HP cases do not show these features. Typical areas of subacute HP may also be evident (Figs. 12.26 and 12.27) but often are not present and are not required for the diagnosis of chronic HP. Apart from areas of subacute HP, some cases of chronic HP show a moderately intense chronic interstitial inflammatory infiltrate, which typically is mostly lymphocytes with a few plasma cells and eosinophils, but chronic HP may also be quite paucicellular.

Unless giant cells, granulomas, or Schaumann bodies are found, the fibrotic NSIP-like form (Figs. 12.21 and 12.22)

is indistinguishable from fibrotic NSIP of other etiologies (see Chapter 7). Similarly, a proportion of chronic HP cases with a UIP pattern have giant cells, granulomas, Schaumann bodies, or areas of subacute HP (Figs. 12.24 to 12.27), but some cases cannot be morphologically separated from UIP/IPF (see Chapter 6, and see section Differential Diagnosis). Fibroblast foci are common in the UIP-like pattern of chronic HP. A finding that supports a diagnosis of chronic HP is the presence of peribronchiolar metaplasia affecting a large proportion of bronchioles (Figs. 12.35 and 12.36); when more

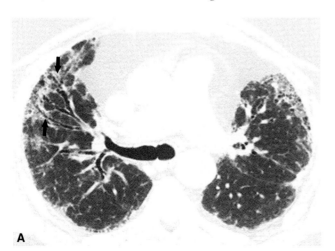
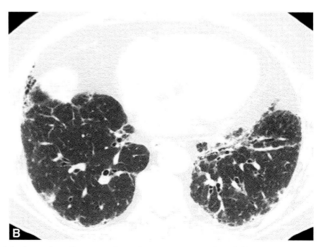

FIGURE 12.32. A: Chronic HP. HRCT image at the level of the right upper lobe bronchus shows moderately extensive subpleural fibrosis. Also note central peribronchial fibrosis (*arrows*), a finding that would be unusual for UIP/IPF. **B:** HRCT image at the level of the basal segments of the lower lobes in the same case shows mild, patchy peripheral reticulation. The relative sparing of the lung bases favors chronic HP over UIP/IPF.

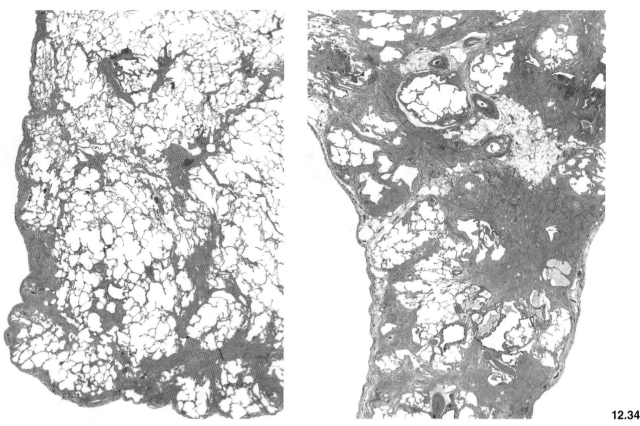

12.33

12.34

FIGURES 12.33 and 12.34. Chronic HP. Same case as Figure 12.32. In this example, the lower lobe biopsy (**Fig. 12.33**) shows predominantly peribronchiolar fibrosis with minimal subpleural fibrosis, whereas the upper lobe biopsy (**Fig. 12.34**) is indistinguishable from UIP/IPF. The pattern seen in Figure 12.33 mitigates against a diagnosis of UIP/IPF, as does the CT imaging. (Reprinted from Churg A, Bilawich A, Wright JL. Pathology of chronic hypersensitivity pneumonitis what is it? what are the diagnostic criteria? why do we care? *Arch Pathol Lab Med.* 2018;142:109–119 with permission from Archives of Pathology & Laboratory Medicine. Copyright 2018 College of American Pathologists.)

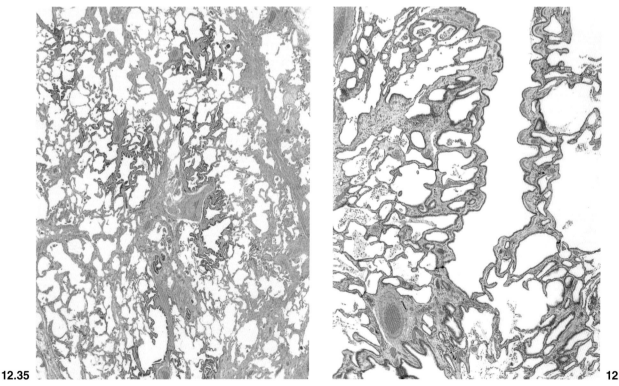

12.35

12.36

FIGURES 12.35 and 12.36. Chronic HP. Note the peribronchiolar metaplasia involving all of the bronchioles in **Figure 12.35** and florid peribronchiolar metaplasia in **Figure 12.36**. Peribronchiolar metaplasia involving more than half of the sampled bronchioles favors a diagnosis of chronic HP. These cases also had granulomas (not illustrated).

128

than half the bronchioles are involved, chronic HP is the most likely diagnosis, but peribronchiolar metaplasia affecting only an occasional bronchiole is not helpful because it can be seen in various forms of ILD[27] (see Chapter 24).

In some cases of chronic HP, peribronchiolar (centrilobular) fibrosis is the only morphologic abnormality and these lesions frequently have associated fibroblast foci. Such cases may show a mixture of typical subacute HP, involving a proportion of bronchioles, and peribronchiolar fibrosis, involving other bronchioles. Chronic HP cases may have delicate fibrous bridges that link bronchioles and the pleura or the interlobular septa (Figs. 12.37 and 12.38), but the reliability of this finding as a distinguishing feature from UIP/IPF decreases as the amount of fibrosis in the periphery of the lobule increases. Coarse fibrous bridges are much less helpful because are frequent in advanced UIP/IPF when fibrosis overruns the whole lobule (Fig. 12.34, and see Chapter 6). It is common to find a mixture of peribronchiolar fibrosis and subpleural fibrosis that resembles UIP/IPF to a greater or lesser extent (Figs. 12.33 and 12.34).

In most cases of chronic HP with centrilobular involvement, the fibrotic tissue has overlying reactive alveolar lining cells or, more commonly, just nonreactive type 1 and 2 cells. Yousem and Dacic[28] described an entity labeled "idiopathic bronchiolocentric interstitial fibrosis"—a fibrosing interstitial pneumonia in which there is fine fibrosis that radiates out from the bronchovascular bundle, following alveolar walls (Fig. 12.39). Characteristically this fibrosis is covered in whole or in part by metaplastic bronchiolar epithelium (Fig. 12.40). Yousem's cases did neither have HRCT nor serologic evidence of HP, but we believe such cases are variants of chronic HP.

ACUTE EXACERBATIONS OF HP

Patients with chronic HP can develop acute exacerbations,[29,30] which are particularly associated with a UIP/IPF-like pattern of fibrosis.[30] Like acute exacerbations of UIP, these consist of a morphologic picture of diffuse alveolar damage or OP superimposed on an underlying fibrotic interstitial pneumonia. Biopsies of putative acute HP should be carefully examined to make sure that there is no old underlying fibrosis.[22]

OTHER ANATOMIC LESIONS IN HP

There appears to be an increased incidence of emphysema in HP[2,31]; this occurs in both smokers and nonsmokers and is associated with airflow obstruction. Some of these cases fall within the general category of combined pulmonary

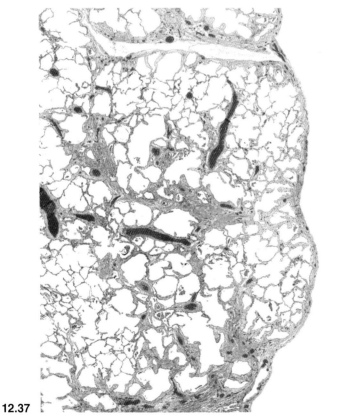
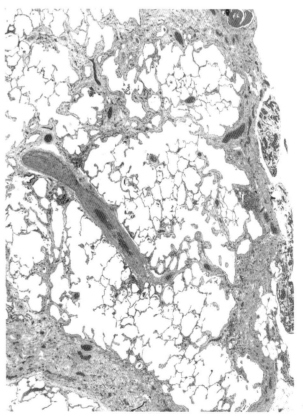

12.37   **12.38**

FIGURES 12.37 and 12.38. Two different cases of chronic HP with delicate fibrous bands extending from the peribronchiolar region to the pleura and interlobular septa. When the fibrosis is mostly centrilobular, this pattern favors chronic HP over UIP/IPF, but its utility decreases as the amount of subpleural and paraseptal fibrosis increases and the bridges become coarse (i.e., the fibrosing process overwhelms the whole lobule).

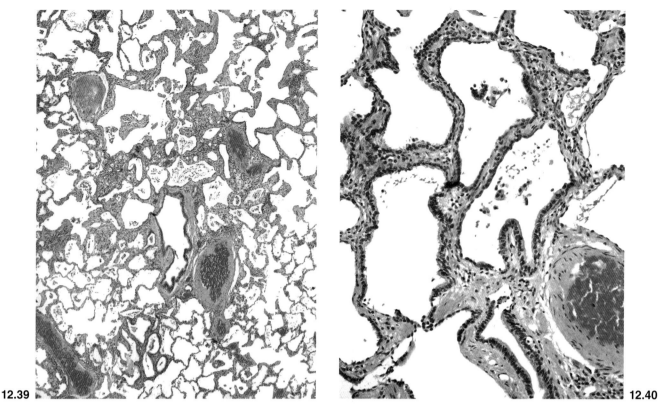

12.39   12.40

FIGURES 12.39 and 12.40. Chronic HP with a pattern of so-called bronchiolocentric interstitial fibrosis. Note the extensive bronchiolar epithelial metaplasia, a characteristic finding in this variant of chronic HP. Patient worked on a farm and had positive serology for avian proteins. (Reproduced by permission from Fenton ME, Cockcroft DW, Wright JL, et al. Hypersensitivity pneumonitis as a cause of airway centered interstitial fibrosis. *Ann Allergy Asthma Immunol.* 2007;99:465–466.)

fibrosis with emphysema (see Figs. 9.7 to 9.10). Pleuroparenchymal fibroelastosis (PPFE) has been reported in patients with chronic HP[31] (see Chapter 24 for descriptions of PPFE).

HOT TUB LUNG

Hot tub lung is caused by atypical mycobacteria and, in rare cases, by other organisms that colonize hot tubs, jacuzzis, saunas, and occasionally showers. Some believe that hot tub lung is really an infectious process requiring antimicrobial therapy, but most view it as a peculiar form of HP[32]; the fact that patients respond to cleaning of the contaminated environment and/or steroids supports the idea that this is really a variant of HP.

HRCT of patients with hot tub lung typically shows bilateral ground-glass opacities and centrilobular nodular opacities, often with air trapping, and is indistinguishable from HP of other causes (Fig. 12.41).

The pathologic findings in hot tub lung can resemble those of ordinary subacute HP, but typically the granulomas are large and numerous and the interstitial inflammatory infiltrate relatively minor (Fig. 12.42).[32] Areas of OP are sometimes present. Around 10% of cases have granulomas with necrosis, something that is never seen

in ordinary HP. Another unusual feature is the presence of granulomas within the lumens of respiratory bronchioles (Figs. 12.42 and 12.43). Granulomas in the lumens of respiratory bronchioles are sometimes seen in aspiration,

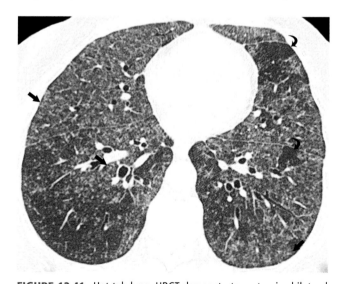

FIGURE 12.41. Hot tub lung. HRCT demonstrates extensive bilateral ground-glass opacities, poorly defined centrilobular nodules (*straight arrows*), and localized areas of decreased attenuation and vascularity (*curved arrows*). The patient was a 68-year-old woman.

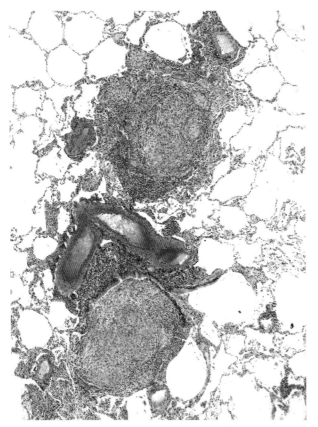

FIGURE 12.42. Hot tub lung. Hot tub lung typically has large granulomas and minimal interstitial infiltrates, as here. Note the granuloma in a bronchiolar lumen, a characteristic (but inconstant) finding in hot tub lung.

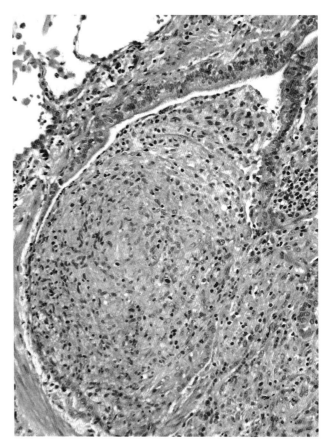

FIGURE 12.43. Hot tub lung. Another example of a large granuloma in a bronchiolar lumen.

but they are never as large as in hot tub lung, and are extremely rare to nonexistent in other conditions. In hot tub lung, mycobacteria can usually be demonstrated by staining or culture. Rarely contaminated hot tub exposure can lead to a picture of chronic HP.

DIFFERENTIAL DIAGNOSIS

DIFFERENTIAL DIAGNOSIS OF ACUTE HP

Organic toxic dust syndrome (OTDS) is caused by massive exposures to moldy hay or grains containing large amounts of endotoxin, fungi, or actinomycetes; it is also seen in workers exposed to textiles contaminated with Fusarium species. Clinically, it is characterized by an acute, febrile, self-limited process that is very similar to acute HP. However, patients with OTDS are not sensitized and do not have serum antibodies against the offending organisms. The pathologic features are poorly defined, but acute bronchiolitis with numerous visible fungal organisms has been reported.[33]

DIFFERENTIAL DIAGNOSIS OF SUBACUTE HP

The important differential diagnoses for subacute HP are sarcoid (see Chapter 13) and lymphocytic interstitial pneumonia (see Chapter 19), and the important separating features are shown in Table 12.6.

DIFFERENTIAL DIAGNOSIS OF CHRONIC HP

Cases of chronic HP with a pure peribronchiolar fibrosis pattern are relatively uncommon; the differential diagnosis includes CVD-ILD, airway-centered interstitial fibrosis, which itself may be a form of chronic HP (see Chapter 24) and microaspiration/gastroesophageal reflux disease (GERD)[34,35] (Table 12.7).

The major differential diagnoses of chronic HP are UIP/IPF, CVD-ILD, and fibrotic NSIP. Fibrotic NSIP is simply one possible pattern of chronic HP, and if giant cells/granulomas/Schaumann bodies are not present, then only clinical and radiologic information can point to the correct diagnosis.

Table 6.6 (see Chapter 6) shows features that help to distinguish chronic HP with a UIP pattern from UIP/

Table 12.6

Differential diagnosis of subacute HP

Subacute HP	Sarcoid	Lymphocytic interstitial pneumonia
Interstitial inflammation always present, usually mild and the predominant feature	Interstitial inflammation very uncommon; granulomas are the predominant feature	Interstitial inflammation always present and marked, often producing widening of alveolar walls to the point of confluence
Interstitial inflammation usually around bronchovascular bundles (centrilobular)		Inflammation diffuse
Granulomas/giant cells in about two-thirds of cases	Granulomas in all, except completely burnt-out disease	Granulomas often present, but usually inconspicuous
Granulomas not necrotizing (except hot tub lung)	Granulomas occasionally necrotizing	Granulomas not necrotizing
Granulomas never show concentric fibrosis	Concentric fibrosis around granulomas common	Granulomas never show concentric fibrosis, except in common variable immunodeficiency
Granulomas usually centrilobular, often in walls of bronchioles	Granulomas follow bronchovascular bundles, interlobular septa, pleura	Granulomas random
No cysts	No cysts	Cysts sometimes present

IPF and CVD-ILD with a UIP pattern. CVD-ILD morphologically overlaps chronic HP and can have UIP-like fibrosis, a pattern of cellular or fibrotic NSIP, or isolated centrilobular fibrosis (see Fig. 21.8). A high ratio of interstitial plasma cells to lymphocytes (1:1 or greater) (see Fig. 21.9), follicular bronchiolitis, or the presence of numerous lymphoid aggregates or lymphoid aggregates containing germinal centers (see Figs. 7.10 to 7.12) favors CVD-ILD, although a few lymphoid aggregates without germinal centers certainly can be seen in chronic HP and

UIP/IPF.[27] These features need to be evaluated away from areas of honeycombing because honeycombing usually shows considerable chronic inflammation and may have lymphoid aggregates. Granulomas and giant cells are not entirely specific because they can also be found in CVD-ILD[27] (see Fig. 21.13), but their presence is against a diagnosis of UIP/IPF. Clinical data (serologic testing, known CVD) is important, but in one sense is less useful than might be supposed, because patients with overt CVD are not usually biopsied; however, positive serology can

Table 12.7

Differential diagnosis of chronic HP with a pure peribronchiolar pattern

Entity	Distinguishing features
Chronic HP	Granulomas/giant cells/Schaumann bodies may be present Peribronchiolar metaplasia around a high fraction of bronchioles Some bronchioles with a subacute HP pattern Fibroblast foci may be present
CVD-ILD	High ratio of plasma cells to lymphocytes Follicular bronchiolitis Numerous lymphoid aggregates Lymphoid aggregates with germinal centers Granulomas/giant cells may be present
Microaspiration/GERD	Granulomas/giant cells may be present Giant cells often foreign body type Presence of aspirated material Fibroblast foci usually not present

suggest a diagnosis of interstitial pneumonia with autoimmune features (see Chapter 21).

An important and recurring problem in the diagnosis of chronic HP is the separation from UIP/IPF when giant cells/granulomas/Schaumann bodies, areas of subacute HP, or numerous bronchioles with peribronchiolar metaplasia are not present. This is currently a disputed issue in the literature.[25,26] The major question is how much peribronchiolar fibrosis (if any) is permitted in UIP/IPF and, if peribronchiolar fibrosis is accepted as a part of UIP/IPF, must the fibrosis be connected to the pleura/interlobular septae or can it be isolated to the bronchioles? Table 6.6 lists what at present appear to be strong and weak morphologic features for making this separation, but there are some chronic HP cases that morphologically cannot be distinguished from UIP/IPF (see also discussion of this topic in Chapter 6). Imaging is often extremely helpful in this situation (Fig. 12.32), but clinical information is typically less helpful, because a patient with compatible clinical features and a known antigen exposure, for example, a pet bird, is unlikely to be biopsied.

DIAGNOSTIC MODALITIES

Occasionally a conventional forceps transbronchial biopsy will show a combination of chronic interstitial inflammation and interstitial giant cells/granulomas/Schaumann bodies in a patient with clinical and imaging features of HP (Figs. 12.44 and 12.45). In this situation, such a biopsy is diagnostic. However, if all that is present is chronic interstitial inflammation, we advise reporting such biopsies as nondiagnostic because chronic interstitial inflammation alone in transbronchial biopsies is both common and nonspecific.

Cryobiopsy can also be used to diagnose HP,[36] but this statement applies primarily to subacute HP; whether cryobiopsy can be used to separate chronic HP from UIP/IPF has not been investigated. In our view, video-assisted thoracoscopic surgery biopsy is the procedure of choice, particularly for suspected chronic HP where evaluation of low-power architecture, airway fibrosis, peribronchiolar metaplasia, and a large enough tissue sample to find giant cells/granulomas are crucial.

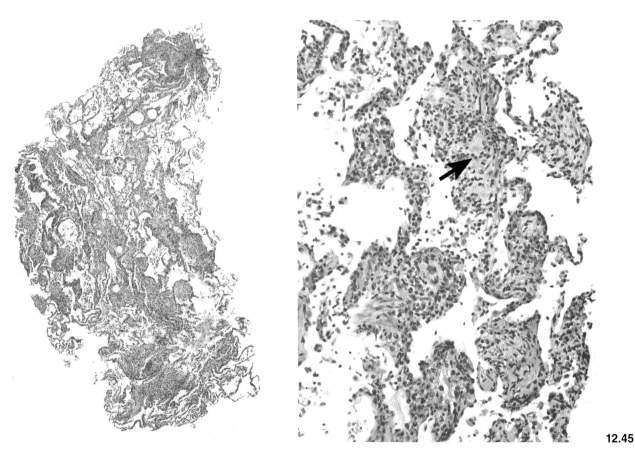

12.44

12.45

FIGURES 12.44 and 12.45 Subacute HP diagnosed on transbronchial biopsy. Note the giant cell (*arrow*) in Figure 12.45. HP can occasionally be diagnosed on transbronchial biopsy, but interstitial giant cells or granulomas are required. Interstitial inflammation by itself is completely nonspecific in transbronchial biopsies. Patient was exposed to birds and clinically and radiologically was thought to have HP.

TREATMENT AND PROGNOSIS

The treatment and prognosis of HP depends on the type of disease (acute, subacute, or chronic). Most authors believe that acute or subacute disease resolves completely with steroid therapy. For chronic HP, immunosuppression with steroids, mycophenolate, or azathioprine are recommended.[9] It is commonly stated that avoidance of the antigen is crucial for resolution, but some authors report that cases in which no antigen can be identified seem to do as well as those with a known antigen,[13,37] whereas others find that identification of an antigen is associated with improved survival in chronic HP.[38] The issue of antigen exposure can be subtle: Tsutsui et al.[39] showed that in patients with chronic HP caused by bird exposures, the amount of residual bird antigens in the house after removal of the bird correlated negatively with prognosis. Whether chronic HP, particularly chronic HP with a UIP pattern, is a self-perpetuating disease in the absence of continuing antigen exposure is not known.

It is clear from radiologic studies that the prognosis of HP with fibrosis on imaging is considerably worse than that in cases without fibrosis[6]; it has also been suggested that cases diagnosed as chronic HP without radiologic honeycombing have a better prognosis than those believed to be UIP without radiologic honeycombing, whereas when honeycombing is present, the prognosis is equally poor for both conditions.

The prognosis of chronic HP probably also depends on the underlying pathologic pattern. Cases with UIP-like fibrosis on biopsy overall have a poor prognosis with time to death or transplantation on the order of 3 to 4 years in most studies (reviewed in Churg et al.[26]), but Chiba et al.[18] reported that patients with a UIP pattern and very low numbers of fibroblast foci had a much better survival than those with numerous fibroblast foci. The prognosis for the other chronic HP patterns is difficult to establish because of small numbers of cases and contradictory data in the literature (reviewed in Churg et al.[26]). Nunes et al.[40] concluded that a fibrotic NSIP pattern in chronic HP had a worse outcome than CVD-associated NSIP, and our experience is that such patients do as badly as those with chronic HP and a UIP pattern.[13] Pure peribronchiolar fibrosis may have a much better prognosis.[13] One study[41] has reported that after lung transplantation, patients with chronic HP had a considerable better prognosis than patients with UIP/IPF in large measure because the chronic HP patients did not develop bronchiolitis obliterans.

REFERENCES

1. Lacasse Y, Selman M, Costabel U, et al.; HP Study Group. Classification of hypersensitivity pneumonitis: a hypothesis. *Int Arch Allergy Immunol.* 2009;149:161–166.
2. Selman M, Pardo A, King TE Jr. Hypersensitivity pneumonitis: insights in diagnosis and pathobiology. *Am J Respir Crit Care Med.* 2012;186:314–324.
3. Vasakova M, Morell F, Walsh S, et al. Hypersensitivity pneumonitis: perspectives in diagnosis and management. *Am J Respir Crit Care Med.* 2017;196(6):680–689.
4. Hanak V, Golbin JM, Hartman TE, et al. High-resolution CT findings of parenchymal fibrosis correlate with prognosis in hypersensitivity pneumonitis. *Chest.* 2008;134:133–138.
5. Churg A, Ryerson CJ. The many faces of hypersensitivity pneumonitis. *Chest.* 2017;152(3):458-460. doi:10.1016/j.chest.2017.03.024.
6. Salisbury ML, Gu T, Murray S, et al. Hypersensitivity pneumonitis: radiologic phenotypes are associated with distinct survival time and pulmonary function trajectory. *Chest.* 2019;155(4):699–711. doi:10.1016/j.chest.2018.08.1076.
7. Walsh SLF, Wells AU, Desai SR, et al. Multicentre evaluation of multidisciplinary team meeting agreement on diagnosis in diffuse parenchymal lung disease: a case-cohort study. *Lancet Respir Med.* 2016;4(7):557–565.
8. Morell F, Villar A, Montero MÁ, et al. Chronic hypersensitivity pneumonitis in patients diagnosed with idiopathic pulmonary fibrosis: a prospective case-cohort study. *Lancet Respir Med.* 2013;1(9):685–694.
9. Morisset J, Johannson KA, Vittinghoff E, et al. Use of mycophenolate mofetil or azathioprine for the management of chronic hypersensitivity pneumonitis. *Chest.* 2017;151(3):619–625.
10. Morisset J, Johannson KA, Jones KD, et al.; HP Delphi Collaborators. Identification of diagnostic criteria for chronic hypersensitivity pneumonitis: an international modified delphi survey. *Am J Respir Crit Care Med.* 2018;197(8):1036–1040.
11. Morell F, Villar A, Ojanguren I, et al. Hypersensitivity pneumonitis: challenges in diagnosis and management, avoiding surgical lung biopsy. *Semin Respir Crit Care Med.* 2016;37(3):395–405.
12. Hanak V, Golbin JM, Ryu JH. Causes and presenting features in 85 consecutive patients with hypersensitivity pneumonitis. *Mayo Clin Proc.* 2007;82:812–816.
13. Churg A, Sin DD, Everett D, et al. Pathologic patterns and survival in chronic hypersensitivity pneumonitis. *Am J Surg Pathol.* 2009; 33:1765–1770.
14. Morell F, Roger A, Reyes L, et al. Bird fancier's lung: a series of 86 patients. *Medicine (Baltimore).* 2008;87:110–130.
15. Singh S, Collins BF, Sharma BB, et al. Interstitial lung disease in India. Results of a prospective registry. *Am J Respir Crit Care Med.* 2017;195(6):801–813.
16. Adegunsoye A, Vij R, Noth I. Integrating genomics into management of fibrotic interstitial lung disease. *Chest.* 2019;155:1026–1040. doi:10.1016/j.chest.2018.12.011.
17. Ley B, Newton CA, Arnould I, et al. The MUC5B promoter polymorphism and telomere length in patients with chronic hypersensitivity pneumonitis: an observational cohort-control study. *Lancet Respir Med.* 2017;5(8):639–647.
18. Chiba S, Tsuchiya K, Akashi T, et al. Chronic hypersensitivity pneumonitis with a usual interstitial pneumonia-like pattern: correlation between histopathologic and clinical findings. *Chest.* 2016;149(6):1473–1481.
19. Silva CI, Churg A, Müller NL. Hypersensitivity pneumonitis: spectrum of high-resolution CT and pathologic findings. *AJR Am J Roentgenol.* 2007;188:334–344.
20. Silva CI, Müller NL, Lynch DA, et al. Chronic hypersensitivity pneumonitis: differentiation from idiopathic pulmonary fibrosis and nonspecific interstitial pneumonia by using thin-section CT. *Radiology.* 2008;246:288–297.

21. Salisbury ML, Gross BH, Chughtai A, et al. Development and validation of a radiological diagnosis model for hypersensitivity pneumonitis. *Eur Respir J.* 2018;52. pii: 1800443.

22. Hariri LP, Mino-Kenudson M, Shea B, et al. Distinct histopathology of acute onset or abrupt exacerbation of hypersensitivity pneumonitis. *Hum Pathol.* 2012;43:660–668.

23. Grunes D, Beasley MB. Hypersensitivity pneumonitis: a review and update of histologic findings. *J Clin Pathol.* 2013;66:888–895.

24. Castonguay MC, Ryu JH, Yi ES, et al. Granulomas and giant cells in hypersensitivity pneumonitis. *Hum Pathol.* 2015;46:607–663.

25. Hashisako M, Tanaka T, Terasaki Y, et al. Interobserver agreement of usual interstitial pneumonia diagnosis correlated with patient outcome. *Arch Pathol Lab Med.* 2016;140:1375–1382.

26. Churg A, Bilawich A, Wright JL. Pathology of chronic hypersensitivity pneumonitis what is it? what are the diagnostic criteria? why do we care? *Arch Pathol Lab Med.* 2018;142:109–119.

27. Churg A, Wright JL, Ryerson CJ. Pathologic separation of chronic hypersensitivity pneumonitis from fibrotic connective tissue disease-associated interstitial lung disease. *Am J Surg Pathol.* 2017;41:1403–1409.

28. Yousem SA, Dacic S. Idiopathic bronchiolocentric interstitial pneumonia. *Mod Pathol.* 2002;15:1148–1153.

29. Costabel U, Bonella F, Guzman J. Chronic hypersensitivity pneumonitis. *Clin Chest Med.* 2012;33:151–163.

30. Miyazaki Y, Tateishi T, Akashi T, et al. Clinical predictors and histologic appearance of acute exacerbations in chronic hypersensitivity pneumonitis. *Chest.* 2008;134:1265–1270.

31. Jacob J, Odink A, Brun AL, et al. Functional associations of pleuroparenchymal fibroelastosis and emphysema with hypersensitivity pneumonitis. *Respir Med.* 2018;138:95–101.

32. Hanak V, Kalra S, Aksamit TR, et al. Hot tub lung: presenting features and clinical course of 21 patients. *Respir Med.* 2006;100:610–615.

33. Perry LP, Iwata M, Tazelaar HD, et al. Pulmonary mycotoxicosis: a clinicopathologic study of three cases. *Mod Pathol.* 1998;11:432–436.

34. Bois MC, Hu X, Ryu JH, et al. Could prominent airway-centered fibroblast foci in lung biopsies predict underlying chronic microaspiration in idiopathic pulmonary fibrosis patients? *Hum Pathol.* 2016;53:1–7.

35. Kuranishi LT, Leslie KO, Ferreira RG, et al. Airway-centered interstitial fibrosis: etiology, clinical findings and prognosis. *Respir Res.* 2015;16:55.

36. Ussavarungsi K, Kern RM, Roden AC, et al. Transbronchial cryobiopsy in diffuse parenchymal lung disease: retrospective analysis of 74 cases. *Chest.* 2017;151:400–408.

37. Coleman A, Colby TV. Histologic diagnosis of extrinsic allergic alveolitis. *Am J Surg Pathol.* 1988;12:514–518.

38. Fernández Pérez ER, Swigris JJ, Forssén AV, et al. Identifying an inciting antigen is associated with improved survival in patients with chronic hypersensitivity pneumonitis. *Chest.* 2013;144:1644–1651.

39. Tsutsui T, Miyazaki Y, Kuramochi J, et al. The amount of avian antigen in household dust predicts the prognosis of chronic bird-related hypersensitivity pneumonitis. *Ann Am Thorac Soc.* 2015;12:1013–1020.

40. Nunes H, Schubel K, Piver D, et al. Nonspecific interstitial pneumonia: survival is influenced by the underlying cause. *Eur Respir J.* 2015;45:746–755.

41. Kern RM, Singer JP, Koth L, et al. Lung transplantation for hypersensitivity pneumonitis. *Chest.* 2015;147:1558–1565.

Sarcoid

EPIDEMIOLOGY

The prevalence of sarcoid varies widely across the world, with local rates from 10 to 400/1,000,000 persons.[1] In North America, the reported numbers are approximately 100/1,000,000 in whites and roughly three times this number in Blacks. In Europe, sarcoid is much more common in northern countries, particularly in Scandinavia. The reported numbers may be underestimates because a proportion of sarcoid patients are asymptomatic and many cases remit spontaneously. Most cases present under age 40 and particularly in the 20 to 29 age range.[1]

CLINICAL FEATURES

Probably one-third of sarcoid patients who come to medical attention are asymptomatic and disease is picked up as an incidental finding on chest imaging. Another one-third have fever, malaise, and weight loss, and an equal proportion have shortness of breath, cough, and sometimes chest pain. Pulmonary function varies by radiologic stage (see section Imaging). Low-stage disease patients may have normal pulmonary function, but airflow obstruction because sarcoid granulomas can narrow the large and small airways[2] (see below) and restriction are also seen. High-stage (i.e., diffuse fibrotic) disease shows a restrictive pattern with decreased diffusing capacity; pulmonary hypertension may also be present.[3,4]

Sarcoid is a systemic disease that can affect any organ. Extrapulmonary manifestations are beyond the scope of this book, but the reader is referred to volume 38 (2017) of *Seminars in Respiratory and Critical Care Medicine* for recent reviews.

IMAGING

The most common and characteristic radiologic manifestation of sarcoidosis is symmetric bilateral hilar and right paratracheal lymph node enlargement (Fig. 13.1). Based on the findings on the radiograph, pulmonary sarcoidosis has traditionally been classified into five stages.[5]

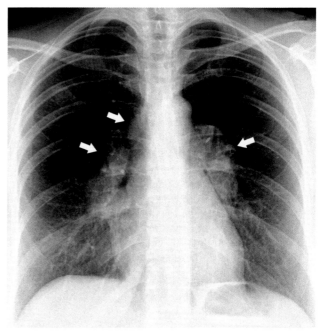

FIGURE 13.1. Sarcoidosis. Chest radiograph shows symmetric bilateral hilar and right paratracheal lymph node enlargement (*arrows*). The lungs are normal. The patient was a 37-year-old woman.

Stage 0: No demonstrable radiographic abnormality
Stage I: Hilar and mediastinal lymph node enlargement without radiographic parenchymal abnormality
Stage II: Hilar and mediastinal lymph node enlargement plus parenchymal abnormality
Stage III: Parenchymal abnormality alone
Stage IV: Advanced fibrosis.

These so-called "stages" do not indicate degrees of disease chronicity but simply radiographic patterns, the main utility of which is predicting outcome. Spontaneous remissions occur in 55% to 90% of patients with Stage I disease, in 40% to 70% of those with Stage II, in 10% to 20% with Stage III disease, and in 0% with Stage IV sarcoidosis.[5] At presentation, the chest radiograph is abnormal in approximately 90% of patients, the most common and characteristic finding being symmetric bilateral hilar and mediastinal lymphadenopathy.[1] An upper lobe predominant small nodular or

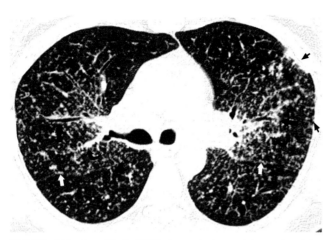

FIGURE 13.2. Sarcoidosis. HRCT demonstrates nodules and nodular thickening along the bronchi (*straight black arrows*), vessels (*curved arrows*), interlobular septa (*arrowheads*), interlobar fissures (*straight white arrows*), and along the costal pleura (*small arrows*).

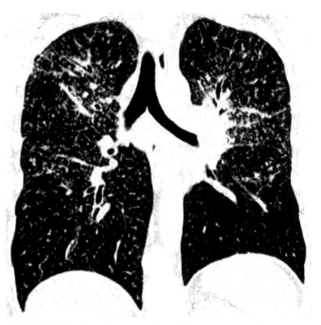

FIGURE 13.3. Coronal reformation of the same case shows upper lobe predominance. The patient was a 38-year-old woman.

reticulonodular pattern is seen in 20% to 50% of patients.[1] The classification of pulmonary sarcoidosis into stages is being used less commonly since the introduction of high-resolution computed tomography (HRCT).[1]

HRCT is much more sensitive than the radiograph in detecting the intrathoracic manifestations of sarcoidosis and, in the proper clinical context, it can be virtually diagnostic.[1,6] It is therefore performed routinely in patients with suspected sarcoidosis.[1] The HRCT manifestations of pulmonary sarcoidosis closely reflect the histologic findings and typically consist of small nodules in a perilymphatic distribution, that is, mainly adjacent to the bronchi, pulmonary arteries and veins, and along the interlobular septa, interlobar fissures, and costal subpleural regions, and result in nodular thickening of these structures (e.g., Figs. 13.2 and 13.3).[1,7] The nodules and the nodular thickening reflect confluence of microscopic granulomas. The nodules may have smooth or irregular margins, are typically well defined, and most commonly measure 2 to 5 mm in diameter. Confluence of granulomas may also result in large nodules or masses measuring 1 to 4 cm in diameter, seen in 15% to 25% of patients.[7] Fibrosis results in irregular linear opacities (reticulation), irregular septal thickening, traction bronchiectasis, and, occasionally, honeycombing. The fibrosis, similar to the nodules, involves mainly the peribronchovascular regions of the upper lobes and typically results in cephalad displacement of the hila and compensatory overinflation of the lower lobes.

PATHOLOGIC FEATURES

Features of sarcoid granulomas

Sarcoid granulomas are always well defined and fairly well circumscribed interstitial collections of giant cells, epithelioid histiocytes, and variable numbers of chronic

inflammatory cells (Fig. 13.4) (Table 13.1). Sarcoid granulomas are often surrounded by fine concentric layers of hyaline collagen (Fig. 13.5), and this feature is helpful in diagnosis because it is never seen in hypersensitivity

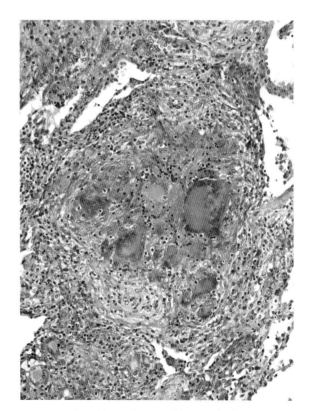

FIGURE 13.4. Sarcoid granuloma. In this example, there are a moderate number of admixed lymphocytes.

Table 13.1

General pathologic features of sarcoid

Generally non-necrotizing, well-defined interstitial granulomas
  Small amounts of necrosis occasionally present
Often concentric layers of fine fibrosis around the granulomas
Granulomas may contain asteroid bodies, Schaumann bodies, or birefringent crystals of calcium oxalate or phosphate. These findings are not specific to sarcoid.
Granulomas follow lymphatic routes
  Along bronchovascular bundles
  Along interlobular septa
  Along pleura
Usually no interstitial infiltrate
Organizing pneumonia usually not a feature of sarcoid
Granulomas may aggregate and develop hyaline scars with eventual replacement of granulomas by scar
Granulomas may be replaced by irregular linear scars

pneumonitis (HP) and is rare in infectious granulomas; however, it can be found in patients with common variable immunodeficiency (see Chapter 14). In our experience, this pattern of fibrosis is seen in sarcoid that is progressing to scar formation (see below).

Although the traditional teaching is that sarcoid granulomas are non-necrotizing, this is not always true. Small amounts of necrosis are occasionally seen in ordinary sarcoid (Fig. 13.6), and by definition are present in necrotizing sarcoid (see below). Whether special stains for organisms are required in every case of sarcoid is controversial (see below), but they should always be carried out if any necrosis is present.

Another common fallacy is that asteroid bodies (Fig. 13.7) and Schaumann bodies are specific features of sarcoid. Asteroid bodies may be seen in giant cells or granulomas of any cause, as may Schaumann bodies, although they are much less common in infectious granulomas, probably because infectious granulomas tend not to persist for long periods of time. Schaumann bodies are much more frequent in HP than in sarcoid. Sometimes the granulomas of sarcoid disappear, leaving only Schaumann bodies as "tombstones," but this same phenomenon is seen in HP (see Figs. 12.19 and 12.20).

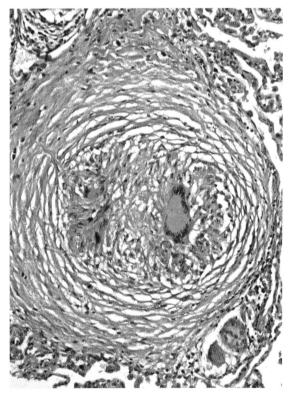

FIGURE 13.5. Sarcoid granuloma with prominent concentric lamellar fibrosis. This pattern is typical of sarcoid granulomas and rare in granulomas of other causes, except common variable immunodeficiency. Concentric lamellar fibrosis tends to be seen in sarcoid that is progressing to scarring.

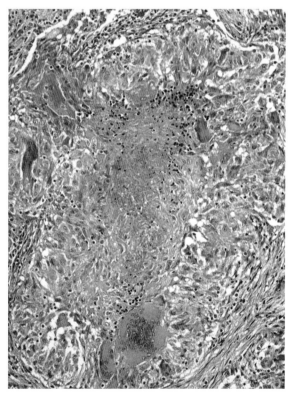

FIGURE 13.6. Necrosis in a sarcoid granuloma. Small amounts of central necrosis are not uncommon in sarcoid granulomas but stains to rule out infection are required in this situation.

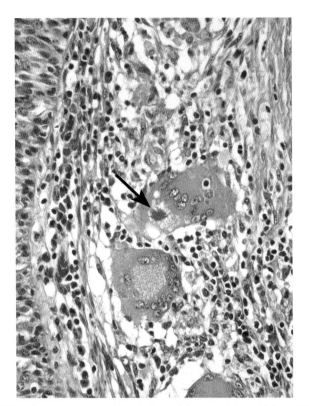

FIGURE 13.7. An asteroid body (*arrow*) in an endobronchial sarcoid granuloma. Asteroid bodies may be seen in granulomas or giant cells of any etiology (although they are rare in HP) and have no diagnostic specificity.

Granulomas of any cause, including sarcoid granulomas, may contain birefringent crystals of calcium oxalate or calcium phosphate (Figs. 13.8 and 13.9). These are endogenous products of macrophage metabolism and do not represent inhaled material.[8]

Distribution of sarcoid granulomas

Sarcoid granulomas characteristically show a lymphatic (lymphangitic) distribution; that is, they are present around the bronchovascular bundles in the centers of the lobules, along interlobular septa, and in the pleura (Figs. 13.10 to 13.15). This distribution is extremely helpful in diagnosis: infectious granulomas tend to be randomly scattered in the parenchyma, and although the granulomas of HP are often centrilobular, they are not present along interlobular septa and usually not in the pleura.

Sarcoid granulomas may be present in such numbers that they cause narrowing of the lumen of small airways (Figs. 13.14 and 13.15), and may also be present in the mucosa of large airways (Fig. 13.16). Granulomatous narrowing of small airways and endobronchial granulomas are never seen in HP.

Sarcoid as a rule does not have an interstitial inflammatory infiltrate away from the granulomas, so that the intervening parenchyma is typically normal (Figs. 13.12 and 13.13) and the granulomas are the dominant feature, as opposed to HP, where there is always an interstitial

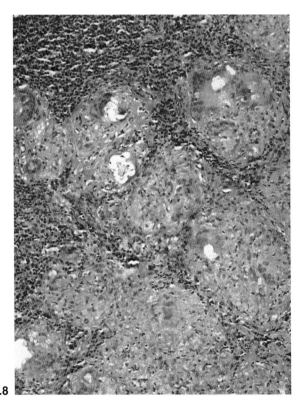
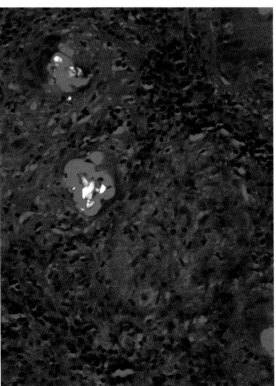

13.8 **13.9**

FIGURES 13.8 and 13.9. Crystalline inclusions (calcium oxalate or calcium carbonate) in sarcoid granulomas in a hilar lymph node under plain and polarized light. Similar crystals may be found in parenchymal granulomas. These crystals are numerous in some cases of sarcoid, but their presence has no diagnostic significance, and similar crystals can be seen in any granulomatous disease.

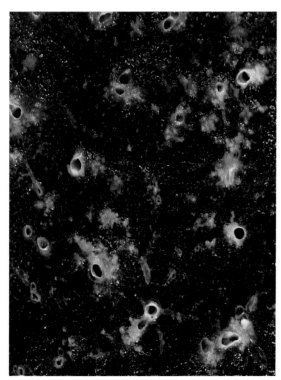

FIGURE 13.10. Gross view of active sarcoid showing granulomas distributed around the bronchovascular bundles.

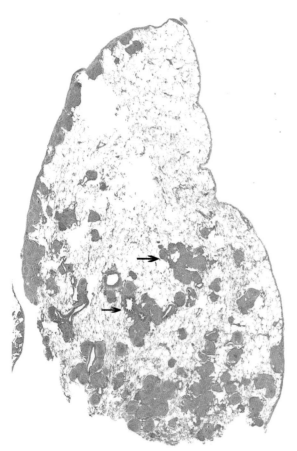

FIGURE 13.11. Low power view of a case of active sarcoid. Granulomas are found around bronchovascular bundles (*arrows*) and along the pleura.

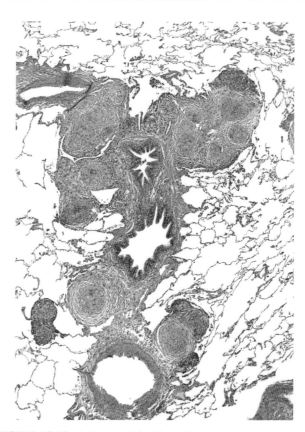

FIGURE 13.12. Active sarcoid with multiple granulomas around a bronchovascular bundle. The granulomas also aggregate to form small nodules. Note the absence of interstitial inflammation, as opposed to HP where there is prominent interstitial inflammation and far fewer and more inconspicuous granulomas.

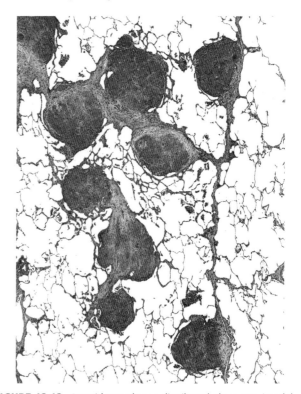

FIGURE 13.13. Sarcoid granulomas distributed along two interlobular septa and a small vessel.

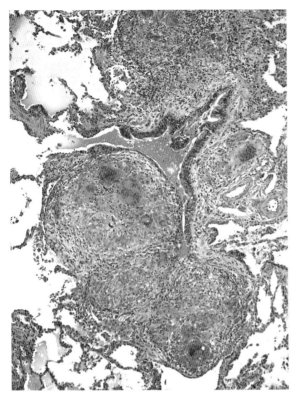

FIGURE 13.14. Granulomas surrounding and compressing a bronchiole. This process can lead to airflow obstruction.

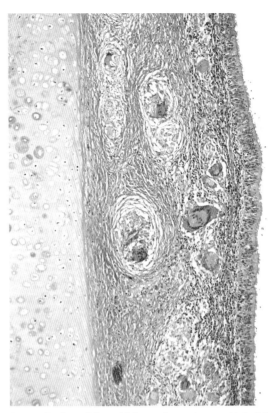

FIGURE 13.16. Endobronchial granulomas in sarcoid. Endobronchial granulomas produce small nodules visible on bronchoscopy and biopsy of such lesions is often diagnostic of sarcoid.

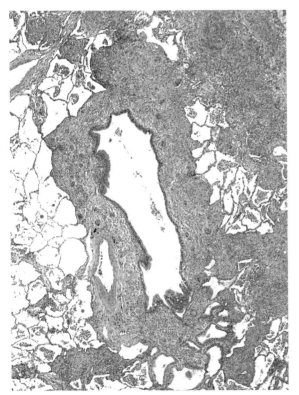

FIGURE 13.15. Granulomas completely surrounding a small airway. Because sarcoid granulomas tend to show a peribronchovascular distribution, the diagnostic yield is high on transbronchial biopsies.

inflammatory process and granulomas can be sparse or nonexistent (see Chapter 12).

Vascular involvement ("Vasculitis")

Sarcoid granulomas may involve vessels (Figs. 13.17 and 13.18). This finding is extremely common (visible in probably 70% of large biopsies) and some authors have referred to it as "vasculitis." As noted above, some patients with sarcoid develop pulmonary hypertension, but it is unclear whether this process reflects granulomatous involvement of vessels or fibrotic obliteration of vessels.[4] Some patients with sarcoid and pulmonary hypertension respond to steroids,[3] suggesting that in at least a portion of cases, granulomatous vasculitis has functional consequences.

Nodule formation and scarring in sarcoid

Sarcoid granulomas may aggregate over time to form nodular collections (Figs. 13.19 and 13.20 and see below). Although this phenomenon was thought to be rare before the days of CT imaging, it is now recognized as in fact quite common.

Sarcoid may resolve spontaneously or with treatment, or it may scar. The most common pattern of scarring is progressive hyalinization of nodules containing aggregated granulomas (Figs. 13.19 to 13.23). Because sarcoid

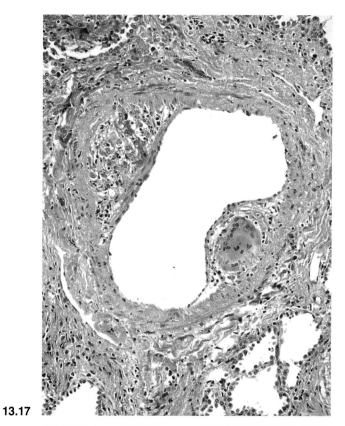

13.17

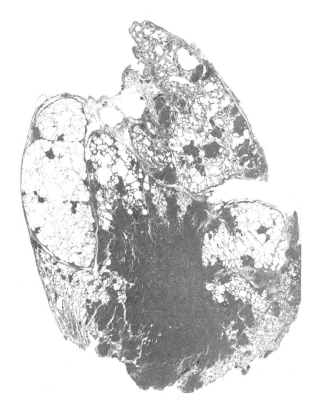

FIGURE 13.19. Nodular sarcoid. Nodules formed by aggregated granulomas are common in sarcoid; if the nodules are larger than 1 cm, the disease is classified as "nodular sarcoid." In this example, the large nodule is cellular and individual granulomas are still present.

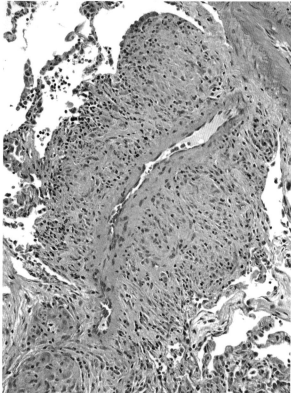

13.18

FIGURES 13.17 and 13.18. Granulomatous vasculitis in sarcoid in an artery (**Fig. 13.17**) and a vein (**Fig. 13.18**). Granulomatous vasculitis is visible in most cases of sarcoid if a large lung biopsy is available for review and is invariably present in nodular and necrotizing sarcoid. The granulomas may be on the intimal or adventitial side of the vessel.

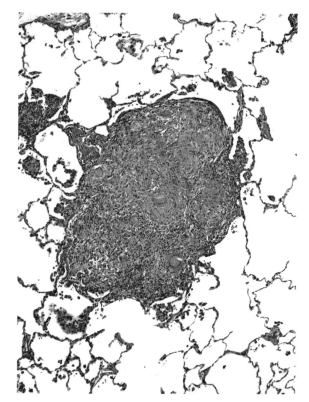

FIGURE 13.20. A cellular nodule formed by aggregation of sarcoid granulomas.

granulomas tend to be present along the bronchovascular bundles, nodules are frequently centrilobular in distribution (Fig. 13.22). Occasionally, nodules of aggregated granulomas also contain a marked chronic inflammatory infiltrate (Fig. 13.24); this is more common with very large nodules (nodular sarcoid). Unless they are very large (see section Nodular and Necrotizing Sarcoid), the presence of nodules does not change the pathologic diagnosis, and they do not need to be explicitly acknowledged in the diagnosis.

A less common pattern of scarring is the formation of linear or stellate scars (Figs. 13.25 to 13.27), often centered on or incorporating the bronchovascular bundles (Fig. 13.27). If the granulomas completely vanish, this type of scarring may not be distinguishable from old scarred Langerhans cell histiocytosis (see Figs. 10.22 and 10.23). Occasionally, scarred sarcoid produces a pattern mimicking fibrotic nonspecific interstitial pneumonia (Fig. 13.28 and see Chapter 7).

Sarcoid can progress to extensive, typically upper zone, scarring (Fig. 13.29). At the time of transplantation, some, but not all, such cases will still have granulomas.[9,10] Others show only dense scarring, which is more typically central than peripheral and can have a lymphangitic pattern. Honeycombing is present in some cases and may be central rather than peripheral, and small numbers of fibroblast foci may also be found.[9,10]

The upper zone distribution of fibrosis is a helpful guide to diagnosis in a completely scarred biopsy, but

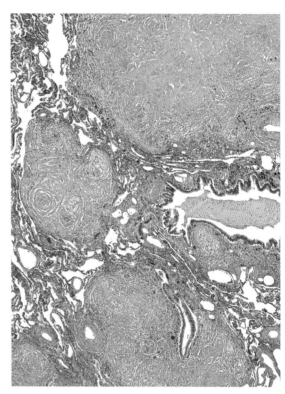

FIGURE 13.22. Nodular sarcoid. In this case, the nodules are largely hyalinized and only a few individual granulomas remain. Formation of hyalinized nodules is one form of scarring in sarcoid.

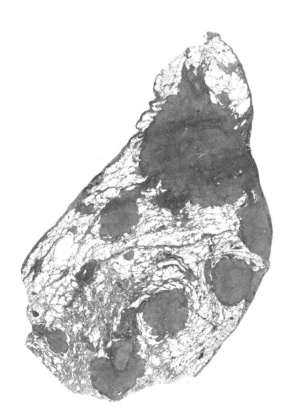

FIGURE 13.21. Nodular sarcoid with multiple hyalinized nodules.

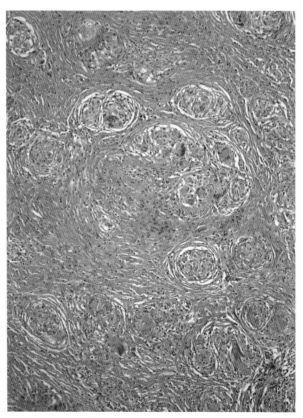

FIGURE 13.23. Higher power view of a nodule in sarcoid showing a mixture of granulomas and dense hyalinized collagen.

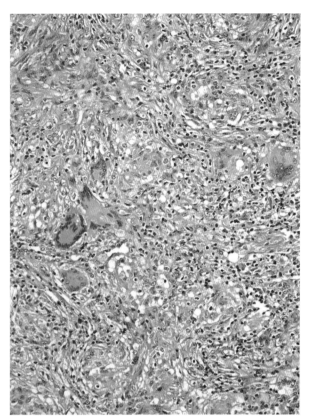

FIGURE 13.24. A sarcoid nodule in which there is considerable chronic inflammation but no fibrosis.

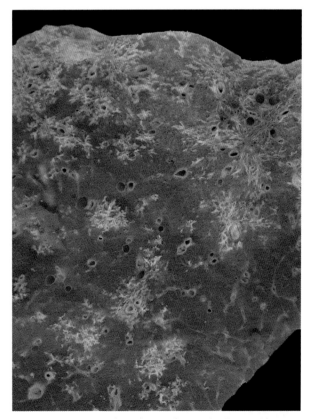

FIGURE 13.25. Fine peribronchovascular scarring in sarcoid.

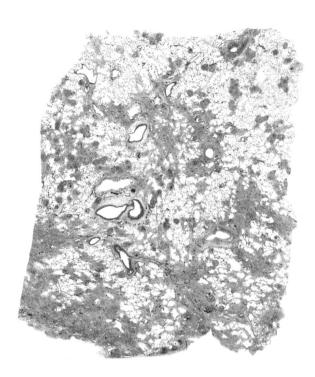

FIGURE 13.26. Sarcoid showing irregular more or less linear scars mixed with individual granulomas.

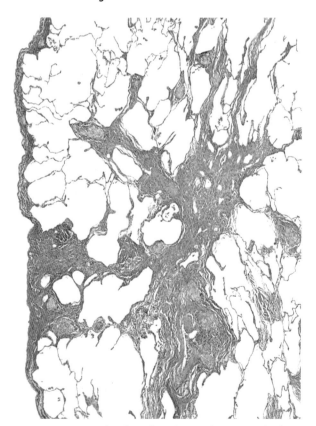

FIGURE 13.27. Sarcoid with peribronchovascular scars and a few residual small granulomas. Peribronchovascular scarring in sarcoid is less common than the formation of nodules, and this pattern of scarring can also be seen in chronic HP and Langerhans cell histiocytosis (which lacks granulomas).

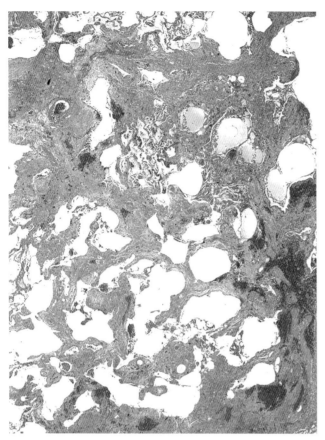

FIGURE 13.28. Diffuse scarring in sarcoid mimicking fibrotic NSIP.

Langerhans cell histiocytosis, some cases of chronic HP, and old tuberculosis (TB) or fungal infections can also produce upper zone scarring. Scarring that spares the lung bases is strongly against a diagnosis of usual interstitial pneumonia.

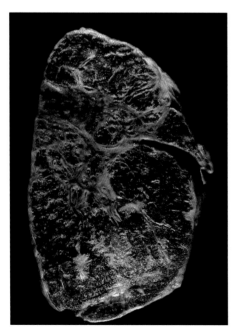

FIGURE 13.29. Gross view of end-stage (Stage IV) scarring in sarcoid showing the typical mid to upper zonal distribution.

Nodular and necrotizing sarcoid

Nodular sarcoid (Table 13.2) is a term that dates from the pre-CT era when nodules in sarcoid were considered to be unusual. In its original meaning, nodular sarcoid referred to sarcoid in which nodules were visible on plain chest radiograph, but today nodular sarcoid simply means sarcoid with nodules greater than or equal to 1 cm in diameter visible on imaging. The major clinical significance of nodular (and necrotizing) sarcoid was that, on imaging, the nodules carried a primary differential diagnosis of malignancy. This is occasionally still true, but because nodular and necrotizing sarcoid often have typical findings of sarcoid on HRCT, the distinction from ordinary sarcoid is not as sharp as it once was.

Table 13.2

Features of nodular and necrotizing sarcoid

Large nodules formed by aggregated granulomas
Central hyalinization in nodular sarcoid
Necrosis in nodules in necrotizing sarcoid
Small nodules and/or individual granulomas present away from the large nodules
Granulomatous vascular involvement always present

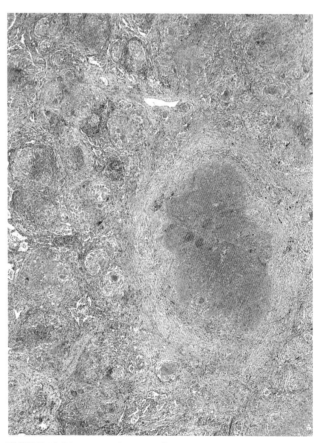

FIGURE 13.30. Necrotizing sarcoid. In this example, an area of necrosis has appeared in the midst of aggregated granulomas.

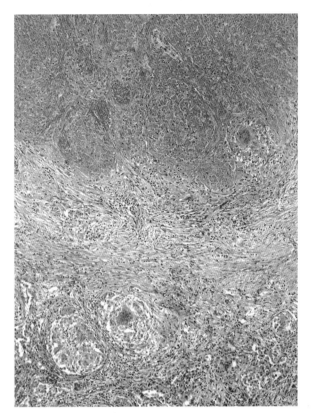

FIGURE 13.31. Necrotizing sarcoid. Higher power view of the same case as Figure 13.30. Stains for acid-fast organisms and fungi are mandatory in this setting because TB and fungal infections can produce an identical morphologic picture.

In nodular sarcoid, the lesions consist of aggregated granulomas that undergo hyaline scarring in a fashion identical to that seen in the small nodules common in ordinary sarcoid (Figs. 13.19 to 13.23); the only distinction is the size of the nodules. Necrotizing sarcoid is similar (Table 13.2), except that small or large areas of necrosis are present in the aggregated granulomas (Figs. 13.30 and 13.31), but this finding mandates careful examination of stains for acid-fast bacilli and fungi, because infectious processes can be microscopically identical. Nodular and necrotizing sarcoid always have smaller nodules or individual granulomas away from the large nodules. Both nodular and necrotizing sarcoid are invariably associated with granulomatous vascular involvement, but granulomas in vessel walls are equally common with TB and fungal infections, so that this finding is not a useful diagnostic tool.

Whether necrotizing sarcoid is simply a variant of sarcoid or a completely different entity has been debated in the literature. A recent review[11] points out that the clinical, radiologic, and pathologic features of ordinary sarcoid, nodular sarcoid, and necrotizing sarcoid show extensive overlap. As well, extrapulmonary granulomatous disease is seen in 20% to 30% of necrotizing sarcoid cases,[12] with eye, skin, central nervous system sites, liver, and gastrointestinal tract being the most common sites of involvement.

These are typical locations for extrapulmonary involvement in ordinary sarcoid, and this phenomenon supports the idea that necrotizing sarcoid is simply a morphologically somewhat unusual form of sarcoid.

Special stains in sarcoid

Whether special stains for organisms always need to be performed in cases that clinically and morphologically are typical sarcoid is controversial. Although it is very rare to find organisms in this setting, we believe that the stains should be performed nonetheless because atypical mycobacteria do not always produce necrotizing granulomas (see below), and even the granulomas of ordinary TB can be non-necrotizing for a short period.

ETIOLOGY AND PATHOGENESIS

Sarcoid appears to represent an abnormal granulomatous response that persists in the absence of a clearly identifiable pathogen.[13] Although viable organisms cannot be cultured from or directly identified in sarcoid granulomas, molecular testing has shown the presence of microbial DNA in some cases, particularly DNA from mycobacteria and *Propionibacterium* species, and mycobacterial catalase-peroxidase has also been found. Some additional support for this idea comes from two small studies in which treatment with an anti-TB antibiotic regime produced improvements in cutaneous and pulmonary sarcoid.[14,15]

Granuloma formation in sarcoid has been extensively studied, and in part consists of a feedback loop in which production of interferon-γ, normally a response to an infectious agent, induces production of tumor necrosis factor-α (TNF-α), as well as interleukin (IL)-12 and IL-23, and TNF-α in turn causes inflammatory cells to secrete more interferon-γ. Further details are available in Le and Crouser.[13]

There are no molecular diagnostic tests for sarcoid, but blocking the actions of the various cytokines just described potentially can be used as a treatment regime. Different TNF-α alleles may be associated with therapeutic responses (see below).

DIAGNOSTIC MODALITIES

Transbronchial biopsies (Fig. 13.32) are commonly performed for the diagnosis of sarcoid and have a high yield, in large part because the peribronchovascular distribution of sarcoid granulomas (Figs. 13.11 to 13.15) means that the biopsy forceps sample the optimum region of the lung. If no granulomas are seen in the original cuts and the clinical impression is sarcoid, additional slides should be prepared because the yield improves with up to seven deeper levels.[16] Endobronchial biopsies similarly have a high yield in sarcoid, particularly if the endoscopist observes

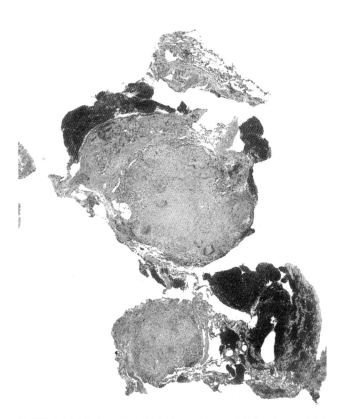

FIGURE 13.32. Transbronchial biopsy in sarcoid showing multiple granulomas.

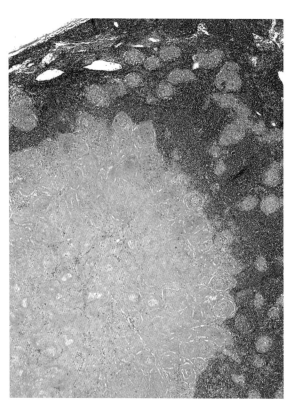

FIGURE 13.34. Individual granulomas and a large hyalinized nodule in a mediastinal lymph node. Nodal granulomas in sarcoid can coalesce to form nodules in the same fashion as parenchymal granulomas.

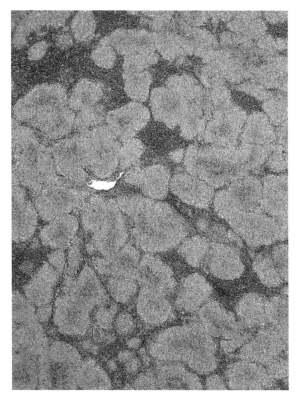

FIGURE 13.33. Sarcoid granulomas in a mediastinal lymph node. Some of these granulomas have small amounts of central necrosis. Sarcoid granulomas in hilar and mediastinal lymph nodes are distinct circumscribed structures and are not located in nodal sinuses, as opposed to sinus histiocytes.

nodularity in the bronchial mucosa (Fig. 13.16). Cryobiopsy is also effective as a diagnostic approach, although not necessarily better than conventional transbronchial forceps biopsy or endobronchial ultrasound (EBUS) biopsy of a mediastinal lymph node.[1,17]

Sarcoid can involve any organ, and hilar and mediastinal nodes typically are filled with granulomas; such nodes occasionally contain hyalinized nodules derived from aggregated granulomas (Figs. 13.33 and 13.34). Sometimes histiocytes in lymph node sinuses mimic granulomas, but real granulomas in sarcoid do not show a sinus distribution and are usually packed together (Fig. 13.33).

Mediastinoscopic and EBUS biopsies (Figs. 13.35 and 13.36) of hilar or mediastinal lymph nodes produce a very high yield,[18] probably better than that of transbronchial biopsy,[1] and extrathoracic sites such as skin are sometimes also suitable for a biopsy diagnosis. Slit lamp examination may show characteristic features of ocular sarcoid and obviate the need for biopsy.

DIFFERENTIAL DIAGNOSIS

The major differential diagnoses of sarcoid are HP and infections, and to a much lesser extent, chronic beryllium disease (Fig. 13.37). The distinction of sarcoid from HP has been referred to above and is presented in more detail in Chapter 12 (see particularly Table 12.7). Table 13.3

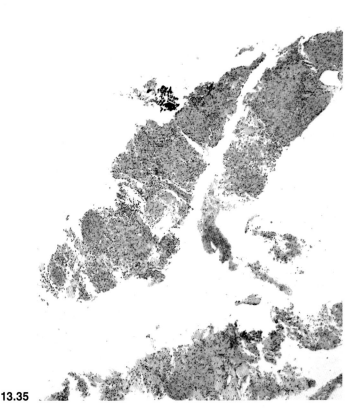

13.35

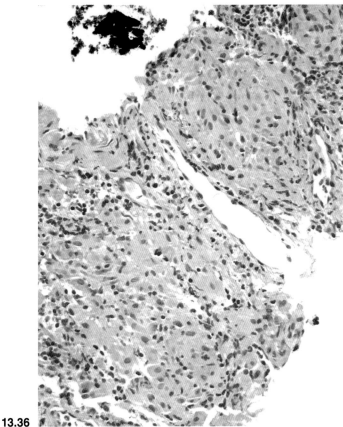

13.36

FIGURES 13.35 and 13.36. Sarcoid granulomas in an EBUS core of a mediastinal lymph node.

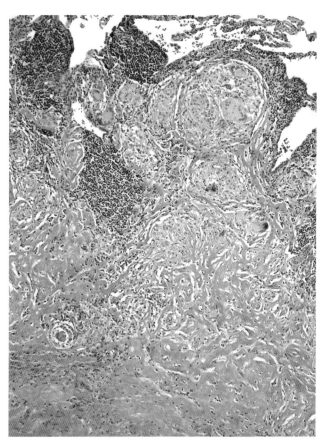

FIGURE 13.37. Chronic beryllium disease (chronic berylliosis). Image shows the edge of a nodular lesion composed of granulomas and hyalinized collagen. Morphologically, chronic berylliosis is indistinguishable from sarcoid.

shows the features of sarcoid compared to fungal and mycobacterial infections. Particular note should be made of non-necrotizing granulomas that look like sarcoid granulomas in the walls of *ectactic* bronchioles or bronchi, because this pattern is very characteristic of atypical mycobacterial infections and not of sarcoid (Figs. 13.38 and 13.39).

Chronic beryllium disease (chronic berylliosis) is morphologically identical to sarcoid in the lung and forms individual non-necrotizing granulomas as well as aggregated granulomas (Fig. 13.37). In practice, berylliosis is very rare and patients with berylliosis almost invariably give a history of beryllium exposure. In questionable cases, beryllium lymphocyte blast transformation testing can be used[19] and it is also possible to demonstrate beryllium by energy dispersive x-ray spectroscopy in histologic sections[20] or by various chemical analysis of lung tissue.[21]

Some drugs can produce a granulomatous reaction in the lung (see Chapter 18). With methotrexate the granulomas are scattered and the process can mimic HP, but anti-TNF agents, interferon therapy, and immune checkpoint inhibitor therapy[21–24] can cause the formation of multiple,

Table 13.3

Comparison of sarcoid and infectious granulomas

Sarcoid	TB and fungal infections	Atypical mycobacterial infections
Granulomas usually but not always non-necrotizing	Granulomas usually but not always necrotizing	Granulomas may be non-necrotizing or necrotizing
Granulomas follow lymphatic routes	Granulomas random in parenchyma	Granulomas random or in walls of *ectatic* bronchioles or bronchi
Aggregated granulomas scar to hyalinized nodules	Aggregated granulomas usually show necrosis	
Granulomas often surrounded by concentric bands of hyalinized collagen	Concentric hyalinization rare	Concentric hyalinization rare
Schaumann bodies occasionally present	Schaumann bodies rare	Schaumann bodies rare
No organisms demonstrable	Organisms often demonstrable	Organisms often demonstrable

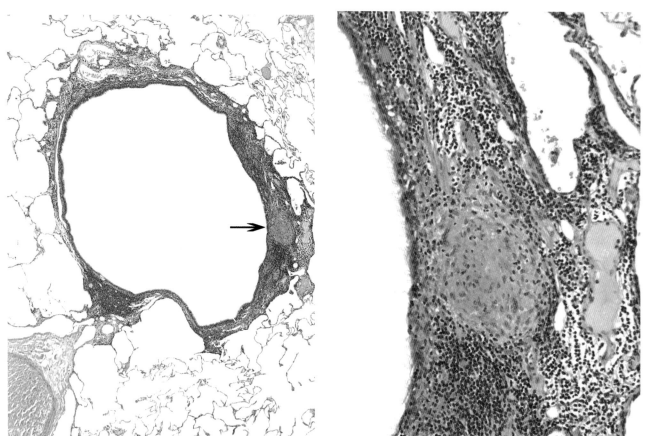

13.38

13.39

FIGURES 13.38 and 13.39. Mycobacterium avium intracellulare (MAC) infection. There is a non-necrotizing granuloma in the wall of an ectactic bronchiole (*arrow* and shown at higher power in Fig. 13.39). Bronchiectactic and bronchiolectatic airways with granulomas in the wall are not features of sarcoid, but are very typical of MAC and other atypical mycobacterial infections. MAC granulomas are often non-necrotizing.

sometimes aggregated, pulmonary granulomas (see Figs. 18.14 and 18.15). This phenomenon is often, albeit incorrectly, referred to in the clinical literature as "sarcoidosis."[22–25] However, in our experience, such granulomas do not have concentric fibrosis nor they are distributed along lymphatic routes. At least for anti-TNF agents the granulomas disappear if the drug is stopped,[25] indicating that this is really a drug reaction.

Sarcoid-type granulomas are a common finding in lungs that harbor tumors, and the hilar and mediastinal lymph nodes from such cases may also contain granulomas. In most such cases, the number of granulomas is much fewer than in sarcoid, the massive aggregates of granulomas seen in lymph nodes with true sarcoid are not present, and there are no radiologic findings to suggest sarcoid.

TREATMENT

Steroids are the first line of treatment but are usually reserved for those with life-threatening or organ-threatening disease or an impaired quality of life.[1] If disease progresses despite steroid therapy, or for steroid sparing, antimetabolites and nonsteroidal agents including azathioprine methotrexate, mycophenolate, and leflunomide have been used. TNF-α antagonists are effective in some patients, particularly those with the TNF-α 308G allele, but carry a risk of tuberculous infection.

PROGNOSIS

As noted above, the prognosis of sarcoid depends to a large extent on the radiologic stage. The higher the stage, the lower the chance of remission (remission is seen in up to 90% of Stage I cases and no Stage IV cases), but even with high stage the disease can be quite slowly progressive; a study of Stage IV sarcoid patients reported a 10-year survival of 84% from the time of diagnosis.[26] Overall remission, with or without treatment, is seen in about 70% of cases. Only 1% to 5% of cases are fatal, and this number may be exaggerated because such cases tend to get referred to academic centers and enumerated. The mortality rate for sarcoid in the United States has been estimated at 2.8/1,000,000.[1] Neurosarcoid and cardiac sarcoid carry a worse prognosis, as does the presence of pulmonary hypertension.[1,4,27,28]

It has been suggested that sarcoid is associated with a slightly increased risk of extrapulmonary malignancy, but apparently not an increased risk of lung cancer.[1] Mycetomas occur in a small percentage of sarcoid patients, almost always those with Stage IV disease.[1]

Nodular and necrotizing sarcoid appear to behave as low-stage disease with a good prognosis.[27] Sarcoid can recur in transplanted lungs, but usually does not cause clinically significant disease.[29]

REFERENCES

1. Spagnolo P, Rossi G, Trisolini R, et al. Pulmonary sarcoidosis. *Lancet Respir Med.* 2018;6:389–402.
2. Morgenthau AS, Teirstein AS. Sarcoidosis of the upper and lower airways. *Expert Rev Respir Med.* 2011;5:823–833.
3. Shigemitsu H, Nagai S, Sharma OP. Pulmonary hypertension and granulomatous vasculitis in sarcoidosis. *Curr Opin Pulm Med.* 2007;13:434–438.
4. Shlobin OA, Baughman RP. Sarcoidosis-associated pulmonary hypertension. *Semin Respir Crit Care Med.* 2017;38:450–462.
5. Baughman RP, Culver DA, Judson MA. A concise review of pulmonary sarcoidosis. *Am J Respir Crit Care Med.* 2011;183:573–581.
6. Naidich D. Are CT findings of pulmonary sarcoidosis ever sufficient for a presumptive diagnosis? *Lancet Respir Med.* 2018;6(9):e43.
7. Criado E, Sánchez M, Ramírez J, et al. Pulmonary sarcoidosis: typical and atypical manifestations at high-resolution CT with pathologic correlation. *Radiographics.* 2010;301:567–586.
8. Visscher D, Churg A, Katzenstein AL. Significance of crystalline inclusions in lung granulomas. *Mod Pathol.* 1988;1:415–419.
9. Xu L, Kligerman S, Burke A. End-stage sarcoid lung disease is distinct from usual interstitial pneumonia. *Am J Surg Pathol.* 2013;37(4):593–600.
10. Zhang C, Chan KM, Schmidt LA, et al. Histopathology of explanted lungs from patients with a diagnosis of pulmonary sarcoidosis. *Chest.* 2016;149:499–507.
11. Rosen Y. Four decades of necrotizing sarcoid granulomatosis: what do we know now? *Arch Pathol Lab Med.* 2015;139:252–262.
12. Karpathiou G, Batistatou A, Boglou P, et al. Necrotizing sarcoid granulomatosis: a distinctive form of pulmonary granulomatous disease. *Clin Respir J.* 2018;12:1313–1319.
13. Le V, Crouser ED. Potential immunotherapies for sarcoidosis. *Expert Opin Biol Ther.* 2018;18:399–407.
14. Drake WP, Oswald-Richter K, Richmond BW, et al. Oral antimycobacterial therapy in chronic cutaneous sarcoidosis: a randomized, single-masked, placebo-controlled study. *JAMA Dermatol.* 2013;149:1040–1049.
15. Drake WP, Richmond BW, Oswald-Richter K, et al. Effects of broad-spectrum antimycobacterial therapy on chronic pulmonary sarcoidosis. *Sarcoidosis Vasc Diffuse Lung Dis.* 2013;30:201–211.
16. Takayama K, Nagata N, Miyagawa Y, et al. The usefulness of step sectioning of transbronchial lung biopsy specimen in diagnosing sarcoidosis. *Chest.* 1992;102:1441–1443.
17. Aragaki-Nakahodo AA, Baughman RP, Shipley RT, et al. The complimentary role of transbronchial lung cryobiopsy and endobronchial ultrasound fine needle aspiration in the diagnosis of sarcoidosis. *Respir Med.* 2017;131:65–69.
18. Colt HG, Davoudi M, Murgu S. Scientific evidence and principles for the use of endobronchial ultrasound and transbronchial needle aspiration. *Expert Rev Med Devices.* 2011;8:493–513.
19. Santo Tomas LH. Beryllium hypersensitivity and chronic beryllium lung disease. *Curr Opin Pulm Med.* 2009;15:165–169.
20. Butnor KJ, Sporn TA, Ingram P, et al. Beryllium detection in human lung tissue using electron probe X-ray microanalysis. *Mod Pathol.* 2003;16:1171–1177.

21. Balmes JR, Abraham JL, Dweik RA, et al; ATS Ad Hoc Committee on Beryllium Sensitivity and Chronic Beryllium Disease. An official American Thoracic Society statement: diagnosis and management of beryllium sensitivity and chronic beryllium disease. *Am J Respir Crit Care Med.* 2014;190:e34–e59.

22. Cousin S, Italiano A. Pulmonary sarcoidosis or post-immunotherapy granulomatous reaction induced by the anti-PD-1 monoclonal antibody pembrolizumab: the terminology is not the key point. *Ann Oncol.* 2016;27:1974–1975.

23. Marzouk K, Saleh S, Kannass M, et al. Interferon-induced granulomatous lung disease. *Curr Opin Pulm Med.* 2004;10:435–440.

24. Tong D, Manolios N, Howe G, et al. New onset sarcoid-like granulomatosis developing during anti-TNF therapy: an under-recognised complication. *Intern Med J.* 201;42:89–94.

25. Cathcart S, Sami N, Elewski B. Sarcoidosis as an adverse effect of tumor necrosis factor inhibitors. *J Drugs Dermatol.* 2012;11:609–612.

26. Nardi A, Brillet PY, Letoumelin P, et al. Stage IV sarcoidosis: comparison of survival with the general population and causes of death. *Eur Respir J.* 2011;38:1368–1373.

27. Lynch JP 3rd, Ma YL, Koss MN, et al. Pulmonary sarcoidosis. *Semin Respir Crit Care Med.* 2007;28:53–74.

28. Sayah DM, Bradfield JS, Moriarty JM, et al. Cardiac involvement in sarcoidosis: evolving concepts in diagnosis and treatment. *Semin Respir Crit Care Med.* 2017;38:477–498.

29. Milman N, Burton C, Andersen CB, et al. Lung transplantation for end-stage pulmonary sarcoidosis: outcome in a series of seven consecutive patients. *Sarcoidosis Vasc Diffuse Lung Dis.* 2005;22:222–228.

Miscellaneous Granulomatous Interstitial Lung Diseases

COMMON VARIABLE IMMUNODEFICIENCY AND SELECTIVE IgA IMMUNODEFICIENCY

Clinical features

Common variable immunodeficiency (CVID) is a somewhat heterogeneous primary immunodeficiency syndrome characterized by low-serum IgG with variably low IgA or IgM, and associated low levels of antibody production, secondary to a failure of B-cell differentiation into antibody-producing plasma cells.[1] In about 50% of cases there is also abnormal T-cell function.[2] The prevalence of CVID is 1 in 25,000 to 1 in 50,000 persons. Specific mutations in genes encoding B and T cells function have been described in around 5% of cases, but in most patients the underlying molecular abnormality is not known.[3] Selective IgA deficiency (IgAD) is actually more common than CVID and differs in that at IgA levels are decreased, often to the point of being undetectable, whereas IgG and IgM levels are by definition normal[4]; however, some cases that start as IgAD evolve into CVID.[5,6]

Infections, particularly recurrent upper and lower respiratory tract infections, are the most common initial manifestation of CVID and IgAD. Both CVID and IgAD patients can have a variety of systemic autoimmune conditions including autoimmune cytopenias such as autoimmune thrombocytopenic purpura and autoimmune hemolytic anemia; rheumatic autoimmune diseases such as juvenile rheumatoid arthritis and adult rheumatoid arthritis[7]; enteropathy including a picture of inflammatory bowel disease; hepatitis/hepatomegaly; splenomegaly; lymphadenopathy; meningitis/encephalitis; and in a small proportion of cases, lymphomas, and other malignancies.[3,4,7,8] The incidence of asthma is also increased. Interstitial lung disease is seen in 10% to 20% of CVID patients.[3]

Some patients initially diagnosed with CVID or whose clinical/immunologic picture resembles CVID have in fact turned out to have much rarer forms of immunodeficiency characterized by specific genetic abnormalities, for example, combined immunodeficiency with RAG mutations,[9] CTLA4 mutations, and PI3KCD mutations.[2]

Imaging

The majority of patients with CVID have pulmonary abnormalities evident on high-resolution computed tomography (HRCT), the most frequent being bronchiectasis.[10,11] The bronchiectasis involves mainly the right middle lobe followed by the lower lobes. The severity of bronchiectasis correlates with the frequency of previous lower respiratory tract infections.[11] Other common findings are ground-glass opacities and one or more pulmonary nodules.[10]

The characteristic HRCT manifestations of granulomatous-lymphocytic interstitial lung disease (GLILD) consist of multiple small ground-glass or solid nodules, interlobular septal thickening, hilar and mediastinal lymph node enlargement, and splenomegaly[10,12] (Figs. 14.4 and 14.5).

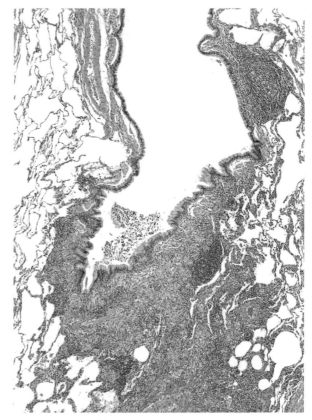

FIGURE 14.1. Bronchiectasis in CVID.

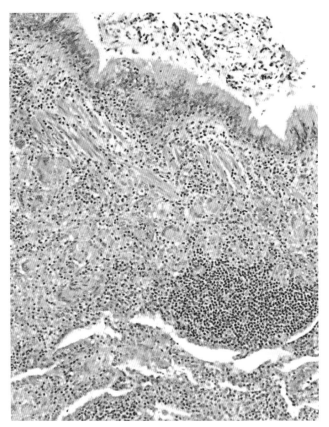

FIGURE 14.2. Higher power view of Figure 14.1 showing granulomas in the wall of the bronchiectactic airway.

The nodules have a perilymphatic distribution and reflect the presence of lymphoid hyperplasia.[10] The abnormalities tend to involve mainly the lower lobes and may wax and wane over time.[10] Areas of consolidation occur in a small percentage of patients.[12]

Pathologic features

The reported pathologic findings in CVID and IgAD (Table 14.1) are very variable and the literature in this area is confused by definitional issues of pathologic lesions, undoubted misclassification of CVID versus IgAD in some instances, and small numbers of cases.

Chronic lung disease is seen in around 30% of CVID patients,[13] of which bronchiectasis (Figs. 14.1 and 14.2), presumed to be the sequela of repeated infections, is probably the most common finding. Bronchiectasis occurs in IgAD as well.[4]

Isolated or aggregated granulomas have been reported in up to 20% of CVID patients, not only in the lung (Figs. 14.3 to 14.6) but also in the lymph nodes, spleen, and less frequently in other organs.[14] The granulomas in the lung are usually, but not invariably, non-necrotizing,[3] and stains for organisms are typically unrewarding. The granulomas sometimes have concentric lamellar fibrosis of the type seen in sarcoid granulomas (Fig. 14.3), but typically do

Table 14.1

Pathologic findings in common variable and selective IgA immunodeficiency

Feature	CVID	IgAD
Bronchiectasis/bronchiolectasis	+	+
Isolated granulomas	+	?
Organizing pneumonia (BOOP, COP)	+	+
Granulomatous-lymphocytic interstitial lung disease	+	?
Follicular bronchiolitis	+	?
Lymphocytic interstitial pneumonia	+	+
Cellular NSIP	+	?
Interstitial fibrosis	+	?

not show the lymphatic distribution characteristic of sarcoid.[15] Although granulomas are not described as features of IgAD, we have seen occasional cases with granulomas, independent of lymphocytic interstitial pneumonia (LIP).

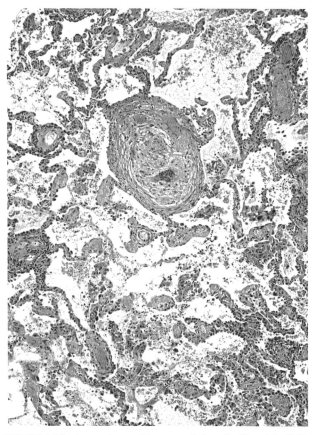

FIGURE 14.3. A granuloma with concentric lamellar fibrosis in CVID.

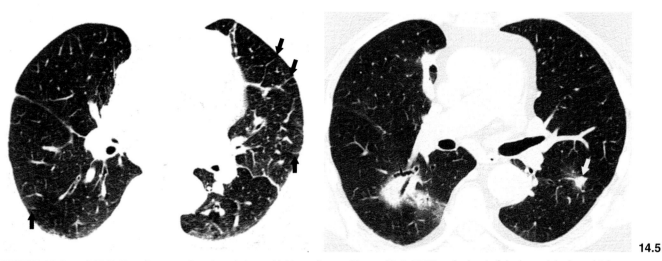

14.4   14.5

FIGURES 14.4 and 14.5. Granulomatous-lymphocytic interstitial lung disease. **Figure 14.4:** HRCT at the level of the lower lobe bronchi demonstrates mild smooth interlobular septal thickening (*black arrows*) mainly in the lingula. **Figure 14.5:** HRCT performed 4 months after Figure 14.1 at the level of the left upper lobe bronchus shows focal peribronchial consolidation and ground-glass opacities in the right lower lobe and a nodule in the left lower lobe (*white arrow*).

Organizing pneumonia (OP) is also common, as is what has been described as nonspecific interstitial pneumonia (NSIP), and sometimes follicular bronchiolitis or LIP.

GLILD (Figs. 14.4 to 14.7) is a form of CVID characterized by a variable combination of non-caseating interstitial granulomas with follicular bronchiolitis (see Chapter 19), lymphoid hyperplasia, mild chronic

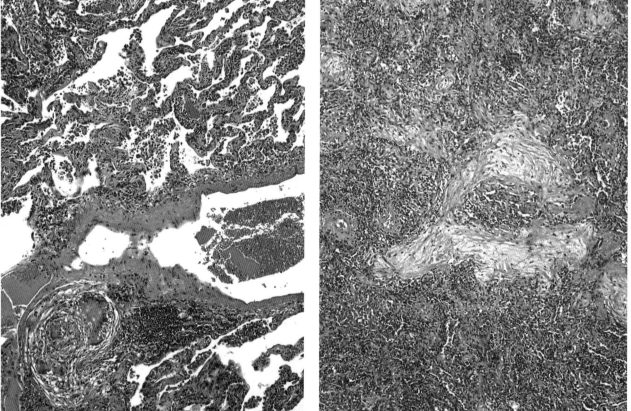

14.6   14.7

FIGURES 14.6 and 14.7. Biopsy of the case shown in Figures 14.4 and 14.5. **Figure 14.6** shows a granuloma and mild chronic interstitial inflammation, whereas **Figure 14.7** shows an area of organizing pneumonia.

interstitial inflammation, or LIP (Chapter 20). The granulomas may be associated with the lymphoid infiltrates or may be separated from them. In the largest published GLILD pathology series,[2] OP was also present in 14/16 cases, and interstitial fibrosis, ranging from minimal to extensive fibrosis with honeycombing, was seen in 12/16 cases. Oddly, patients with CVID/GLILD tend to have low numbers of circulating B cells but tissue biopsies nonetheless show CD20-positive B cells in considerable numbers. It is not clear whether GLILD occurs in IgAD, although LIP certainly does.

Whether GLILD is actually a specific entity or is really just a variety of forms of ILD, particularly LIP, in patients with CVID is also not entirely clear (see Chapter 20). However, in our experience and in illustrations in the literature, the granulomas of GLILD are much larger and better defined than those of LIP; may not be spatially associated with the lymphoid infiltrates in contradistinction to LIP; and sometimes have concentric lamellar fibrosis, something that is not seen in the granulomas of LIP. OP is not a concomitant of most cases of LIP. These findings suggest that GLILD probably is different from LIP.

Granulomas or GLILD has been described in other rare forms of immunodeficiency, such as patients with CTLA4 mutations, and lipopolysaccharide-responsive beige-like anchor protein deficiency[2] (see Rose et al.[14] for a more detailed listing).

Diagnostic modalities

In a patient known to have CVID, GLILD might be diagnosable on transbronchial biopsy; however, the diagnosis requires a combination of findings that are unlikely to all be present in a transbronchial biopsy. Isolated granulomas on a small biopsy can be confused with sarcoid, but sarcoid patients typically do not have a history of recurrent infections and often have polyclonal hypergammaglobulinemia rather than hypogammaglobulinemia. The diagnosis of LIP and bronchiectasis/bronchiolectasis in CVID or IgAD ordinarily requires a video-assisted thoracoscopic biopsy; the value of cryobiopsy is not known.

Differential diagnosis

CVID and IgAD are difficult to diagnose without an appropriate history because many of the pathologic patterns are common to other forms of ILD including OP (Chapter 5), NSIP (Chapter 7), hypersensitivity pneumonitis (Chapter 12), follicular bronchiolitis (Chapter 19), lymphoid hyperplasia (Chapter 20), and LIP (Chapter 20). A combination of granulomas and interstitial inflammatory infiltrates can be seen in hypersensitivity pneumonitis and LIP of other etiologies, and granulomas plus OP are often seen as a manifestation of aspiration (Chapter 19). However, a history of repeated pulmonary infections should raise a question of CVID or IgAD.

Treatment and prognosis

The use of exogenous immunoglobulin has greatly decreased the incidence of pulmonary infections in CVID. A wide variety of agents have been employed for refractory/systemic diseases including prednisone, rituximab, azathioprine, cyclophosphamide, hydroxchloroquine, and cyclosporin A. Overall, patients with GLILD have a worse prognosis than those without interstitial lung disease.[3,16] Antibiotics and exogenous immunoglobulin are also recommended for IgAD patients with recurrent infections.[4]

PRIMARY BILIARY CHOLANGITIS (PRIMARY BILIARY CIRRHOSIS) IN THE LUNG

Primary biliary cholangitis (PBC), formerly known as primary biliary cirrhosis, is a form of autoimmune liver disease in which there is serologic evidence of cholangitis, antimitochondrial antibodies in almost all cases, and microscopic evidence of a nonsuppurative cholangitis with progressive loss of small bile ducts. Non-necrotizing granulomas are found associated with the inflamed bile duct in about one-third of cases (so-called florid duct lesions).[17] In some patients, the disease progresses to cirrhosis.

Although PBC is not rare in terms of inflammatory liver diseases, involvement of the lung appears to be quite uncommon and there is relatively little information available about imaging or pathologic changes. The largest series[18] to date describes 16 cases. On CT imaging, bilateral ground-glass opacities were the most common finding, but reticulation, and, occasionally, honeycombing were seen in some patients (Fig. 14.8). Coexisting autoimmune

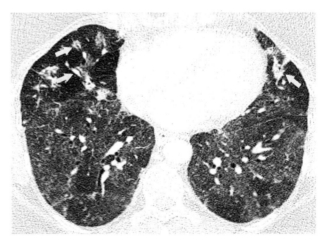

FIGURE 14.8. HRCT image in a patient with PBC shows extensive bilateral ground-glass opacities. Also noted are a few poorly defined small nodules mainly in the lower lobes and focal areas of peribronchial consolidation in the right middle lobe and lingula (*arrows*). Surgical lung biopsy demonstrated peribronchial lymphoid infiltrates with granulomas. These presumably accounted for the peribronchial areas of consolidation. The histologic findings responsible for the ground-glass opacities in this patient are not known.

diseases (myasthenia gravis, systemic sclerosis, and cutaneous lupus) were present in some cases.

On biopsy, lymphocytic infiltration of the peribronchiolar stroma and interstitium was seen in 15/16 cases with a tendency to a peribronchiolar/lymphangitic pattern, but in some instances there was more diffuse interstitial spread (Fig. 14.9). Granulomas, typically but not always poorly formed, were seen in the interstitium, peribronchiolar tissues, airspaces, and pleura and occasionally in bronchiolar walls in 13/16 cases (Fig. 14.10); one case had only granulomas but no interstitial infiltrate. None of the granulomas was necrotizing. Other pathologic features included an eosinophilic infiltrate in six cases, and various patterns of fibrosis (NSIP-like, usual interstitial pneumonia [UIP]-like, and unclassifiable) in seven cases. In our experience, granulomas may also be found in hilar lymph nodes.

Differential diagnosis

The differential diagnosis is wide and includes subacute hypersensitivity pneumonitis (see Chapter 12), LIP (Chapter 20), NSIP (Chapter 7), UIP (Chapter 6), Crohn disease (CD) (see below), and granulomatous drug reactions (Chapter 18). Morphologically, these entities may be impossible to sort out, although hypersensitivity pneumonitis and LIP typically do not show the large numbers of granulomas found in some cases of PBC in the lung. In a patient with a history of PBC, or at least positive antimitochondrial antibodies, these various forms of ILD are most likely a manifestation of the PBC.

CD AND ULCERATIVE COLITIS IN THE LUNG

Overt pulmonary disease in CD and ulcerative colitis (UC) is very infrequent, although it has been claimed that airflow obstruction is present in a significant proportion of patients, especially CD patients, if looked for,[19] suggesting that subclinical pathologic abnormalities in the airways may actually be fairly common. In most cases, pulmonary disease occurs in patients with established diagnoses of CD and UC, but pulmonary disease may occasionally be the initial clinical presentation, and in some patients colectomy seems to precipitate overt pulmonary disease. Flares of bowel and pulmonary disease may occur in parallel.[20]

A wide variety of abnormalities are found in the lungs in both CD and UC (Figs. 14.11 to 14.18). The most common abnormalities on HRCT are bronchial wall thickening and bronchiectasis (Fig. 14.16), both of which are more common in UC than in CD.[21,22] HRCT findings of small airway disease are less common and include centrilobular nodules, tree in bud pattern, and mosaic attenuation on

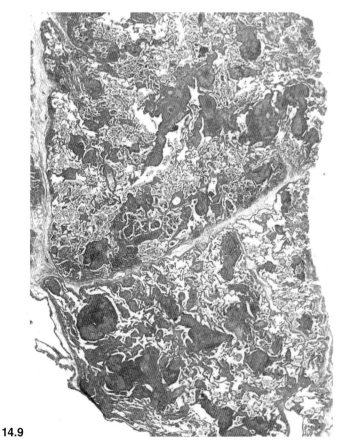

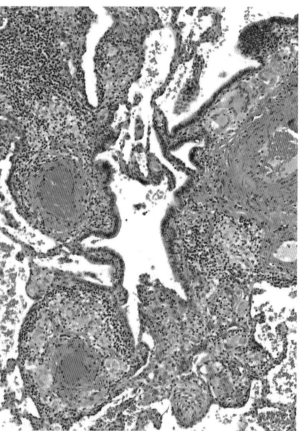

14.9

14.10

FIGURES 14.9 and 14.10. Low- and medium-power views of PBC in the lung. Lymphoid infiltrates with interstitial granulomas surround many airways. (Reprinted from Lee HE, Churg A, Ryu JH, et al. Histopathologic findings in lung biopsies from patients with primary biliary cholangitis. *Hum Pathol.* 2018;82:177–186 with permission from Elsevier.)

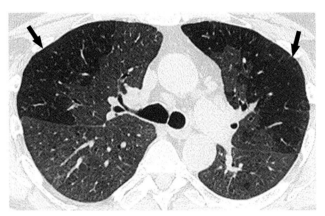

FIGURE 14.11. Crohn disease. HRCT demonstrates extensive bilateral areas of decreased attenuation and vascularity (*arrows*) characteristic of obstructive small airway disease. Blood flow redistribution to normal lung results in areas of increased attenuation and vascularity. This combination of findings is known as mosaic attenuation and perfusion.

inspiratory images and air trapping on expiratory images[22] (Fig. 14.11). Multifocal peribronchial and peripheral areas of consolidation may be caused by OP secondary to the inflammatory bowel disease or, probably more commonly, be caused by infection or drug reaction.[21,22]

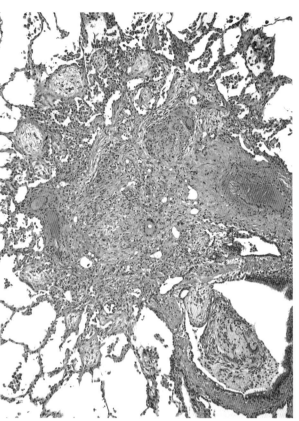

14.13

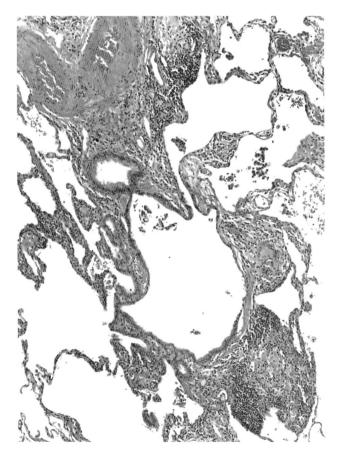

FIGURE 14.12. Granulomatous bronchiolitis in CD. This image has a wide differential including aspiration and hypersensitivity pneumonitis and requires a history of CD for accurate diagnosis.

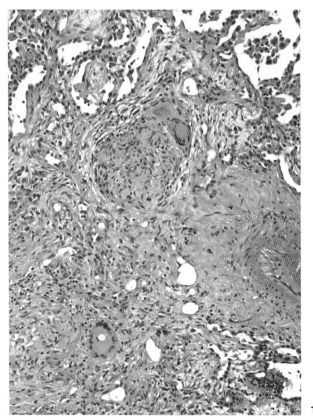

14.14

FIGURES 14.13 and 14.14. Peribronchial inflammatory nodule in CD. There is a mixture of organizing pneumonia, inflammatory cells, and granulomas.

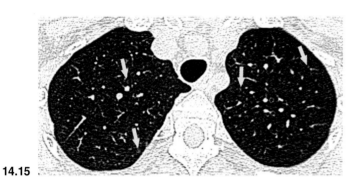
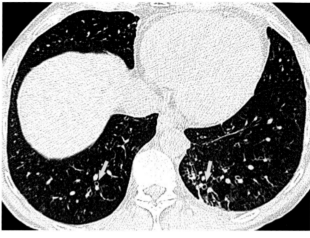

14.15   14.16

FIGURES 14.15. and 14.16. Ulcerative colitis. **Figure 14.15:** HRCT at the level of the lung apices shows scattered bilateral poorly defined centrilobular nodules. **Figure 14.16:** HRCT at the level of the basal segments of the lower lobes demonstrates bilateral bronchial wall thickening and mild left lower lobe bronchiectasis (*arrows*). Also noted are a few centrilobular nodules, mild patchy ground-glass opacities, and linear areas of atelectasis or scarring.

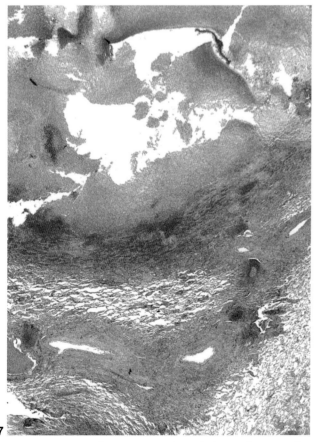
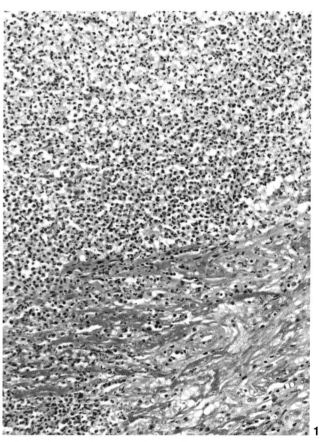

14.17   14.18

FIGURES 14.17 and 14.18. UC involving the lung. A large necrobiotic nodule (sterile abscess) occupies the top of image in **Figure 14.17**, and there is peribronchovascular inflammation in the lower half of the field. At higher power (**Fig. 14.18**) the necrotic biotic nodule contains sheets of neutrophils.

Pathologic findings

Table 14.2 lists pathologic lesions that have been described in CD and UC (Figs. 14.12 to 14.14, 14.17, and 14.18), although the relative frequencies shown in Table 14.2 are based on a small number of cases and are really approximations. Most of the lesions listed in Table 14.2 arc relatively nonspecific in terms of etiology, and a history of inflammatory bowel disease is usually necessary for accurate diagnosis.

Pulmonary lesions may involve the large and small airways as well as the parenchyma. Granulomatous bronchiolitis and OP (BOOP/COP) with granulomas are particularly characteristic of CD[23] (Figs. 14.12 to 14.14); the granulomas are usually non-necrotizing. In rare cases, the granulomas are sufficiently numerous that the process somewhat mimics sarcoid.[24] Acute/necrotizing bronchiolitis can be seen in both CD and UC, as can peri-airway inflammatory collections without granulomas. Sterile necrobiotic nodules that look microscopically like abscesses are more common in UC (Figs. 14.17 and 14.18).

Some of the patterns listed in Table 14.2 are probably drug reactions rather than direct manifestations of CD and UC; for example, salicylates causing eosinophilic pneumonias (see Chapter 18, Case 3), azathioprine or methotrexate causing interstitial inflammation (and granulomas with methotrexate, see Fig. 18.7), and anti-tumor necrosis factor (TNF) agents causing a sarcoid-like pattern of granulomas (see Chapter 18, Case Study 1). Because CD and UC patients are frequently treated with steroids or anti-TNF agents, stains for organisms should be performed before attributing granulomas to CD or drugs.

Treatment and prognosis

Most of the lesions listed in Table 14.2 respond surprisingly well to steroid therapy. Possible exceptions are the various forms of bronchiolitis, including constrictive bronchiolitis, where the literature on outcome is contradictory and difficult to interpret.[19,20,23]

Table 14.2		
Relative frequency of pathologic lesions in the lung in CD and UC		
Pathologic lesion	**CD**	**UC**
Tracheal inflammation or stenosis	+	++
Neutrophilic large airway inflammation	+/−	++
Bronchiectasis	+	++
Granulomatous bronchiolitis with chronic inflammation	+	−
Acute bronchiolitis/ bronchopneumonia	+	+
Morphologic picture of diffuse panbronchiolitis	−	+
Constrictive bronchiolitis	−	+
Organizing pneumonia (BOOP, COP)	+/−	++
Organizing pneumonia with granulomas	+	−
Granulomatous interstitial inflammation	++	+/−

Modified from Camus P, Colby TV. The lung in inflammatory bowel disease. *Eur Respir J.* 2000;15:5–1; Casey MB, Tazelaar HD, Myers JL, et al. Noninfectious lung pathology in patients with Crohn's disease. *Am J Surg Pathol.* 2003;27:213–219.

REFERENCES

1. Resnick ES, Cunningham-Rundles C. The many faces of the clinical picture of common variable immune deficiency. *Curr Opin Allergy Clin Immunol.* 2012;12:595–601.
2. Rao N, Mackinnon AC, Routes JM. Granulomatous and lymphocytic interstitial lung disease: a spectrum of pulmonary histopathologic lesions in common variable immunodeficiency—histologic and immunohistochemical analyses of 16 cases. *Hum Pathol.* 2015;46:1306–1314.
3. Prasse A, Kayser G, Warnatz K. Common variable immunodeficiency-associated granulomatous and interstitial lung disease. *Curr Opin Pulm Med.* 2013;19:503–509.
4. Yazdani R, Azizi G, Abolhassani H, et al. Selective IgA deficiency: epidemiology, pathogenesis, clinical phenotype, diagnosis, prognosis and management. *Scand J Immunol.* 2017;85:3–12.
5. Español T, Catala M, Hernandez M, et al. Development of a common variable immunodeficiency in IgA-deficient patients. *Clin Immunol Immunopathol.* 1996;80(3, pt 1):333–335.
6. Aghamohammadi A, Mohammadi J, Parvaneh N, et al. Progression of selective IgA deficiency to common variable immunodeficiency. *Int Arch Allergy Immunol.* 2008;147:87–92.
7. Azizi G, Tavakol M, Rafiemanesh H, et al. Autoimmunity in a cohort of 471 patients with primary antibody deficiencies. *Expert Rev Clin Immunol.* 2017;13:1099–1106.
8. Gathmann B, Mahlaoui N, Ceredih GL, et al; European Society for Immunodeficiencies Registry Working Party. Clinical picture and treatment of 2212 patients with common variable immunodeficiency. *J Allergy Clin Immunol.* 2014;134:116–126.

9. Buchbinder D, Baker R, Lee YN, et al. Identification of patients with RAG mutations previously diagnosed with common variable immunodeficiency disorders. *J Clin Immunol.* 2015;35:119–124.

10. Maglione PJ, Overbey JR, Radigan L, et al. Pulmonary radiologic findings in common variable immunodeficiency: clinical and immunological correlations. *Ann Allergy Asthma Immunol.* 2014;113:452–459.

11. Bang TJ, Richards JC, Olson AL, et al. Pulmonary manifestations of common variable immunodeficiency. *J Thorac Imaging.* 2018;33:377–383.

12. Torigian DA, LaRosa DF, Levinson AI, et al. Granulomatous-lymphocytic interstitial lung disease associated with common variable immunodeficiency: CT findings. *J Thorac Imaging.* 2008;23:162–169.

13. Resnick ES, Moshier EL, Godbold JH, et al. Morbidity and mortality in common variable immune deficiency over 4 decades. *Blood.* 2012;119:1650–1657.

14. Rose CD, Neven B, Wouters C. Granulomatous inflammation: the overlap of immune deficiency and inflammation. *Best Pract Res Clin Rheumatol.* 2014;28:191–212.

15. Bouvry D, Mouthon L, Brillet PY, et al; Groupe Sarcoïdose Francophone. Granulomatosis-associated common variable immunodeficiency disorder: a case-control study versus sarcoidosis. *Eur Respir J.* 2013;41:115–122.

16. Bates CA, Ellison MC, Lynch DA, et al. Granulomatous-lymphocytic lung disease shortens survival in common variable immunodeficiency. *J Allergy Clin Immunol.* 2004;114:415–421.

17. Carey EJ, Ali AH, Lindor KD. Primary biliary cirrhosis. *Lancet.* 2015;386:1565–1575.

18. Lee HE, Churg A, Ryu JH, et al. Histopathologic findings in lung biopsies from patients with primary biliary cholangitis. *Hum Pathol.* 2018;82:177–186.

19. Majewski S, Piotrowski W. Pulmonary manifestations of inflammatory bowel disease. *Arch Med Sci.* 2015;11:1179–1188.

20. Camus P, Colby TV. The lung in inflammatory bowel disease. *Eur Respir J.* 2000;15:5–10.

21. Olpin JD, Sjoberg BP, Stilwill SE, et al. Beyond the bowel: extraintestinal manifestations of inflammatory bowel disease. *Radiographics.* 2017;37:1135–1160.

22. Cozzi D, Moroni C, Addeo G, et al. Radiological patterns of lung involvement in inflammatory bowel disease. *Gastroenterol Res Pract.* 2018;2018:5697846.

23. Casey MB, Tazelaar HD, Myers JL, et al. Noninfectious lung pathology in patients with Crohn's disease. *Am J Surg Pathol.* 2003;27:213–219.

24. Thao C, Lagstein A, Allen T, et al. Crohn's disease-associated interstitial lung disease mimicking sarcoidosis: a case report and review of the literature. *Sarcoidosis Vasc Diffuse Lung Dis.* 2016;33:288–291.

Eosinophilic Pneumonias

NOMENCLATURE ISSUES

Eosinophilic pneumonias are conventionally separated into simple eosinophilic pneumonia (Loeffler syndrome), acute eosinophilic pneumonia (AEP), a process that clinically sometimes resembles acute respiratory distress syndrome (ARDS) or a community-acquired pneumonia, and chronic eosinophilic pneumonia (CEP), which has a much longer time course and typically does not result in respiratory failure. However, these distinctions are sometimes not sharp and cases can be found that, at least morphologically, are borderline between acute and CEP.[1-4] Because treatment is the same (high-dose steroids), the distinction is usually not crucial.

CAUSES OF EOSINOPHILIC PNEUMONIAS

Table 15.1 lists causes of eosinophilic pneumonias. AEP is relatively uncommon; the most frequent causes are drugs (prescribed or inhaled recreational) and cigarette smoke, typically in those who start smoking or take it up after a hiatus.[3,5] More than 120 drugs have been reported to produce eosinophilic pneumonias.[6] Eosinophilic pneumonia may be the only manifestation of Churg–Strauss syndrome (eosinophilic granulomatosis with polyangiitis, EGPA)[7] or allergic bronchopulmonary aspergillosis (ABPA),[8] but usually these diseases show a variety of other features. A more detailed listing of etiologies for AEP is available in De Giacomi et al.[3] and an extensive listing of drugs associated with eosinophilic pneumonias in Bartal et al.,[6] as well as at pneumotox.com.

CLINICAL FEATURES

Simple Eosinophilic Pneumonia (Loeffler Syndrome)

Simple eosinophilic pneumonia is characterized by fleeting migratory pulmonary infiltrates on imaging in the absence of pulmonary symptoms or with minimal symptoms. Patients typically have a peripheral blood eosinophilia. Most cases of Loeffler syndrome are believed to be caused by pulmonary passage of intestinal parasites, most commonly *Ascaris*,[1] but some cases don't have an identifiable cause.

Table 15.1

Causes of eosinophilic pneumonias

Idiopathic
Drug reactions
  Prescribed medications, especially antibiotics, nonsteroidal anti-inflammatory agents, and antiepileptic agents[3-6] (see Chapter 20)
  Inhaled recreational drugs (heroin, marijuana, cocaine, crystal methamphetamine)
Inhaled organic antigens
Churg–Strauss syndrome (EGPA)
Fungal hypersensitivity (ABPA/mycosis)
- Infections
- Loeffler syndrome (fleeting airspace infiltrates, often due to *Ascaris* or other intestinal parasites)
- Parasites
- Fungal infections, especially *Coccidioides*
- Pneumocystis
- Tuberculosis
- HIV infection
- Viral infections, especially respiratory syncytial virus

Unusual response to cigarette smoke (AEP and occasionally CEP)
  First-time smoking
  Resumption of cigarette smoking
  Change of cigarette brand or increased smoking amount
Malignancies
Collagen vascular disease (particularly rheumatoid arthritis)
Inflammatory bowel disease
Hypereosinophilic syndrome (>1,500 eosinophils/mm^3 for 6 months or longer)

Acute Eosinophilic Pneumonia

AEP (Table 15.2) is characterized by an abrupt onset, with symptoms present by definition for less than 1 month, but often for less than 7 days. Although the initial descriptions

<table>
<tr><td colspan="2">

Table 15.2

Features of AEP

Acute respiratory illness of <1 month and often <7 days duration

Severity varies from mild and self-limited to acute respiratory failure

Frequently systemic symptoms including fevers, night sweats, myalgias, chills, and pleuritic chest pain

Diffuse ground-glass opacities and/or consolidation on HRCT

Smooth interlobular septal thickening on HRCT

Pleural effusions common

>25% eosinophils on bronchoalveolar lavage

In most cases, no peripheral eosinophilia at presentation, but peripheral eosinophilia may develop over time

Pathologic diffuse alveolar damage (acute or organizing phase) with eosinophils or eosinophilic pneumonia on biopsy

Responds dramatically to steroids

</td><td>

Table 15.3

Features of CEP

Often long history (months) before diagnosis

Systemic symptoms (fever, night sweats, weight loss) common

History of asthma or atopy in many cases

Blood eosinophilia in 90% of cases

Peripheral consolidation, often migratory, on imaging

Pathologic patterns:

Classic form (sheets of eosinophils and macrophages)
- May have eosinophil necrosis with giant cells or granulomatous response
- Noncaseating granulomas seen in a small percentage of cases

OP with eosinophils

Cellular NSIP-like pattern with eosinophils

Acute fibrinous pneumonia and OP pattern with eosinophils

Irregular scarring with eosinophils

Minor degrees of vascular infiltration by eosinophils

</td></tr>
</table>

Note: Eosinophils may be relatively few in all but the classic form, especially if the patient has been treated with steroids before biopsy.

of AEP emphasized the rapid onset of respiratory failure, more recent studies have shown that the process varies from mild disease that may spontaneously remit to severe disease requiring mechanical ventilation. There appear to be differences in presentation/severity with different inciting agents; in particular, AEP related to cigarette smoking is often severe.[5] As opposed to CEP, patients with AEP typically are not asthmatic.

Systemic symptoms/signs in the form of fevers, night sweats, chills, and myalgias may be present. In the majority of patients, peripheral eosinophilia is not found at presentation, although blood eosinophilia may develop over time. By definition, the patient must have more than 25% eosinophils on bronchoalveolar lavage or an eosinophilic lung disease on biopsy.[1–4,9]

AEP is often, clinically, very similar to ARDS or a community-acquired pneumonia, and it is often only the presence of eosinophils on lavage or biopsy that indicates the correct diagnosis.

Chronic Eosinophilic Pneumonia

Most cases of CEP (Table 15.3) have an insidious onset and a longtime course of symptoms, often many months before diagnosis.[4] In addition to cough and shortness of breath, systemic symptoms (fever, weight loss, night sweats) are common. A history of asthma is present in 25% to 75% of patients, and in some instances overt asthma only develops after the onset of CEP.[4] Some patients have elevated serum immunoglobulin E (IgE) levels. Blood eosinophilia is seen in 90% of cases and eosinophils are frequently the

majority of white cells. Pulmonary function testing can show an obstructive or restrictive defect. Recurrences of CEP are common, often with the infiltrates in new areas of the lung.

IMAGING

Simple pulmonary eosinophilia (Loeffler syndrome) is characterized by transient and migratory areas of consolidation that typically clear spontaneously within 1 month (Figs. 15.1 and 15.2).[10] The areas of consolidation may be single or multiple and tend to have ill-defined margins on the radiograph. CT demonstrates patchy areas of consolidation and ground-glass opacities that usually have a predominantly peripheral distribution.[11] The main radiologic differential diagnosis includes pulmonary hemorrhage, organizing pneumonia (OP), and recurrent aspiration.

The radiographic and high-resolution computed tomography (HRCT) manifestations of AEP usually consist of extensive bilateral ground-glass opacities, patchy areas of consolidation, interlobular septal thickening, thickening of bronchovascular bundles, and bilateral pleural effusions without cardiomegaly[12] (Fig. 15.3, and see section Diagnostic Modalities) The radiologic differential diagnosis includes hydrostatic pulmonary edema, ARDS, and bacterial or viral pneumonia.

The classic description of the radiograph of CEP is that of peripheral airspace consolidation ("photographic negative shadow of pulmonary edema") involving mainly the upper lobes (Fig. 15.4).[10] It should be noted, however,

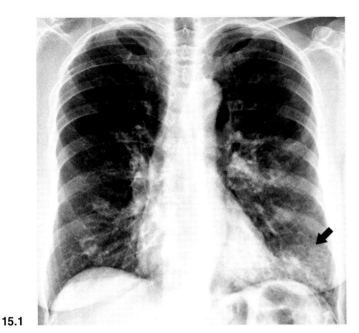
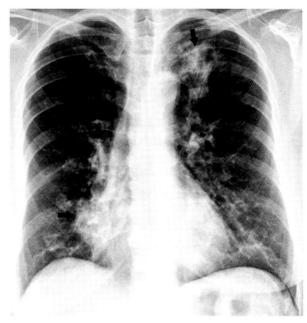

15.1

15.2

FIGURES 15.1 and 15.2. Simple pulmonary eosinophilia. **Figure 15.1:** Chest radiograph shows ill-defined areas of consolidation (*arrows*) in the left lower lobe. **Figure 15.2:** Chest radiograph 6 days later demonstrates new areas of consolidation (*arrows*) in the left upper and right middle lobes and almost complete resolution of the left lower lobe consolidation. The patient was a 54-year-old woman.

that this finding is present in fewer than 50% of cases. In the remaining patients, the peripheral distribution is not apparent on the radiograph, but it is usually present on HRCT, which demonstrates a peripheral predominance of consolidation and ground-glass opacities in more than 90% of cases (Fig. 15.5). The main radiologic differential diagnosis is with OP and Churg–Strauss syndrome (EGPA).

Rarely CEP may result in pulmonary fibrosis (Fig. 15.6).

PATHOLOGIC FEATURES

Simple eosinophilic pneumonia

Few cases are biopsied, but the morphologic picture is that of CEP (see below).

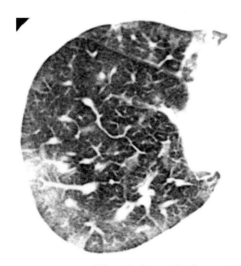

FIGURE 15.3. AEP. View of the right lower lobe from a HRCT shows diffuse ground-glass opacities, extensive thickening of the interlobular septa, and small foci of consolidation. Similar findings were present throughout both lungs. (Courtesy of Dr. Kiminori Fujimoto, Kurume, Japan.)

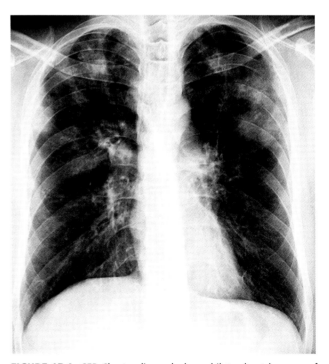

FIGURE 15.4. CEP. Chest radiograph shows bilateral patchy areas of consolidation mainly in the peripheral regions of the upper lobes. The patient was a 32-year-old man.

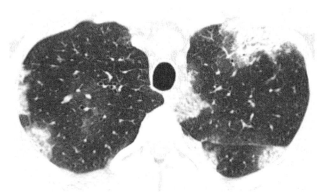

FIGURE 15.5. Chronic eosinophilic pneumonia. HRCT demonstrates peripheral consolidation and ground-glass opacities in the apical regions of the upper lobes. The patient was a 31-year-old woman.

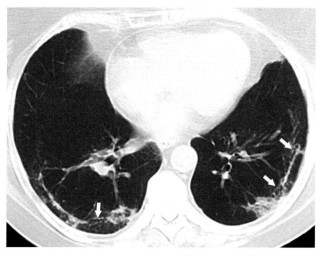

FIGURE 15.6. Fibrotic CEP. Conventional CT image at the level of the lower lung zones shows focal areas of peripheral reticulation and traction bronchiectasis (*arrows*) consistent with fibrosis. Also noted are peripheral band-like opacities and focal ground-glass opacities. Surgical biopsy demonstrated interstitial fibrosis with eosinophils.

Acute Eosinophilic Pneumonia

In its most severe form, AEP looks morphologically like diffuse alveolar damage but with added eosinophils[2] (Figs. 15.7 to 15.9) (Table 15.2). In ordinary diffuse alveolar damage/ARDS/acute interstitial pneumonia (AIP), eosinophils are extremely rare to nonexistent, so the finding of even a few is noteworthy and should suggest a diagnosis of AEP. The diffuse alveolar damage can be in the acute phase with hyaline membranes or demonstrates any morphologic pattern of organization typically seen in diffuse alveolar damage (DAD) (Figs. 15.7 and 15.8 and see Chapter 4). Eosinophils are usually fairly sparse, but occasionally are quite numerous, and the picture resembles more that of CEP with a few hyaline membranes, or sometimes simply CEP without evidence of diffuse alveolar damage.

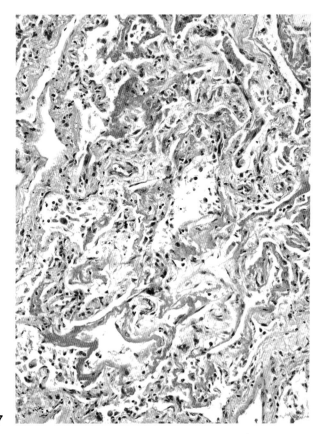

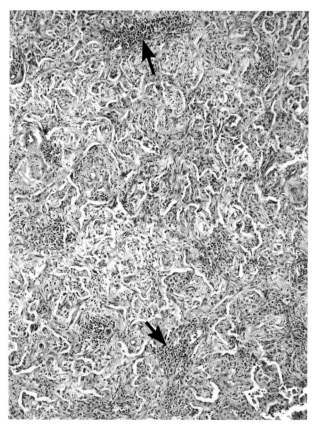

15.7

15.8

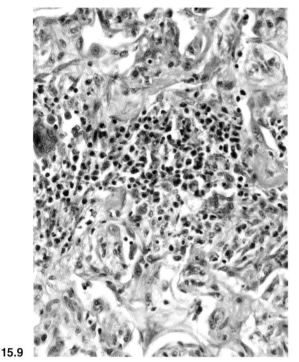

15.9

FIGURES 15.7 to 15.9. AEP. **Figures 15.7** and **15.8** show what at first appears to be ordinary acute and organizing diffuse alveolar damage. However, there are collections of eosinophils present in **Figures 15.8** (*arrows*) and **15.9**, indicating that this is actually AEP. Patient had received chemotherapeutic agents and developed acute respiratory failure.

Chronic Eosinophilic Pneumonia

CEP shows a considerable variety of morphologic patterns (Table 15.3). The classic form consists of sheets of eosinophils filling alveolar spaces (Figs. 15.10 and 15.11), that is, it looks like a bacterial pneumonia with eosinophils substituted for neutrophils. In our experience, this form is seen as the only pattern in a minority of cases. More frequently, there are large numbers of alveolar macrophages mixed with variable numbers of eosinophils (Figs. 15.12 and 15.13).

Areas of OP are extremely common in CEP (see Figs. 5.25, 5.26, 15.14 15.15, 18.20, and 18.21), and some cases look like OP at low power (see Fig. 18.20). Idiopathic OP can have occasional eosinophils, but once eosinophils are readily found (several per high-power field in multiple fields, or sheets of eosinophils) in what appears to be OP, a diagnosis of CEP is more likely.

Some cases of CEP demonstrate a fibrinous and organizing pneumonia picture[13] picture consisting of large amounts of alveolar fibrin mixed to a greater or lesser degree with OP-like granulation tissue (Figs. 15.16 and 15.17 and see Chapter 5 for a description of the fibrinous and organizing pneumonia pattern), whereas others mimic cellular nonspecific interstitial pneumonia (NSIP) (Fig. 15.18). Again, the presence of eosinophils indicates the correct diagnosis.

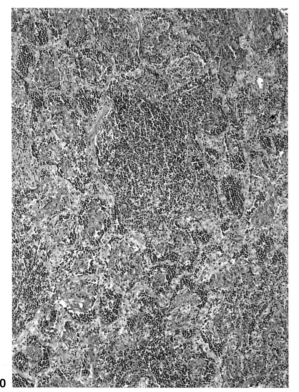

15.10

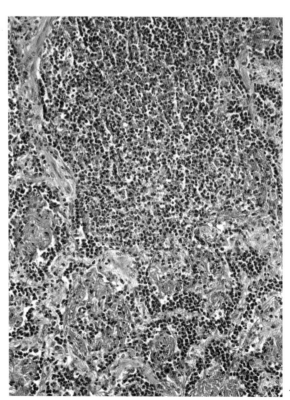

15.11

FIGURES 15.10 and 15.11. Classic pattern of CEP showing sheets of eosinophils filling airspaces. Patient cultivated mushrooms and mushroom exposure was believed clinically to be the source of his disease.

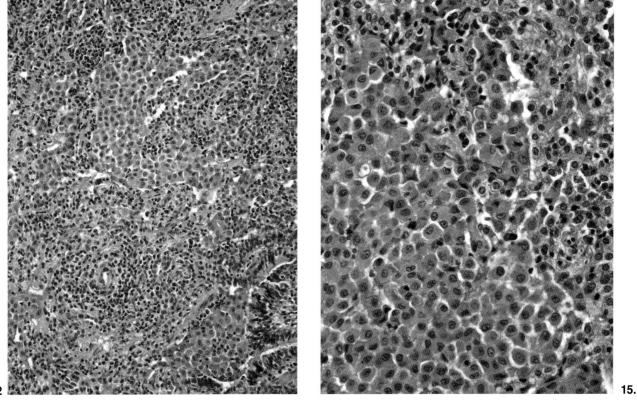

15.12   15.13

FIGURES 15.12 and 15.13. Pattern of CEP in which there are numerous airspace macrophages. Taken out of context, **Figure 15.13** could be mistaken for DIP because DIP typically has a few eosinophils; however, CEP and DIP are completely different on imaging, and DIP never has the number of eosinophils seen in **Figure 15.12**. Patient developed shortness of breath and consolidation after taking erythromycin.

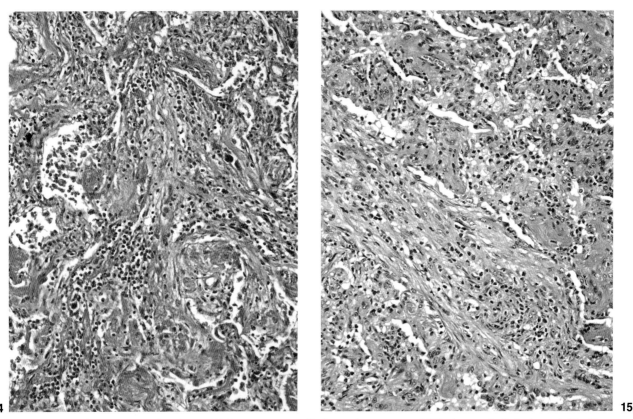

15.14   15.15

FIGURES 15.14 and 15.15. Areas of OP in CEP. This is a very common finding and some cases of CEP microscopically look mostly like OP.

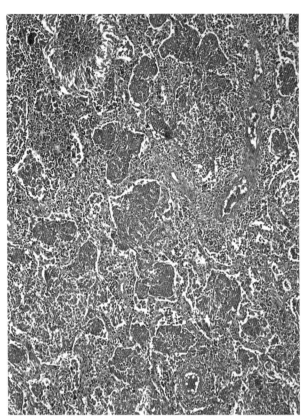 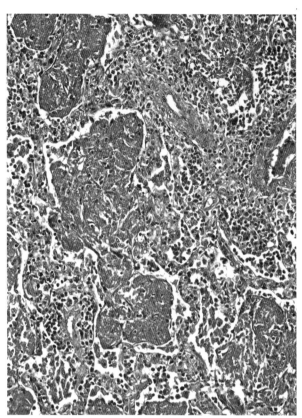

15.16   15.17

FIGURES 15.16 and 15.17. Marked airspace fibrin deposition in CEP (fibrinous and organizing pneumonia pattern). Cases like this should be simply reported as CEP.

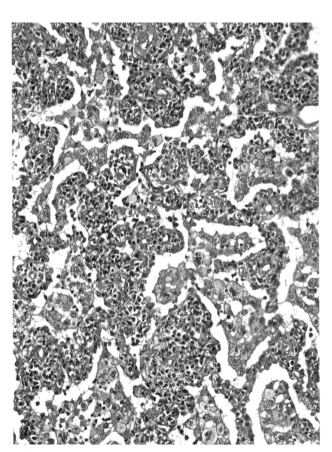

Noncaseating granulomas are found in 10% to 20% of CEP cases (Fig. 15.19). Necrosis of eosinophils (Fig. 15.20) with a giant cell or epithelioid histiocyte response producing a granulomatous pattern (Figs. 15.21 and 15.22) is seen in about 15% of cases.[14] This pattern is not, per se, indicative of underlying Churg–Strauss syndrome.[7] Minor degrees of infiltration of vessels by eosinophils and chronic inflammatory cells (Fig. 15.23) in the midst of areas of CEP are a frequent finding and also are not indicative of Churg–Strauss syndrome (EGPA) or underlying vasculitis.

CEP tends to wax and wane and appears in different areas of the lung over time; however, if disease keeps recurring in the same area, it can lead to fibrosis. There is very little in the literature on the patterns of fibrosis in CEP; in our experience, such cases can look more or less like fibrotic NSIP or have a patchy pattern of fibrosis somewhat mimicking usual interstitial pneumonia, but mixed with eosinophils. Fibroblast foci may be present.

Effects of Treatment on Morphologic Appearances

Eosinophils are exquisitely sensitive to steroids and undergo apoptosis in a dramatic and rapid fashion. If a biopsy is performed even 1 or 2 days after starting treatment with high-dose steroids, eosinophils may be very sparse. In this situation, a history of migratory peripheral consolidation

FIGURE 15.18. CEP mimicking cellular NSIP.

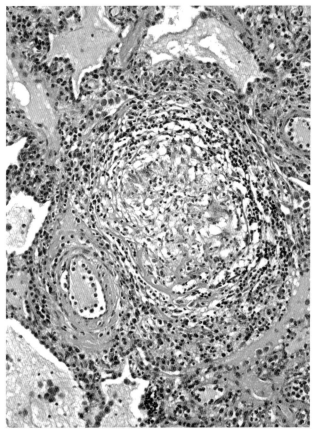

FIGURE 15.19. A noncaseating granuloma in the same case as Figures 15.12 and 15.13.

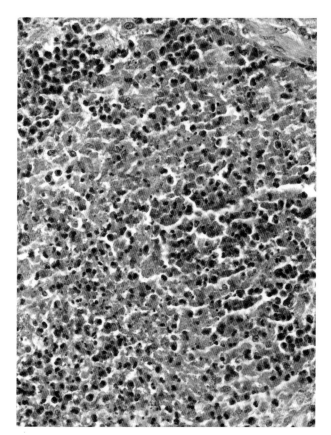

FIGURE 15.20. Early eosinophil necrosis in CEP.

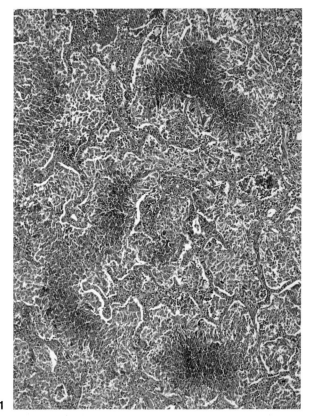

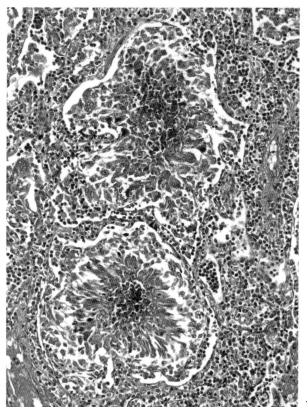

15.21

15.22

FIGURES 15.21 and 15.22. Areas of eosinophil necrosis with a granulomatous response. This is a common finding in CEP and does not change the diagnosis to Churg–Strauss syndrome.

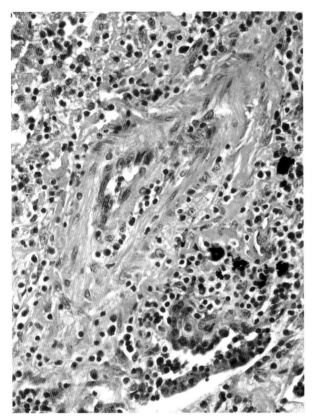

FIGURE 15.23. Vascular infiltration in chronic eosinophilic pneumonia. Minor degrees of vascular infiltration such as this are common and do not indicate a diagnosis of vasculitis.

on imaging or a high lavage or serum eosinophil count prior to steroids are important clues to the correct diagnosis.

Diagnostic Modalities

Given an appropriate clinical and imaging setting, CEP can sometimes be diagnosed without need for a biopsy. Transbronchial biopsy is sometimes diagnostic (see Figs. 18.20 and 18.21), but in most cases video-assisted thoracoscopic surgery (VATS) biopsy is used. As is true of AIP/ARDS, AEP is more difficult to diagnose on transbronchial biopsy because the diagnostic features (eosinophils) may be focal; however, given a patient with a clinical and imaging picture of ARDS, a transbronchial biopsy showing diffuse alveolar damage and eosinophils would allow a definitive diagnosis. Cryobiopsy is suitable for the diagnosis of eosinophilic pneumonias,[15] although the yield versus VATS biopsy is not known. Bronchoalveolar lavage is also a useful diagnostic approach if the clinical and radiologic findings are consistent with an eosinophilic pneumonia; the finding of greater than 25% eosinophils is then considered diagnostic (Figs. 15.24 and 15.25).[4]

DIFFERENTIAL DIAGNOSIS

Major differential diagnoses are listed in Table 15.4. The morphologic distinction between diffuse alveolar damage representing AEP and diffuse alveolar damage representing AIP/ARDS depends entirely on the finding of eosinophils

15.24

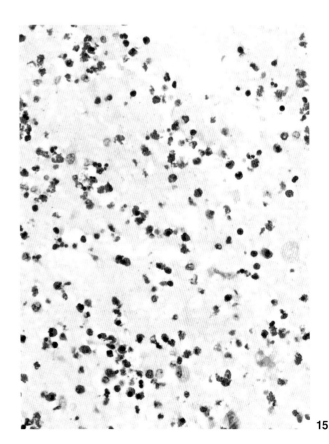

FIGURES 15.24 and 15.25. AEP in a patient given levofloxacin. Administration of the drug was followed by the rapid onset of hypoxic respiratory failure and development of extensive bilateral ground-glass opacities and consolidation involving mainly the dependent lung regions (**Fig. 15.24**). Also noted is interlobular septal thickening (*arrows*). Lavage showed greater than 25% eosinophils (**Fig. 15.25**), thus confirming the diagnosis.

15.25

Table 15.4

Morphologic differential diagnosis of eosinophilic pneumonias

AEP	Diffuse alveolar damage (AIP/ARDS)
CEP	OP
	Langerhans cell histiocytosis
	Hodgkin disease
	Reactive eosinophilic pleuritis
	DIP
	Churg–Strauss syndrome (EGPA)
	ABPA

in the former. The underlying patterns of diffuse alveolar damage are not distinguishable.

The most important differential diagnosis of CEP is OP, and occasionally a VATS biopsy in a patient with peripheral consolidation on imaging shows OP with a small increase in eosinophils but not enough to be overtly diagnosable as CEP. In that setting, we recommend making a comment to the effect that CEP should be considered; this alerts the clinician to look for blood eosinophilia and also for a potential offending agent.

Langerhans cell histiocytosis (Chapter 10) may have numerous eosinophils but the cellular nodules are primarily composed of S-100/CD1a-positive Langerhans cells, there are often smoker's macrophages mixed in, and the nodules center on small airways (see Fig. 10.10).

Classical Hodgkin disease in the lung has a lymphocytic background with a few eosinophils but Reed–Sternberg cells are also present; the lesions are typically nodular and center around the bronchovascular bundles.

Reactive eosinophilic pleuritis (see Figs. 10.40 and 10.41) may also have large numbers of eosinophils, but they are confined to the pleural space and there is no underlying lung disease, or only subpleural and pleural blebs.

Desquamative interstitial pneumonia (DIP; Chapter 8) usually has small numbers of eosinophils mixed with the alveolar macrophages or in the interstitium (see Fig. 8.17), and a given field of DIP and CEP may be indistinguishable (compare Figs. 8.17, 15.12, and 5.13); however, in most cases of CEP, there are areas with considerably greater numbers of eosinophils and in doubtful cases imaging will solve the problem. The separation of CEP, Churg–Strauss syndrome (EGPA), and ABPA is sometimes morphologically problematic because all three conditions can produce a picture of CEP (Table 15.5). Some cases of Churg–Strauss syndrome are difficult to separate from CEP because asthma

Table 15.5

Separation of CEP, Churg–Strauss Syndrome (CSS, EGPA), and ABPA

Feature	CEP	CSS (EGPA)	ABPA
Asthma	25% to 75% of cases	100% of cases	Almost all cases[a]
Blood eosinophilia	>90% of cases	100% of cases	Yes
Elevated IgE	Yes	Yes	Very high
Serum precipitins against *Aspergillus*	No	No	Yes
Cutaneous reaction to injected *Aspergillus* antigen	No	No	Yes
ANCA	Negative	p-ANCA 50% of cases	Negative
Imaging	Consolidation, typically peripheral	Often consolidation, may be peripheral	Central mucoid impaction and bronchiectasis
Pathologic picture of eosinophilic pneumonia	Yes	Often	Usually a minor component[b]
True vasculitis	No[c]	Sometimes	No
Bronchiectasis	No	No	Yes
Mucoid impaction	No	No	Yes[b]
Bronchocentric granulomatosis	No	No	Yes[b]
Cellular bronchiolitis with eosinophils	No	No	Yes[b]

[a]ABPA is also seen in patients with cystic fibrosis who are not asthmatic.
[b]Any of these features may or may not be present in a given case of ABPA.
[c]CEP may show minor degrees of vascular infiltration within the inflammatory lesions.

is present in 100% of Churg–Strauss syndrome patients and many CEP patients, and both conditions are associated with blood eosinophilia (Table 15.5). Many, but not all, Churg–Strauss syndrome patients have evidence of systemic vasculitis and a positive antineutrophil cytoplasmic antibodies (ANCA),[7] findings that do not occur in CEP.

Morphologically, Churg–Strauss syndrome in the lung can be identical to CEP (Fig. 15.26) or it can have a picture of CEP with true vasculitis. Necrosis of eosinophils with or without a granulomatous response is seen in both Churg–Strauss syndrome and ordinary CEP and is not useful as a diagnostic separator. As noted above, minor degrees of vascular infiltration by eosinophils and lymphocytes are common in CEP (Fig. 15.23) and do not constitute vasculitis. Features that suggest a true vasculitis are necrosis of vessel walls, marked infiltration of vessel walls by eosinophils in the midst of CEP-like area, or infiltration of vessel walls by eosinophils away from areas of CEP (Fig. 15.27).

ABPA/mycosis is a hypersensitivity reaction to ambient fungi, and the sensitizing agent is almost always Aspergillus.[8] Most cases of ABPA occur in asthmatics, but some occur in patients with cystic fibrosis who are not asthmatic (Table 15.5). Pathologically, eosinophilic pneumonia, which is morphologically indistinguishable from ordinary

CEP, is one of the features that can be seen in ABPA, but it is usually a minor component and is absent in many cases. Central bronchiectasis with or without mucoid impaction is much more common than eosinophilic pneumonia, and there may also be bronchocentric granulomatosis or bronchiolitis, typically associated with eosinophils.

PROGNOSIS

Simple eosinophilic pneumonia is, more or less by definition, a self-limited process. AEP responds dramatically and rapidly to steroids.[1,4,9] Because most other forms of ARDS/AIP are resistant to steroids, correct identification of AEP on biopsy is crucial to treatment. CEP also responds rapidly to steroids, but a significant proportion of patients have a relapse after steroids are tapered, although most again resolve when steroids are reinstituted.[1,4] The disappearance of clinical symptoms within 2 to 3 days and clearing of imaging infiltrates within a week after initiation of steroid therapy are virtually diagnostic of an eosinophilic pneumonia.

Interleukin-5 (IL-5) is a cytokine that causes eosinophil maturation and leads to increased levels of eosinophils in the blood. In addition, it prolongs eosinophil

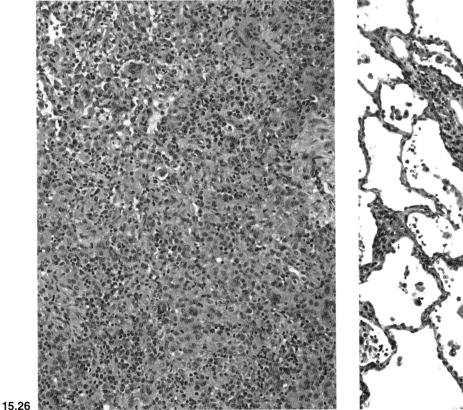

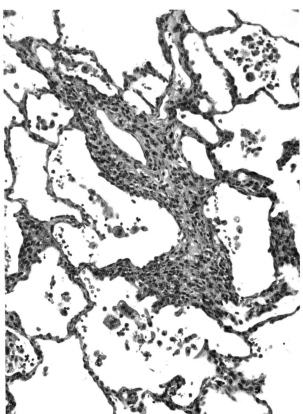

FIGURES 15.26 and 15.27. Churg–Strauss syndrome (EGPA). Parts of the biopsy show a morphologic picture that is indistinguishable from ordinary CEP (**Fig. 15.26**); however, there is also marked infiltration of vessel walls by eosinophils away from areas of eosinophilic pneumonia (**Fig. 15.27**), indicating that the correct diagnosis is Churg–Strauss syndrome.

lifetime in the blood, activates eosinophils, and enhances migration into tissues.[16] Anti-IL-5 drugs (mepolizumab and reslizumab) are now clinically available, and in Churg–Strauss syndrome mepolizumab has been shown to increase remission intervals and increase the number of patients in remission compared to steroids alone.[17] These drugs potentially may be useful as steroid-sparing agents in patients with eosinophilic pneumonias.

REFERENCES

1. Fernández Pérez ER, Olson AL, Frankel SK. Eosinophilic lung diseases. *Med Clin North Am.* 2011;95:1163–1187.
2. Tazelaar HD, Linz LJ, Colby TV, et al. Acute eosinophilic pneumonia: histopathologic findings in nine patients. *Am J Respir Crit Care Med.* 1997;155:296–302.
3. De Giacomi F, Vassallo R, Yi ES, et al. Acute eosinophilic pneumonia. Causes, diagnosis, and management. *Am J Respir Crit Care Med.* 2018;197:728–736.
4. Cottin V. Eosinophilic lung diseases. *Clin Chest Med.* 2016;37:535–556.
5. De Giacomi F, Decker PA, Vassallo R, et al. Acute eosinophilic pneumonia: correlation of clinical characteristics with underlying cause. *Chest.* 2017;152:379–385.
6. Bartal C, Sagy I, Barski L. Drug-induced eosinophilic pneumonia: a review of 196 case reports. *Medicine (Baltimore).* 2018;97:e9688.
7. Churg A. Recent advances in the diagnosis of Churg-Strauss syndrome. *Mod Pathol.* 2001;14:1284–1293.
8. Hogan C, Denning DW. Allergic bronchopulmonary aspergillosis and related allergic syndromes. *Semin Respir Crit Care Med.* 2011;32:682–692.
9. Philit F, Etienne-Mastroïanni B, Parrot A, et al. Idiopathic acute eosinophilic pneumonia: a study of 22 patients. *Am J Respir Crit Care Med.* 2002;166:1235–1239.
10. Jeong YJ, Kim KI, Seo IJ, et al. Eosinophilic lung diseases: a clinical, radiologic, and pathologic overview. *Radiographics.* 2007;27:617–637.
11. Price M, Gilman MD, Carter BW, et al. Imaging of eosinophilic lung diseases. *Radiol Clin North Am.* 2016;54:1151–1164.
12. Daimon T, Johkoh T, Sumikawa H, et al. Acute eosinophilic pneumonia: thin-section CT findings in 29 patients. *Eur J Radiol.* 2008;65:462–467.
13. Beasley MB, Franks TJ, Galvin JR, et al. Acute fibrinous and organizing pneumonia: a histological pattern of lung injury and possible variant of diffuse alveolar damage. *Arch Pathol Lab Med.* 2002;126:1064–1070.
14. Colby TV, Carrington CB. Interstitial lung disease. In: Thurlbeck WM, Churg A, eds. *Pathology of the Lung.* 2nd ed. New York, NY: Thieme Medical Publishers; 1995:668.
15. Ussavarungsi K, Kern RM, Roden AC, et al. Transbronchial cryobiopsy in diffuse parenchymal lung disease: retrospective analysis of 74 cases. *Chest.* 2017;151:400–408.
16. Domingo C. Overlapping effects of new monoclonal antibodies for severe asthma. *Drugs.* 2017;77:1769–1787.
17. Wechsler ME, Akuthota P, Jayne D, et al; EGPA Mepolizumab Study Team. Mepolizumab or placebo for eosinophilic granulomatosis with polyangiitis. *N Engl J Med.* 2017;376:1921–1932.

Pulmonary Alveolar Proteinosis

DEFINITION

Pulmonary alveolar proteinosis (PAP) is an interstitial lung disease in which there is filling of alveolar spaces by lipoproteinaceous material as a result of an abnormality in surfactant homeostasis.[1] PAP is uncommon: the incidence in a recent study from Japan was 0.49 cases per million.[2]

ETIOLOGY AND SUBCLASSIFICATION

Surfactant is secreted by type II cells and normally is degraded by alveolar macrophages and type II cells. The function of surfactant is to lower surface tension, preventing alveolar collapse; surfactant proteins A, B, C, and D also play an important role in innate immunity in the lung.[1,3]

In PAP, surfactant is not degraded but instead accumulates in alveolar spaces where it appears microscopically as coarsely granular eosinophilic material. PAP can be subclassified by the etiology of surfactant accumulation. Alveolar macrophages require granulocyte-macrophage colony-stimulating factor (GM-CSF) for maturation to a fully functional cell that has the ability to degrade surfactant, and 90% of PAP cases are caused by the development of circulating anti-GM-CSF antibodies (called primary or autoimmune PAP) (Fig. 16.1). GM-CSF is also required for the normal immune function of myeloid cells, and neutrophils from PAP patients have impaired antimicrobial properties.[1]

Most of the remaining cases are labeled secondary and have a variety of associations including hematologic disorders, other forms of malignancy, immunosuppression, exposure to exogenous dusts and fumes, and drugs (Table 16.1), all of which are believed to be mediated through impaired macrophage function (Table 16.1).

A very small percentage of cases are caused by mutations that affect the structure and function of surfactant genes, GM-CSF itself, or genes related to GM-CSF signaling; these are referred to as congenital or hereditary PAP (Table 16.1). There are also rare cases in which neither anti-GM-CSF antibodies nor genetic abnormalities are found.[1,4,5]

Normal surfactant secretion and degradation

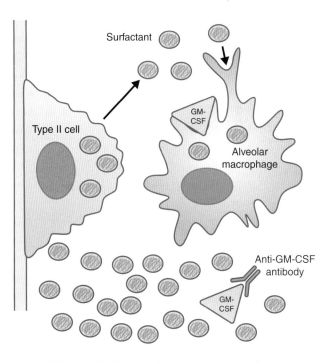

Autoimmune (primary) pulmonary alveolar proteinosis

FIGURE 16.1. Pathogenesis of primary (autoimmune) PAP. Surfactant is secreted by type II cells and is normally phagocytized and degraded by alveolar macrophages; this process requires binding of GM-CSF to the macrophage GM-CSF receptor. In primary (autoimmune) PAP, antibodies to GM-CSF prevent GM-CSF binding to the macrophage receptor, leading to failure of macrophage maturation and accumulation of surfactant as proteinosis material in the airspaces.

CLINICAL FEATURES

The clinical features of PAP are nonspecific and include cough, shortness of breath, malaise, and sometimes chest pain or weight loss, usually developing in an indolent fashion. Chest examination is frequently unremarkable, although crackles, clubbing, and cyanosis have occasionally been reported. There appears to be an association with smoking, and also with dust exposure, even in patients who have autoimmune PAP.[1,6]

Table 16.1

Etiologic Classification and Reported Associations of Pulmonary Alveolar Proteinosis

Primary (also called acquired or autoimmune): caused by anti-GM-CSF antibodies

Secondary

Hematologic malignancies, especially leukemias and myelodysplastic syndromes

Nonhematologic malignancies

Immunodeficiency states

Inhalation of very high levels of very finely divided mineral dust (8[a])

  Silica (called silicoproteinosis or acute silicosis) (9)

  Aluminum (10)

  Indium compounds (11)

  Titanium dioxide (12)

Organic dusts[a] (3) including sawdust, bakery flour, and fertilizer

Earthquake dust (exact agent unclear) (13)

Fumes[a] (3) including chlorine, cleaning products, gasoline, synthetic plastic fumes, paint fumes, varnish fumes, hydrofluoric acid

Drug reactions (1)

  Chemotherapeutic agents, especially busulfan

  Cyclosporin

  Dasatinib

  Imatinib

  Leflunomide

  Mycophenolate mofetil

  Sirolimus

  Inhaled Fentanyl patches (see Figures 18-16 to 18-18)

Occasionally seen in fibrosing interstitial pneumonias as a local phenomenon

Hereditary

  Mutations in *GM-CSF* gene

  Mutations in GM-CSF receptor genes (*CSF2RA, CSF2RB*)

  Mutations in surfactant structure/production genes (*SFTPB, SFTPC, BCA3, TTF1*)

---

[a]Apart from silica and indium, the specific agents listed in this part of Table 16.1 are largely represented in the literature by single case reports and it is not known whether these are actual causes of PAP.

GM-CSF antibody levels are the only established biomarker, and elevated levels are essentially 100% specific and sensitive for autoimmune PAP.[3]

IMAGING

The chest radiograph usually shows patchy bilateral areas of consolidation with relative sparing of the apices and costophrenic angles. The characteristic high-resolution

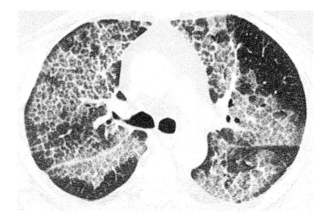

FIGURE 16.2. High-resolution CT scan showing ground-glass opacities and interlobular septal thickening ("crazy paving"), typical of PAP.

computed tomography (CT) manifestation consists of bilateral ground-glass opacities with a superimposed fine linear pattern because of interlobular septal thickening, a combination known as crazy-paving pattern[7] (Fig. 16.2). The areas of crazy-paving pattern often have sharply defined margins with geographic or lobular sparing. Although the crazy-paving pattern is relatively nonspecific, in patients with chronic symptoms, it should raise the possibility of PAP.

PATHOLOGIC FEATURES

Grossly, PAP appears as a yellow homogeneous soft material that fills airspaces; the process can be quite patchy (Fig. 16.3). The characteristic microscopic feature of

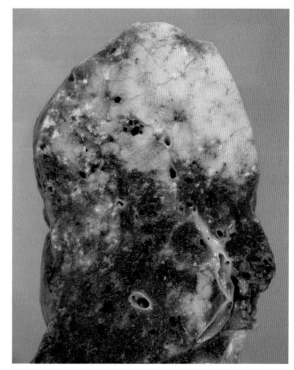

FIGURE 16.3. Gross appearance of PAP characterized by soft yellow material completely filling the airspaces in a localized area. (Case Courtesy Dr. Julia Flint.)

PAP is filling of alveolar spaces by coarsely granular eosinophilic material that frequently contains rounded or elongated dense bodies, probably representing dead macrophages (Figs. 16.4 to 16.6). Cholesterol clefts and small numbers of foamy macrophages may also be present in the granular material. Proteinosis material is strongly digested periodic acid–Schiff (dPAS) positive (Fig. 16.7), and this is useful for distinguishing it from edema fluid that is dPAS negative (see below).

Mild degrees of interstitial inflammation and/or very mild interstitial fibrosis that just slightly thickens alveolar walls are occasionally present, more often, in our experience, in secondary forms of PAP than in primary forms (Figs. 16.8 and 16.9). PAP resulting from exposure to indium compounds is reported to be frequently associated with fibrosis, but the diagnosis of fibrosis has been generally made on imaging, and the pathologic findings in such cases are unclear.[8]

Silicoproteinosis typically has a mild chronic interstitial infiltrate, and polarization may reveal fine pale orange birefringent particles of silica (Fig. 16.10), but in some cases the silica particles are too small to be seen by light microscopy. Other dusts that have been reported to cause proteinosis are often too finely divided to be visible by light microscopy, although they can be detected by electron microscopy (Fig. 16.11).

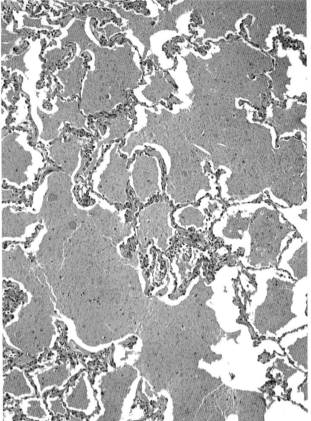

16.5

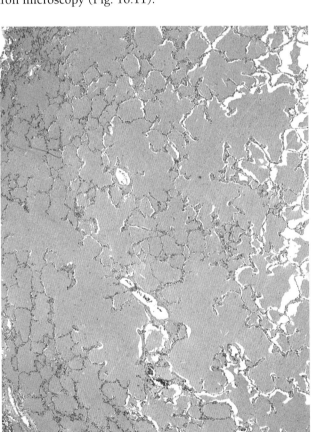

16.4

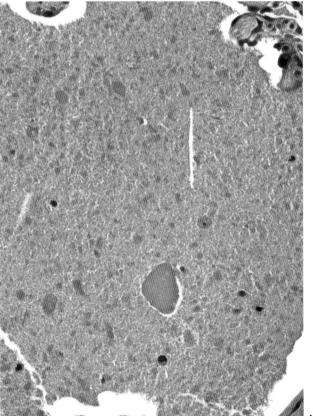

16.6

FIGURES 16.4 to 16.6. PAP showing filling of airspaces by coarsely granular eosinophilic material. Note the absence of interstitial inflammation and interstitial fibrosis: this is the typical finding in most cases of PAP. At high power (**Fig. 16.5**), the proteinosis material is distinctly granular and contains densely eosinophilic structures that may represent the remains of alveolar macrophages.

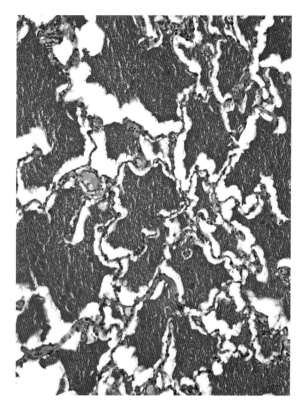

FIGURE 16.7. Digested PAS stain shows intense staining of the proteinosis material. Digested PAS stain is useful for separating PAP from pulmonary edema that is PAS negative (compare Fig. 16.14).

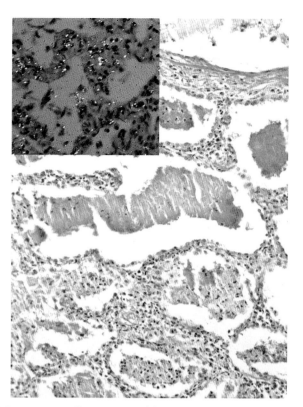

FIGURE 16.10. Silicoproteinosis (also called acute silicosis). In silicoproteinosis, there typically is an interstitial chronic inflammatory infiltrate. Inset shows birefringent silica particles.

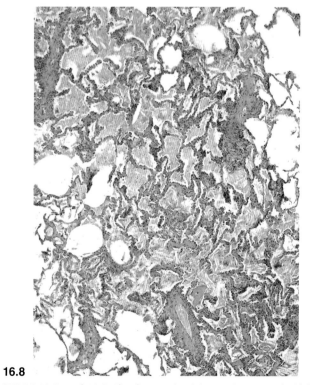

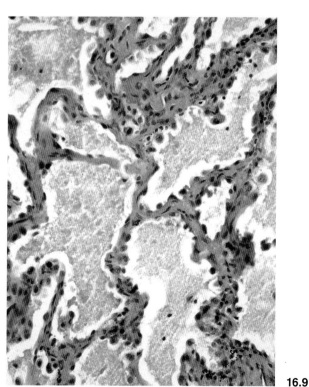

16.8

16.9

FIGURES 16.8 and 16.9. Alveolar proteinosis in a patient treated with busulfan for a hematologic malignancy. In this example, there is fine interstitial fibrosis that may be part of the PAP but may also reflect busulfan toxicity.

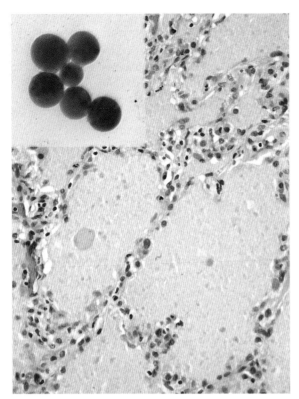

FIGURE 16.11. PAP in a man who ground aluminum metal. PAP is seen in some patients exposed to very high levels of very finely divided dust. Inset: Electron micrograph showing submicron aluminum spheres recovered from a digest of the biopsy. (Reproduced by permission from Miller RR, Churg AM, Hutcheon M, et al. Pulmonary alveolar proteinosis and aluminum dust exposure. *Am Rev Respir Dis.* 1984;130:312–315.)

Verma et al.[9] reported five cases of PAP that also had morphologic changes of hypersensitivity pneumonitis, including bronchiolocentric interstitial inflammation and non-necrotizing granulomas. Three of the patients had bird exposures. The two patients in whom testing was performed did not have anti-GM-CSF antibodies.

DIFFERENTIAL DIAGNOSIS

Edema fills airspaces with eosinophilic material that is smooth or very finely granular rather than coarsely granular as in PAP, may show chatter artifact from cutting, and is dPAS negative (Figs. 16.12 to 16.14).

Pneumocystis is characterized by filling of airspaces by foamy rather than granular eosinophilic material (Fig. 16.15), and organisms are visible on silver stains.

PAP associated with marked interstitial fibrosis or chronic inflammation or distortion of the underlying lung architecture by fibrosis suggests another underlying process such as fibrosis secondary to a chemotherapeutic agent or a fibrosing interstitial pneumonia in which the proteinosis may be a local finding.

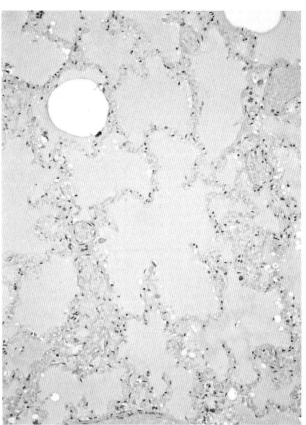

16.12

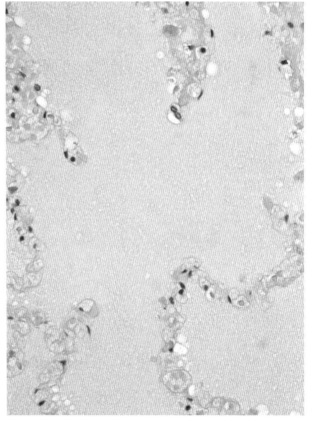

16.13

FIGURES 16.12 to 16.14. See figure legend 6.14.

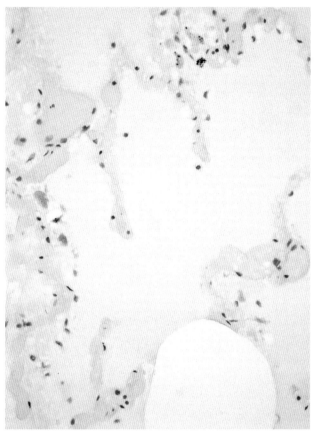

16.14

FIGURES 16.12 to 16.14. Pulmonary edema. In contrast to proteinosis material, edema fluid appears smooth or very finely granular and does not stain with digested PAS (Fig 16.14).

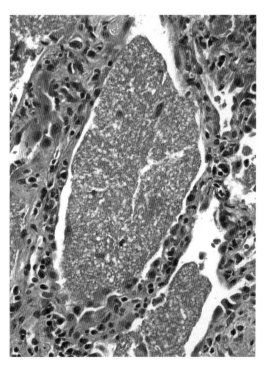

FIGURE 16.15. Pneumocystis pneumonia. In contrast to proteinosis fluid, *Pneumocystis* produces foamy eosinophilic material in which fine dots are often visible.

DIAGNOSTIC MODALITIES

Transbronchial biopsy can be used to diagnose PAP (Figs. 16.16 and 16.17), but areas with PAP can be patchy and may be missed on transbronchial biopsy. Cryobiopsy has

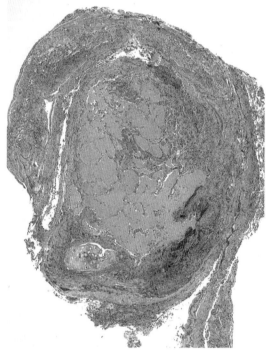

16.16

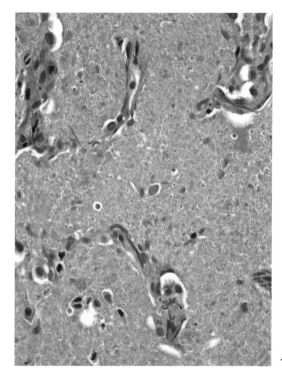

16.17

FIGURES 16.16 and 16.17. PAP in a transbronchial biopsy. PAP is readily diagnosed in transbronchial biopsies if the biopsy samples the lesion, but PAP can be patchy (compare Fig. 16.3) and is often missed by transbronchial biopsy.

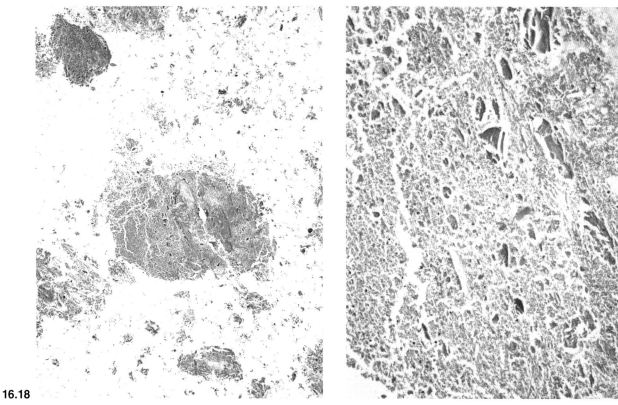

16.18 **16.19**

FIGURES 16.18 and 16.19. Low- and high-power views of proteinosis material in lavage fluid stained with dPAS. The material is essentially identical to what is seen in the alveolar spaces in histologic sections.

been used for the diagnosis of PAP.[10] Microscopic examination of bronchoalveolar lavage fluid can also be employed: the diagnostic finding is granular dPAS-positive material that looks like proteinosis material as seen in histologic sections (Figs. 16.18 and 16.19).

COMPLICATIONS

Infection with opportunistic organisms such as *Nocardia*, *Aspergillus*, *Mycobacterium tuberculosis*, atypical mycobacteria, and *Pneumocystis* can be seen in patients with PAP.[1] This probably reflects defective macrophage and neutrophil killing of organisms, because of lack of GM-CSF or GM-CSF signaling (see section Etiology and Subclassification).

TREATMENT AND PROGNOSIS

A small percentage of patients with primary (autoimmune) PAP have a spontaneous remission, but most require treatment with large-volume (whole-lung) bronchoalveolar lavage. This is effective in most cases in relieving symptoms, but recurrence rates up to 70% have been reported and lavage may need to be repeated. Treatment with injected or aerosolized GM-CSF has also been employed; in one study from Japan[11] 6 months of treatment with inhaled

GM-CSF produced a remission in about two-thirds of patients and the remissions lasted at least 30 months. More recently rituximab has been reported to be effective in a handful of cases.[1]

The prognosis of primary PAP is good, with 5-year survival rates of 85% to 94%,[12,13] but these figures may be biased by inclusion of older cases; in newer material, the survival rate is typically 100%.[3] The prognosis of hereditary PAP depends on the exact mutation; some are lethal. The prognosis of secondary PAP depends on the underlying cause of the process, particularly in patients with underlying malignancies. Recent data suggest the prognosis in such patients is poor.[6] The prognosis of silicoproteinosis is also poor, even with lavage,[14,15] and this may be true of exposure to other mineral dusts, although data are scanty.[15]

Proteinosis as an incidental local finding in a fibrosing interstitial pneumonia probably has no prognostic significance.

REFERENCES

1. Kumar A, Abdelmalak B, Inoue Y, et al. Pulmonary alveolar proteinosis in adults: pathophysiology and clinical approach. *Lancet Respir Med.* 2018;6:554–565. doi:10.1016/S2213-2600(18)30043-2.
2. Inoue Y, Trapnell BC, Tazawa R, et al; Japanese Center of the Rare Lung Diseases Consortium. Characteristics of a large

cohort of patients with autoimmune pulmonary proteinosis in Japan. *Am J Respir Crit Care Med.* 2008;177:752–762.

3. Suzuki T, Trapnell BC. Pulmonary alveolar proteinosis syndrome. *Clin Chest Med.* 2016;37:431–440.

4. Martinez-Moczygemba M, Huston DP. Immune dysregulation in the pathogenesis of pulmonary alveolar proteinosis. *Curr Allergy Asthma Rep.* 2010;10:320–325.

5. Carey B, Trapnell BC. The molecular basis of pulmonary alveolar proteinosis. *Clin Immunol.* 2010;135:223–235.

6. Ishii H, Tazawa R, Kaneko C, et al. Clinical features of secondary pulmonary alveolar proteinosis: pre-mortem cases in Japan. *Eur Respir J.* 2011;37:465–468.

7. Frazier AA, Franks TJ, Cooke EO, et al. From the archives of the AFIP: pulmonary alveolar proteinosis. *Radiographics.* 2008;28:883–899.

8. Cummings KJ, Nakano M, Omae K, et al. Indium lung disease. *Chest.* 2012;141:1512–1521.

9. Verma H, Nicholson AG, Kerr KM, et al. Alveolar proteinosis with hypersensitivity pneumonitis: a new clinical phenotype. *Respirology.* 2010;15:1197–1202.

10. Ussavarungsi K, Kern RM, Roden AC, et al. Transbronchial cryobiopsy in diffuse parenchymal lung disease: retrospective analysis of 74 cases. *Chest.* 2017;151:400–408.

11. Tazawa R, Inoue Y, Arai T, et al. Duration of benefit in patients with autoimmune pulmonary alveolar proteinosis after inhaled granulocyte-macrophage colony-stimulating factor therapy. *Chest.* 2014;145:729–737.

12. Luisetti M, Kadija Z, Mariani F, et al. Therapy options in pulmonary alveolar proteinosis. *Ther Adv Respir Dis.* 2010;4:239–248.

13. Chung MJ, Lee KS, Franquet T, et al. Metabolic lung disease: imaging and histopathologic findings. *Eur J Radiol.* 2005;54:233–245.

14. Souza CA, Marchiori E, Gonçalves LP, et al. Comparative study of clinical, pathological and HRCT findings of primary alveolar proteinosis and silicoproteinosis. *Eur J Radiol.* 2012;81:371–378.

15. Xiao YL, Xu KF, Li Y, et al. Occupational inhalational exposure and serum GM-CSF autoantibody in pulmonary alveolar proteinosis. *Occup Environ Med.* 2015;72:504–512.

16. Bomhard EM. Particle-induced pulmonary alveolar proteinosis and subsequent inflammation and fibrosis: a toxicologic and pathologic review. *Toxicol Pathol.* 2017;45:389–440.

17. Miller RR, Churg AM, Hutcheon M, et al. Pulmonary alveolar proteinosis and aluminum dust exposure. *Am Rev Respir Dis.* 1984;130:312–315.

18. Keller CA, Frost A, Cagle PT, et al. Pulmonary alveolar proteinosis in a painter with elevated pulmonary concentrations of titanium. *Chest.* 1995;108:277–280.

19. Hisata S, Moriyama H, Tazawa R, et al. Development of pulmonary alveolar proteinosis following exposure to dust after the Great East Japan Earthquake. *Respir Invest.* 2013;51:212–216.

Lymphangioleiomyomatosis

NATURE AND PATHOGENESIS

Although lymphangioleiomyomatosis (LAM) is traditionally regarded as a form of interstitial lung disease, there is an emerging consensus that it is actually a neoplastic process that is either an unusual form of PEComa (perivascular epithelioid cell tumor) or is very closely related to PEComas.[1,2] The evidence for a neoplastic process is summarized in Table 17.1. Circulating LAM cells can be found in lung, chylous effusions, and urine (Fig. 17.1), and when LAM recurs in lung transplants, the LAM cells in the transplanted lung show the same mutations as are present in the patient's original lesions. LAM cells show destructive behavior in the lung with inappropriate proliferation, angiogenesis and lymphangiogenesis, and destruction of lung matrix secondary to protease production. Metabolically, LAM cells use aerobic glycolysis (the Warburg effect), a finding typical of many malignant neoplasms. In a

Table 17.1

Evidence supporting the idea that LAM is a neoplasm

Presence of circulating LAM cells in blood, chylous effusions, and urine

Identical mutations found in lung LAM cells, nodal lymphangiomyomas, and angiomyolipomas in a given case, suggesting seeding from a common source

Loss of heterozygosity for TSC genes in lung LAM lesions, angiomyolipomas, and lymphangiomyomas

Inappropriate invasion, proliferation, angiogenesis, lymphangiogenesis, and protease-driven matrix destruction, features common to other malignant neoplasms

LAM cells use aerobic glycolysis (Warburg effect), a finding in many malignant tumors

Recurrent LAM cells in lung transplants have the same genetic abnormalities as are present in the original host LAM cells

Ability to stop progression of LAM by inhibiting mTORC1 signaling

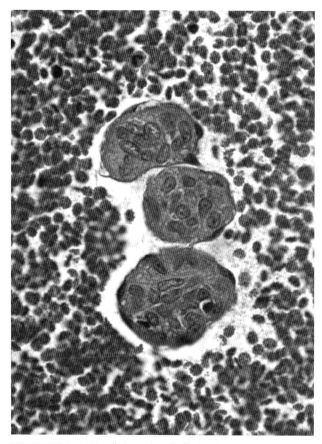

FIGURE 17.1. LAM cells in a pleural effusion (Courtesy Dr. Thomas V Colby).

given patient with LAM and angiomyolipomas or lymphangiomyomas, all lesions show identical mutations, and there is commonly loss of heterozygosity in LAM cells.

LAM may be sporadic or associated with tuberous sclerosis (TSC), and the genetic abnormality in most cases is a mutation in either *TSC1* (tuberous sclerosis 1), which produces a protein called hamartin, thought to have a role in actin cytoskeleton organization, or *TSC2* (tuberous sclerosis 2), which produces tuberin, a protein involved in cell growth and cell cycle/cell proliferation control.[3] Sporadic LAM in general shows biallelic somatic *TSC2* mutations, whereas TSC-associated LAM usually shows *TSC1* germ-line mutations. However, these rules are not absolute and occasional sporadic LAM cases have *TSC1* mutations.[4] Of note, PEComas typically have TSC2 mutations.[1]

Hamartin and tuberin combine with the protein product of *TBC1D7* to form a complex that normally down-regulates mTORC1, the mammalian target of rapamycin complex 1 (Fig. 17.2). mTORC1 itself is a protein complex that functions as a sensor of cell energy/redox status/nutrient status, is driven by growth factors including estrogen, and controls downstream protein synthesis. In LAM, the abnormal *TSC2* or *TSC1* gene protein products allow constitutive mTOR activity, which results in upregulated growth, mobility, and survival of LAM cells[3,5] (Fig. 17.2). Mutations or deletions of *TSC1* and *TSC2* are thus considered driver mutations. Most importantly, mTORC1 signaling can be downregulated by exogenous rapamycin (sirolimus) or related drugs such as everolimus, and this forms the basis for one approach to the treatment of LAM (see section Treatment and Prognosis).

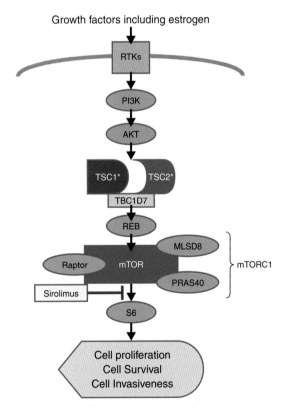

FIGURE 17.2. Simplified schematic of molecular events in LAM. Growth factor signaling through receptor tyrosine kinases (RTKs) activates the TSC1/TSC2/TBC1D7 complex, which normally inhibits mTORC1. In LAM, a mutation in TSC1 or TSC2 (labeled TSC1* and TSC2*) renders the TSC1/TSC2/TBC1D7 complex nonfunctional, leading to constitutive activation of mTORC1 with resulting enhanced proliferation, survival, and invasiveness of LAM cells. mTOR inhibitors such as sirolimus or everolimus block the activity of mTORC1 and hence can be used as a treatment for LAM.

Not all cases of LAM have *TSC1* or *TSC2* mutations, but some have mutations in genes that are related to control of mTORC1 signaling, for example, *PPP2R2B*,[4] and this situation may account for the failure of some patients to respond to mTOR inhibitors.

Because estrogen also drives mTORC1, it has been suggested[5] that proliferation of LAM cells requires a hormonally supportive milieu. In the presence of estrogen, LAM cells express Bcl-2 (B-cell lymphoma 2), which is an antiapoptotic and thus can enhance LAM cell survival. A requirement for estrogen may help explain why sporadic LAM is almost universally a disease of women and why disease progresses more slowly in postmenopausal women.[6]

The idea of LAM as a neoplasm, and particularly a malignant neoplasm,[2] has limitations. Many of the features of LAM as described earlier are typical of malignant neoplasms. However, LAM cells do not show aneuploidy or losses/gains of whole chromosome arms, a very typical finding in malignant neoplasms.[4] It has now become apparent that the natural history of LAM between diagnosis and death or transplantation extends over decades[7] (see section Treatment and Prognosis), again a finding that is not characteristic of most malignant neoplasms. Furthermore, if mTORC1 inhibitors do not work or cannot be tolerated, LAM can be treated by transplantation, even though there are circulating LAM cells, and this is not the usual scenario for malignant neoplasms.

The finding of identical mutations in lung, angiomyolipomas, and lymphangiomyomas implies seeding from a common source. It has been suggested that LAM might arise in the uterus,[8] and small foci of uterine LAM can be found in some patients with pulmonary LAM,[8] but given the ability of LAM cells to circulate widely, this is not proof of a uterine origin. Lymphangiomyomas may be encountered as incidental findings in pelvic lymph nodes in patients undergoing node dissections for treatment of a pelvic malignancy, sometimes without evidence of pulmonary LAM, but it is not clear if such patients will go on to develop LAM.[9,10] At this point, the primary site of LAM is not known.

CLINICAL FEATURES

LAM is seen not only in about one-third of women with TSC[3] but also in women who have no evidence of TSC ("sporadic LAM"), where the incidence has been estimated at 3 to 7.8 per million persons per year.[3] The traditional teaching has been that LAM is a disease of premenopausal women, but in a series of 230 patients accumulated by the National Heart, Lung and Blood Institute LAM Registry,[11] 40% were postmenopausal at presentation. A small number of LAM cases have been reported in males with TSC.[12]

Suggested criteria for the diagnosis of LAM are listed in Table 17.2. Patients with LAM often present with shortness of breath, but pneumothorax (reflecting rupture of

Table 17.2

Criteria for the diagnosis of LAM

An appropriate pattern of diffuse cystic lung disease on HRCT plus at least one of the following findings:
TSC
Renal angiomyolipoma(s) on imaging
Chylothorax
Lymphangiomyoma(s) on imaging
Serum VEGF-D greater than 800 pg/mL
LAM cells in effusions or lymph nodes
Biopsy proof of pulmonary LAM or an extrapulmonary manifestation (angiomyolipoma; lymphangiomyoma)

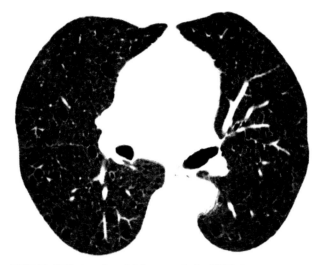

FIGURE 17.3. Lymphangioleiomyomatosis. HRCT demonstrates numerous bilateral thin-walled cysts ranging from approximately 3 to 15 mm in diameter. The parenchyma between the cysts is normal. The patient was a 53-year-old woman.

subpleural cysts) as a presenting complaint is common, and repeated pneumothoraces are seen in some patients. Extrapulmonary manifestations are frequent. Renal angiomyolipomas are found in 30% of sporadic LAM and as many as 90% of TSC-associated LAM; some patients present with a renal angiomyolipoma and are then found to have cysts on chest imaging.[13] Lymphangiomyomas are more common in sporadic LAM[13] and can be found in any lymphatic site but may be more frequent in pelvic lymph nodes.[9,10] Lymphangiomyomas that obstruct the thoracic duct cause chylous pleural effusions, seen in up to 10% of patients, and chylous effusions may also be found in the peritoneal and pericardial spaces. Serious hemoptysis occasionally occurs and is believed to reflect growth of LAM cells into small pulmonary vessels. LAM patients often show elevations in pulmonary artery pressure on exercise, presumably for the same reason.[12] LAM cells also grow into small airways,[8] which is believed to account for the fact that pulmonary function tests may show an obstructive or mixed obstructive–restrictive pattern.

LAM cells secrete serum vascular endothelial growth factor-D (VEGF-D), a substance that drives the formation of lymphatics, and serum levels greater than 800 pg/mL strongly support a diagnosis of LAM. However, many LAM patients do not have high levels of VEGF-D.[3,14,15]

IMAGING

The characteristic high-resolution computed tomography (HRCT) finding of LAM consists of bilateral thin-walled cysts scattered uniformly throughout the lungs and surrounded by normal parenchyma (Fig. 17.3). The cysts tend to have fairly uniform size and shape, measure less than 5 mm in diameter in patients with mild disease but may become larger than 1 cm with severe involvement.[16] Spontaneous pneumothorax occurs in more than 50% of patients and is the primary event that leads to diagnosis in approximately 35% of cases.[11] Although in the proper

clinical setting the HRCT findings may be characteristic enough to strongly suggest the diagnosis, there can be considerable overlap with other cystic lung diseases, particularly Langerhans cell histiocytosis (LCH), lymphocytic interstitial pneumonia, and Birt–Hogg–Dubé syndrome (see section Differential Diagnosis).

The pulmonary manifestations of TSC include LAM and multifocal micronodular pneumocyte hyperplasia (MMPH). Up to one-third of women with TSC have lung cysts characteristic of LAM.[17] MMPH manifests as 1- to 8-mm-diameter ground-glass nodules distributed throughout both lungs, although they may have an upper lobe predominance (Fig. 17.4).[18] MMPH may be seen in isolation or in the presence of LAM.

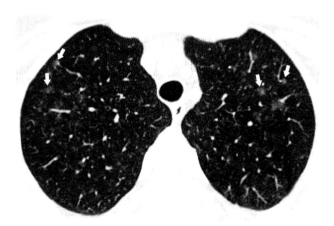

FIGURE 17.4. Multifocal micronodular pneumocyte hyperplasia. HRCT shows multiple bilateral ground-glass nodules (*arrows*). The patient was a 43-year-old woman with TSC.

PATHOLOGIC FEATURES

Gross appearances

Cysts with walls that are, visually, thicker than those of emphysema, but thinner and softer than those of honeycombing, are the characteristic finding in LAM (Fig. 17.5).

MICROSCOPIC FINDINGS

The defining feature of LAM in the lung is the presence of cystic spaces with walls composed of LAM cells. LAM cells typically have a slightly more clear or slightly vacuolated cytoplasm compared to ordinary smooth muscle cells (Fig. 17.6). The number/volume of LAM cells is extraordinarily variable. Textbooks typically illustrate cases in which the LAM cells produce bulky thickening of the entire wall of a cyst with many such cysts in the lung (Figs. 17.7 and 17.8), but in some cases there are only small nodular thickenings in the cyst walls (Figs. 17.9 and 17.10). Still other cases mimic emphysema

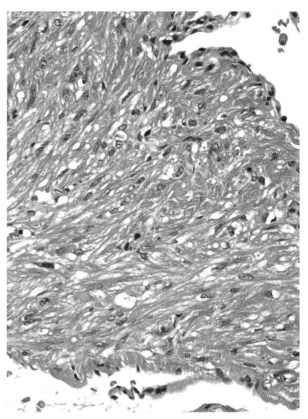

FIGURE 17.6. High-power appearance of LAM cells. Note the typical slightly cleared or vacuolated cytoplasm.

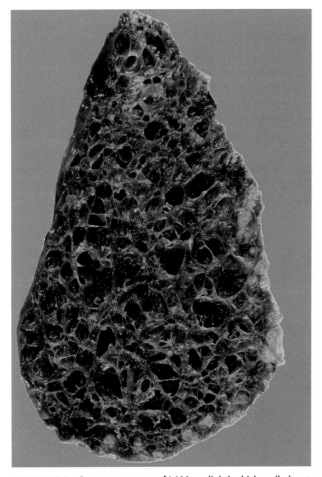

FIGURE 17.5. Gross appearance of LAM as slightly thick-walled cysts that somewhat mimic honeycombing. However, as opposed to honeycombing, the cyst walls are soft on palpation and have no fibrosis in their walls on microscopic examination.

(Figs. 17.11 and 17.12), and only close inspection of one or more cysts reveals the characteristic LAM cells (Fig. 17.12).

LAM cells can grow into small airways, although this is often only obvious on immunohistochemical staining.[8] LAM cells can also grow into blood vessels, and hemosiderin, thought to reflect blood vessel invasion, is present in some cases (Fig. 17.8).

Immunohistochemical staining

LAM cells express muscle markers such as desmin, but in addition are HMB-45 positive. Although studies on LAM frequently illustrate HMB-45 staining of almost every LAM cell in a given lesion, in our experience, it is much more common to find quite focal staining (Fig. 17.13). LAM cells show cytoplasmic staining for β-catenin,[19] and we find that this stain is more diffusely positive and often easier to interpret than HMB-45 (Fig. 17.14). Normal smooth muscle does not stain for β-catenin, although bronchial and bronchiolar epithelium often does. LAM cells in many cases are also positive for estrogen (ER) and progesterone (PR) receptors, which typically show more diffuse staining than HMB-45 (Figs. 17.15 and 17.16).

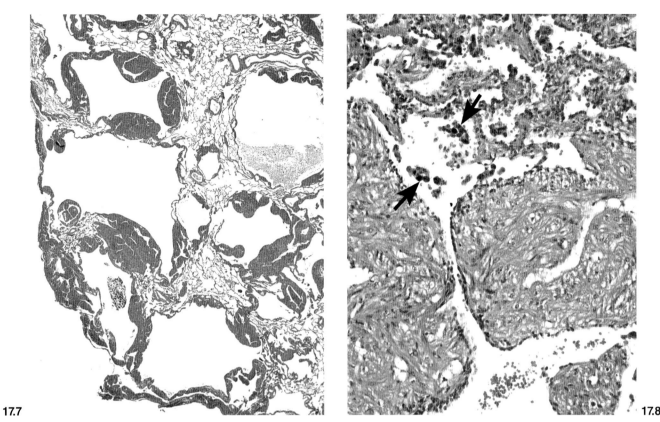

17.7

17.8

FIGURES 17.7 and 17.8. An example of LAM in which there are fairly bulky masses of LAM cells in the cyst walls. Hemosiderin secondary to chronic hemorrhage, a common finding in LAM, is visible in the high-power view (*arrows*).

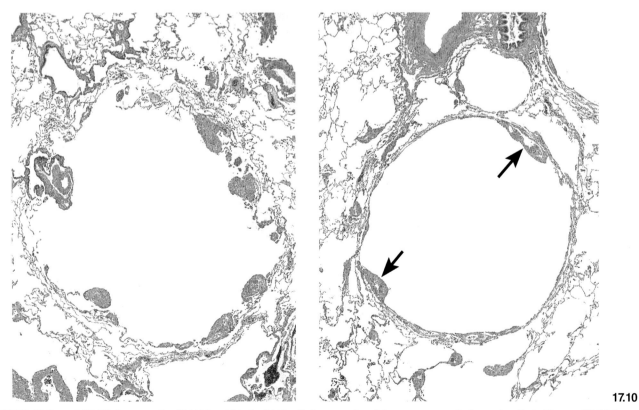

17.9

17.10

FIGURES 17.9 and 17.10. An example of LAM in which the LAM cells form small nodular excrescences in the cyst walls. In **Figure 17.10** the area occupied by LAM cells (*arrows*) is fairly small and the cyst might be mistaken for an emphysematous space at first glance.

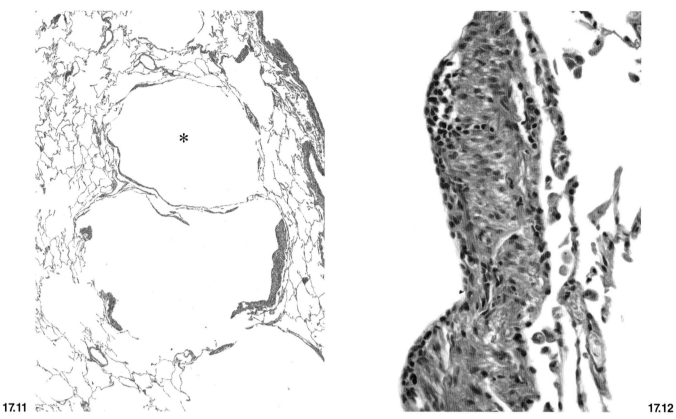

17.11   17.12

FIGURES 17.11 and 17.12. Portions of three LAM cysts in a patient with minimal proliferation of LAM cells. The middle cyst has an area of thickening of the wall by LAM cells (shown at higher power in **Fig. 17.12**), but the adjacent cyst (*) has almost none. Such cysts are difficult to separate from emphysematous spaces or Birt–Hogg–Dubé cysts (compare Fig. 17.26).

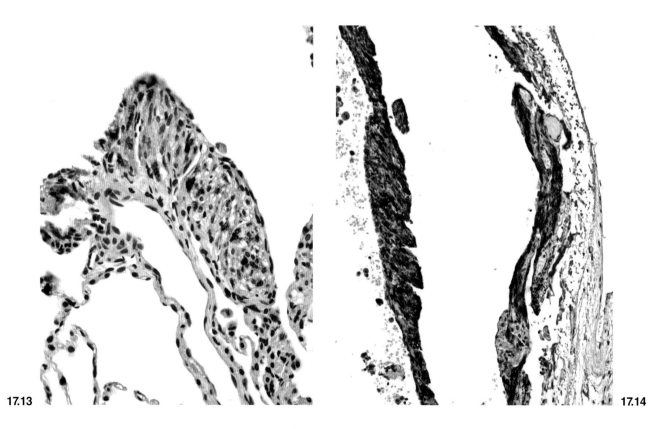

17.13   17.14

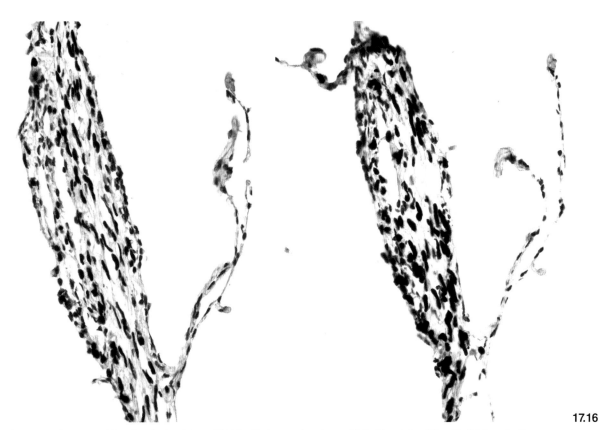

17.15   17.16

FIGURES 17.13 to 17.16. Immunohistochemical staining of LAM cells. In our experience, HMB-45 staining (**Fig. 17.13**) is typically very patchy, whereas b-catenin staining (**Fig. 17.14**) is strong and diffuse. ER (**Fig. 17.15**) and PR (**Fig. 17.16**) staining is not always present but usually stains all or most of the LAM cells when positive.

Lymphangiomyomas

Lymphangiomyomas are composed of LAM cells forming abortive D2-40-positive lymphatic channels (Figs. 17.17 and 17.18); some authors refer to these as lymph node metastases.[9] They are extremely rare in the lung, but can affect any lymph node or lymphatic structure in the thorax. Angiomyolipomas are usually found in the kidneys but rare angiomyolipoma-like lesions have been reported in the lung.

MULTIFOCAL MICRONODULAR PNEUMOCYTE HYPERPLASIA

MMPH is seen in some cases of LAM in patients with TSC, but can also occur without LAM in these patients. It consists of multiple small nodules composed of bland-appearing hyperplastic type 2 cells growing along the alveolar walls with underlying dense interstitial fibrosis confined to the nodules (Figs. 17.19 to 17.21).

DIFFERENTIAL DIAGNOSIS

The major morphologic differential diagnoses of LAM are shown in Table 17.3. Centrilobular emphysema forms cystic spaces with either a very attenuated wall or occasionally

a fibrotic wall (Figs. 17.22 and 17.23). LAM with minimal muscle in the cyst wall can mimic emphysema (Fig. 17.11), but emphysematous spaces never have muscle in their walls. The respiratory bronchiole leading into the emphysematous space has a partially muscularized wall that might be confused with LAM. However, respiratory bronchioles leading into emphysematous spaces are not cystic and they usually have very obvious ciliated epithelium, something that is not a feature of LAM. The smooth muscle in the walls of respiratory bronchioles is HMB-45 and β-catenin negative.

Benign metastasizing leiomyoma is really a very low-grade leiomyosarcoma that has metastasized to the lung; virtually all cases originate in the uterus. Benign metastasizing leiomyoma forms interstitial nodules without cysts, although they often incorporate small spaces lined by metaplastic alveolar epithelium (Figs. 17.24 and 17.25). The cells of benign metastasizing leiomyoma are ER positive, but negative for HMB-45 and β-catenin.

LCH is described in detail in Chapter 10. It can form cystic spaces, but the walls of these spaces are cellular proliferations of Langerhans cells, eosinophils, smoker's macrophages (see Figs. 10.10 and 10.11), or, if the lesions are old, composed of dense fibrous tissue (see Figs. 10.22 to 10.24). Langerhans cells are S-100, CD1a, and cyclin D1 positive (see Figs. 10.29, 10.30, and 10.36) and negative for HMB-45 and β-catenin.

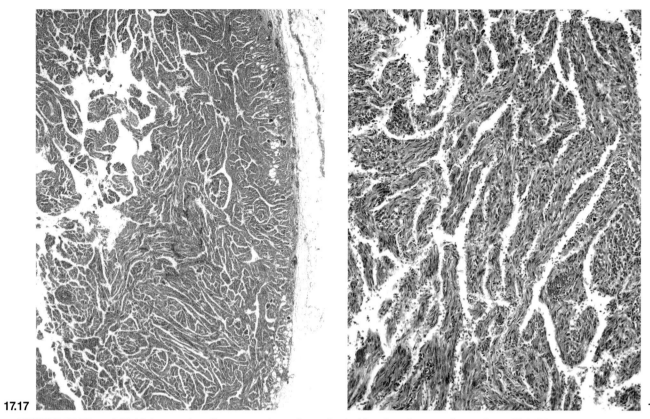

17.17   17.18

FIGURES 17.17 and 17.18. Low- and medium-power views of a mediastinal lymphangiomyoma in a patient with LAM.

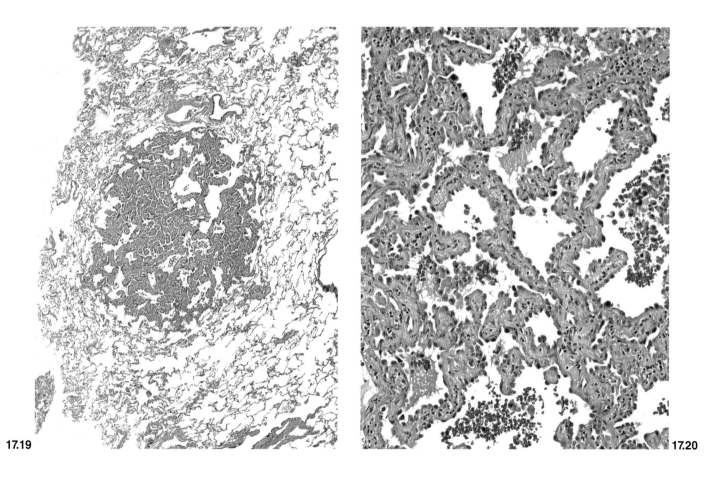

17.19   17.20

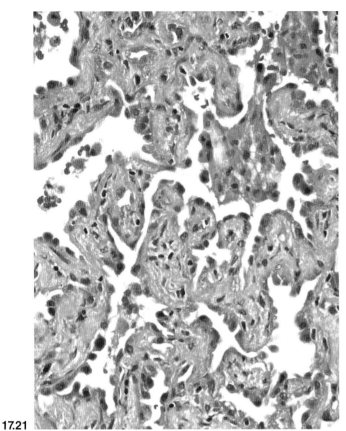

17.21

FIGURES 17.19 to 17.21. MMPH in a patient with LAM. The lesion consists of proliferating type II cells overlying a densely fibrotic interstitium.

Birt–Hogg–Dubé syndrome is an autosomal dominant condition characterized by cutaneous fibrofolliculomas, renal cell carcinomas, lung cysts in 80% of cases,

and, sometimes, pneumothoraces.[20,21] Birt–Hogg–Dubé syndrome is caused by a mutation in the gene encoding folliculin, a protein of unknown function.

On computed tomography, the cysts tend to be variable in size and shape and larger than those seen in LAM and typically involve mainly the lower lung zones, often abutting the mediastinum (Fig. 17.26), whereas those of LAM usually have a random distribution throughout the lungs.[22,23]

Microscopically, the lung cysts usually appear to be formed from keratin-positive thinly stretched alveolar walls, and there is neither aberrant smooth muscle nor fibrous tissue lining the cysts[21,24] (Fig. 17.27); however, some authors have suggested that the cysts tend to abut interlobular septa.[21]

PATHOLOGIC DIAGNOSTIC MODALITIES

Given a proper pattern of cystic lung disease and an elevated VEGF-D, biopsy is not required for a diagnosis of LAM.[24] If tissue is needed, an American Thoracic Society position paper[25] recommends transbronchial biopsy as the first tissue procurement approach. The series described by Koba et al.[26] reported a positive transbronchial biopsy diagnosis in 17/24 cases; generally, cysts are not seen but the typical LAM cells with characteristic staining patterns can be identified. LAM cell aggregates can sometimes be found in cytologic preparations of chylous effusions or ascites (Fig. 17.1). Cryobiopsy should also be efficacious. Video-assisted thoracoscopic surgery biopsies are commonly used in cases that are not clinically/radiologically evident.

Table 17.3

Morphologic differential diagnosis of LAM

Centrilobular emphysema	Benign metastasizing leiomyoma	LCH	Birt–Hogg–Dubé syndrome
Cystic spaces have thin walls or occasionally fibrotic walls, but no muscle	Muscle forms interstitial nodules without cysts. Nodules can incorporate small airspaces with metaplastic alveolar lining	In early disease, cysts have a cellular wall composed of Langerhans cells, eosinophils, and smoker's macrophages	Cyst walls consist of attenuated alveolar parenchyma, no muscle or fibrous tissue (but cysts sometimes abut interlobular septa)
Muscular wall of respiratory bronchioles leading to emphysematous space has an epithelial lining. Muscle of respiratory bronchiole is HMB-45 and β-catenin negative	Muscle cells are ER positive, negative for HMB-45 and β-catenin	Langerhans cells are S-100, CD1a, and cyclin D1 positive, negative for HMB-45 and β-catenin Old LCH has cysts with fibrotic walls	Patients have cutaneous fibrofolliculomas and renal cell carcinomas

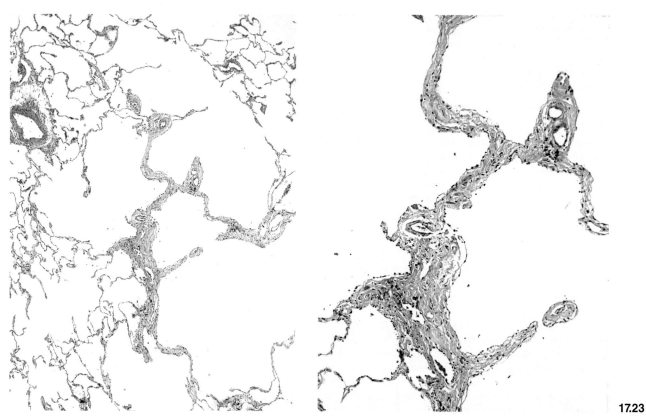

17.22   17.23

FIGURES 17.22 and 17.23. Centrilobular emphysema. The cystic spaces in centrilobular emphysema usually have attenuated walls, but sometimes, as in this example, there is fibrosis of walls of the spaces as well. Emphysematous spaces do not have muscle in the walls.

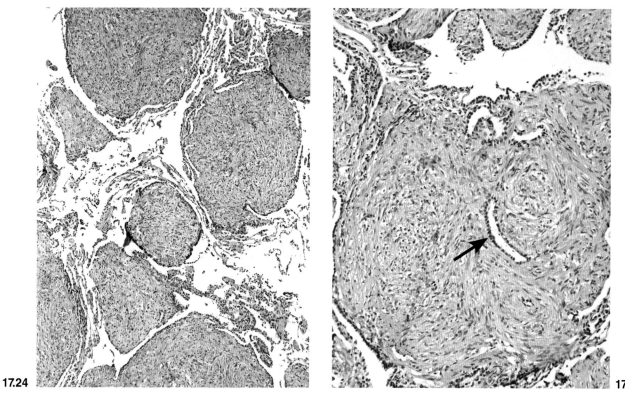

17.24   17.25

FIGURES 17.24 and 17.25. Benign metastasizing leiomyoma. The nodules of muscle in benign metastasizing leiomyoma are actually interstitial and sometimes contain small cyst-like spaces that are really metaplastic residual alveolar epithelium (**Fig. 17.25**, *arrow*). However, cystic spaces of the size seen in LAM are never present, and the muscle is HMB-45 negative but ER positive.

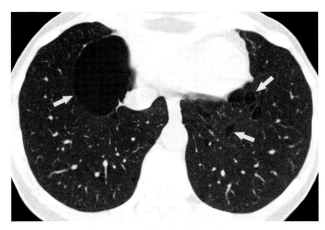

FIGURE 17.26. Birt–Hogg–Dubé (BHD) syndrome. HRCT shows a large thin-walled cyst in the right lower lobe and several smaller cysts of various shapes in the left lower lobe (*arrows*). The larger cyst and several of the smaller ones are in the medial regions of the lung. The patient was a 54-year-old woman with BHD.

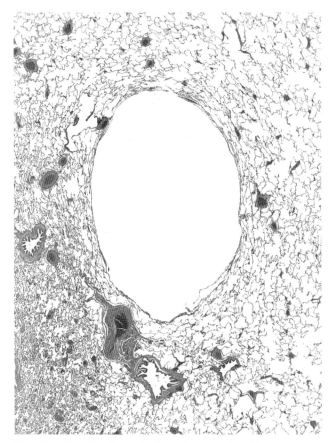

FIGURE 17.27. Birt–Hogg–Dubé syndrome. Cyst wall is composed of attenuated lung parenchyma with no muscle in the wall.

TREATMENT AND PROGNOSIS

When first described, LAM was viewed as an aggressive disease with a poor outcome. However, it has now become apparent that most cases of LAM are in fact slowly progressive. Oprescu et al.[7] reported a transplant-free 10-year survival of 86% in a series of 410 patients; the median transplant-free survival from diagnosis was 23 years, and most of those patients would not have been treated with sirolimus.

There are several possible reasons for this "improvement." First, HRCT will pick up cases of LAM that would have been missed on plain chest radiograph, so the diagnosis will be made earlier. Second, the original descriptions of LAM in the pathology literature reported cases with very extensive muscle (such as Figs. 17.7 and 17.8), but pathologists now recognize much more subtle disease (such as Fig. 17.11), which is either earlier or simply less severe, and Matsui et al.[27] showed that the rate of progression is proportional to the relative number of LAM cells seen in the biopsy. Third, the original descriptions of LAM were all in premenopausal women, but as noted earlier, it's now recognized that a significant proportion of patients present when they are postmenopausal, and postmenopausal women have considerably better survival,[6] which fits with the observation that estrogen drives mTORC1 signaling (see comments on pathogenesis above).

Some cases progress very slowly and may not require treatment. For those that do, inhibition of mTORC1 signaling with sirolimus or everolimus has been shown to stabilize or improve pulmonary function, decrease serum VEGF-D levels, reduce or eliminate chylothorax, and lead to shrinkage of angiomyolipomas and lymphangiomyomas.[3,15,16,28,29] However, these effects only persist as long as the drug is administered. mTORC1 inhibitors produce a variety of toxicities, including immunosuppression, and may not be tolerated. Lung transplantation is the other effective treatment option. Although LAM is driven by estrogen, antiestrogen treatments are not effective.[15,16]

REFERENCES

1. Pan CC, Chung MY, Ng KF, et al. Constant allelic alteration on chromosome 16p (TSC2 gene) in perivascular epithelioid cell tumour (PEComa): genetic evidence for the relationship of PEComa with angiomyolipoma. *J Pathol.* 2008;214:387–393.
2. McCormack FX, Travis WD, Colby TV, et al. Lymphangioleiomyomatosis: calling it what it is: a low-grade, destructive, metastasizing neoplasm. *Am J Respir Crit Care Med.* 2012;186:1210–1212.
3. Harari S, Torre O, Cassandro R, et al. The changing face of a rare disease: lymphangioleiomyomatosis. *Eur Respir J.* 2015;46:1471–1485.
4. Murphy SJ, Terra SB, Harris FR, et al. Genomic rearrangements in sporadic lymphangioleiomyomatosis: an evolving genetic story. *Mod Pathol.* 2017;30:1223–1233.
5. El-Chemaly S, Henske EP. Towards personalised therapy for lymphangioleiomyomatosis: lessons from cancer. *Eur Respir Rev.* 2014;23:30–35.
6. Gupta N, Lee HS, Ryu JH, et al; NHLBI LAM Registry Group. The NHLBI LAM registry: prognostic physiological and radiological biomarkers emerge from a 15-year

prospective longitudinal analysis. *Chest*. 2019;155:288–296. doi:10.1016/j.chest.2018.06.016.

7. Oprescu N, McCormack FX, Byrnes S, et al. Clinical predictors of mortality and cause of death in lymphangioleiomyomatosis: a population-based registry. *Lung*. 2013;191:35–42.

8. Hayashi T, Kumasaka T, Mitani K, et al. Prevalence of uterine and adnexal involvement in pulmonary lymphangioleiomyomatosis: a clinicopathologic study of 10 patients. *Am J Surg Pathol*. 2011;35:1776–1785.

9. Rabban JT, Firetag B, Sangoi AR, et al. Incidental pelvic and para-aortic lymph node lymphangioleiomyomatosis detected during surgical staging of pelvic cancer in women without symptomatic pulmonary lymphangioleiomyomatosis or tuberous sclerosis complex. *Am J Surg Pathol*. 2015;39:1015–1025.

10. Schoolmeester JK, Park KJ. Incidental nodal lymphangioleiomyomatosis is not a harbinger of pulmonary lymphangioleiomyomatosis. *Am J Surg Pathol*. 2015;39:1404–1410.

11. Ryu JH, Moss J, Beck GJ, et al; NHLBI LAM Registry Group. The NHLBI lymphangioleiomyomatosis registry: characteristics of 230 patients at enrollment. *Am J Respir Crit Care Med*. 2006;173:105–111.

12. Meraj R, Wikenheiser-Brokamp KA, Young LR, et al. Lymphangioleiomyomatosis: new concepts in pathogenesis, diagnosis, and treatment. *Semin Respir Crit Care Med*. 2012;33:486–497.

13. Ryu JH, Hartman TE, Torres VE, et al. Frequency of undiagnosed cystic lung disease in patients with sporadic renal angiomyolipomas. *Chest*. 2012;141:163–168.

14. Young LR, Vandyke R, Gulleman PM, et al. Serum vascular endothelial growth factor-D prospectively distinguishes lymphangioleiomyomatosis from other diseases. *Chest*. 2010;138:674–681.

15. McCormack FX, Gupta N, Finlay GR, et al; ATS/JRS Committee on Lymphangioleiomyomatosis. Official American Thoracic Society/Japanese Respiratory Society Clinical Practice Guidelines: lymphangioleiomyomatosis diagnosis and management. *Am J Respir Crit Care Med*. 2016;194:748–761.

16. Abbott GF, Rosado-de-Christenson ML, Frazier AA, et al. From the archives of the AFIP: lymphangioleiomyomatosis: radiologic-pathologic correlation. *Radiographics*. 2005;25:803–828.

17. Avila NA, Dwyer AJ, Rabel A, et al. Sporadic lymphangioleiomyomatosis and tuberous sclerosis complex with lymphangioleiomyomatosis: comparison of CT features. *Radiology*. 2007;242:277–285.

18. Ajlan AM, Bilawich AM, Müller NL. Thoracic tomographic manifestations of tuberous sclerosis in adults. *Can Assoc Radiol J*. 2012;63:61–68.

19. Flavin RJ, Cook J, Fiorentino M, et al. β-Catenin is a useful adjunct immunohistochemical marker for the diagnosis of pulmonary lymphangioleiomyomatosis. *Am J Clin Pathol*. 2011;135:776–782.

20. Menko FH, van Steensel MA, Giraud S, et al; European BHD Consortium. Birt-Hogg-Dubé syndrome: diagnosis and management. *Lancet Oncol*. 2009;10:1199–1206.

21. Koga S, Furuya M, Takahashi Y, et al. Lung cysts in Birt-Hogg-Dubé syndrome: histopathological characteristics and aberrant sequence repeats. *Pathol Int*. 2009;59:720–728.

22. Tobino K, Hirai T, Johkoh T, et al. Differentiation between Birt-Hogg-Dubé syndrome and lymphangioleiomyomatosis: quantitative analysis of pulmonary cysts on computed tomography of the chest in 66 females. *Eur J Radiol*. 2012;81:1340–1346.

23. Gupta S, Kang HC, Ganeshan D, et al. The ABCs of BHD: an in-depth review of Birt-Hogg-Dubé syndrome. *AJR Am J Roentgenol*. 2017;209:1291–1296.

24. Hayashi M, Takayanagi N, Ishiguro T, et al. Birt-Hogg-Dubé syndrome with multiple cysts and recurrent pneumothorax: pathological findings. *Intern Med*. 2010;49:2137–2142.

25. Gupta N, Finlay GA, Kotloff RM, et al; ATS Assembly on Clinical Problems. Lymphangioleiomyomatosis diagnosis and management: high-resolution chest computed tomography, transbronchial lung biopsy, and pleural disease management. An Official American Thoracic Society/Japanese Respiratory Society Clinical Practice Guideline. *Am J Respir Crit Care Med*. 2017;196:1337–1348.

26. Koba T, Arai T, Kitaichi M, et al. Efficacy and safety of transbronchial lung biopsy for the diagnosis of lymphangioleiomyomatosis: A report of 24 consecutive patients. *Respirology*. 2018;23:331–338.

27. Matsui K, Beasley MB, Nelson WK, et al. Prognostic significance of pulmonary lymphangioleiomyomatosis histologic score. *Am J Surg Pathol*. 2001;25:479–484.

28. Taveira-DaSilva AM, Jones AM, Julien-Williams P, et al. Term effect of sirolimus on serum vascular endothelial Growth factor D levels in patients with lymphangioleiomyomatosis. *Chest*. 2018;153:124–132.

29. Takada T, Mikami A, Kitamura N, et al. Efficacy and safety of long-term sirolimus therapy for Asian patients with lymphangioleiomyomatosis. *Ann Am Thorac Soc*. 2016;13:1912–1922.

Drug Reactions Producing Interstitial Lung Disease

GENERAL APPROACH TO DRUG REACTIONS IN THE LUNG AND PLEURA

The diagnosis of drug reactions in the lung and pleura is a difficult area, in part because of the plethora of drugs that produce adverse reactions, and in part because most drug reaction patterns are not specific, so that the diagnosis of drug reactions tends to be exclusionary, and the pathologist often ends up in the position of calling something a "possible" drug reaction. A further source of confusion is the tendency of drug reactions that appear as interstitial lung disease (ILD) to produce unusual patterns or combinations of findings, but this phenomenon is sometimes helpful in making one think about drug toxicity.

Table 18.1 lists some general principles for approaching cases that might represent drug reactions. Knowledge of the temporal sequence between the onset of drug use and the

Table 18.1

General approach to drug reactions

Proper temporal sequence of drug administration and response required

Most drug reactions start fairly close in time to the onset of drug use, but occasionally drug reactions are seen after long-term use of the drug in question or long after the drug has been stopped

Known correlation between drug and pathologic reaction pattern helps establish diagnosis (see www .pneumotox.com for a listing of drugs and published reactions)

An alternate (non-drug) etiology does not better explain the clinical scenario

Disappearance of disease after discontinuing drug is best proof of etiology

Disease reappears after rechallenge with the drug (not often done)

Drug reactions are usually exclusionary diagnoses and *very few* pathologic reaction patterns are pathognomonic of a drug reaction

appearance of intrathoracic disease is crucial. Although most drug reactions start in reasonable time proximity after the onset of drug use, some drugs usually do not produce adverse reactions until a certain dose has been reached (amiodarone is a good example),[1] and some drugs, for example, Asacol[2] (see Case Study 3), can cause a reaction after years of use with no previous ill effects. Other drugs, especially chemotherapeutic agents such as BCNU, may cause interstitial fibrosis long after drug administration has ceased.[3]

One of the most helpful diagnostic aids is information about whether the drug in question is known to cause the imaging/pathologic reaction pattern at hand. The literature on drug reactions is huge and expanding at a rapid rate, but a concise summary can be found at www.pneumotox.com. This site is sponsored by Groupe d'Etudes de la Pathologie Pulmonaire Iatrogène and provides a compilation of pulmonary drug reactions in the literature classified by drug name and also by reaction pattern. One note of caution for pathologists: the pneumotox database is quite good and even has listings for many drugs by specific pathologic patterns, but also has listings based on clinical reports that may not provide accurate indications of the underlying pathology. A further complication is that some adverse drug reaction reports predate current classifications of ILD; in particular, many things were labeled "usual interstitial pneumonia (UIP)" in the past that now would be regarded as something else.

Probably the best proof of a drug reaction is disappearance of the abnormal imaging/pathology after the drug is discontinued (and, even better, reappearance of the lesions with rechallenge, something that is rarely done), but this means that many diagnoses of *definite* drug reactions are really made post hoc by the clinician following the patient. Most often at the time of biopsy all the pathologist can say is "possible" or "probable" drug reaction (see section Case Studies).

CLINICAL FEATURES

There is an extremely broad range of clinical findings in patients with drug reactions. These vary from acute events (anaphylaxis, bronchospasm, pulmonary edema) to processes that take weeks to months to develop (probably the majority of drug reactions) to lesions that are only seen after years, typically fibrotic reactions. Most clinical findings are nonspecific and include shortness of breath, cough, and frequently systemic complaints including fever, fatigue, and weight loss. Blood or lavage eosinophilia is fairly common and helpful in suggesting a drug reaction.

IMAGING

The radiologic manifestations of drug reactions are protean and nonspecific. High-resolution computed tomography (HRCT) allows better assessment of the pattern and distribution of findings than the chest radiograph and may demonstrate abnormalities in patients with normal radiographs. HRCT is therefore the imaging modality of choice in the assessment of patients with suspected drug-induced lung disease.[4] The most common findings on HRCT are bilateral ground-glass opacities with or without areas of consolidation.[4] Reticular opacities occur less commonly. The HRCT patterns of drug reaction, however, are similar to those seen in other interstitial and airspace diseases (Fig. 18.1).[4–6] Furthermore, particularly in patients receiving chemotherapy, pulmonary parenchymal opacities may result from a number of other complications including infection, pulmonary edema, and progression of the underlying disease. Allowing for these limitations, the possibility of drug reaction should be suspected in all patients receiving medications that are known to cause the HRCT pattern being seen. Drug reaction or collagen vascular disease should also be suspected when the HRCT shows findings consistent with two different reaction patterns, most commonly nonspecific interstitial pneumonia (NSIP) and organizing pneumonia (OP).

In a small number of cases, the HRCT findings may be suggestive of a particular drug reaction. The best example is amiodarone, which contains about 37% iodine by weight and therefore has high attenuation on computed tomography (CT). As a consequence, pulmonary abnormalities caused by amiodarone toxicity, particularly when chronic, frequently have high attenuation (80 to 175 Hounsfield units [HU]) on CT[7] (Figs. 18.2 and 18.3). Because amiodarone normally accumulates in the reticuloendothelial system, the liver also typically has high attenuation in patients who take amiodarone. It should be noted that high attenuation of the liver is usually a normal finding in patients who take amiodarone and that the lack of high attenuation of the lung abnormalities does not exclude amiodarone toxicity.

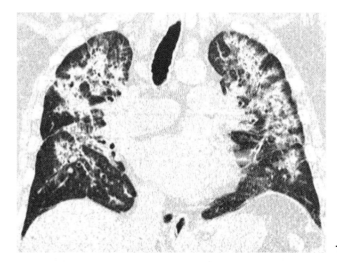

18.2

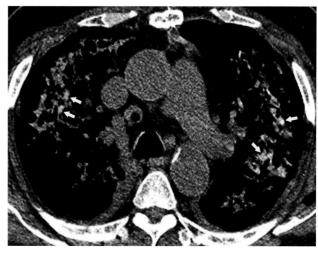

18.3

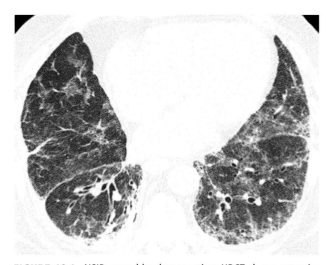

FIGURE 18.1. NSIP caused by drug reaction. HRCT shows extensive bilateral ground-glass opacities and mild peripheral reticulation and traction bronchiectasis. The patient had an NSIP reaction to methotrexate used in the treatment of psoriasis.

FIGURES 18.2 and 18.3. Amiodarone toxicity. **Figure 18.2:** Coronal reformation of a volumetric HRCT shows bilateral peribronchial areas of consolidation mainly in the middle and upper lung zones. **Figure 18.3:** Cross-sectional CT image photographed at soft tissue windows demonstrates regions of high attenuation (*arrows*) within the airspace consolidation, consistent with amiodarone deposition. The patient had an OP-like reaction to amiodarone.

PATHOLOGIC PATTERNS OF DRUG REACTIONS IN THE LUNG AND PLEURA

Drug reactions can affect any structure in the lung and also the pleura (Table 18.2). However, statistically, the vast majority of drug reactions affect the parenchyma and produce patterns that mimic ILD on imaging and biopsy[8–10] (Table 18.2).

A major problem in interpreting potential drug reactions is that some drugs can cause many different reaction patterns, sometimes even in the same biopsy. For example, methotrexate can produce non-necrotizing granulomas, hypersensitivity pneumonitis-like reactions, NSIP-like interstitial pneumonias, OP, acute respiratory distress syndrome (ARDS; diffuse alveolar damage), and UIP-like fibrosis (Figs. 18.4 to 18.7). Conversely, the number of pathologic reaction patterns is limited and a given reaction pattern can be seen with many drugs; thus, as of August 2018, pneumotox.com lists 180 drugs reported to produce eosinophilic pneumonias. Some combinations of drug/agents seem to produce toxicity or increase toxicity beyond that seen with either agent used singly: combinations of chemotherapeutic drugs and radiation are a good example.[8]

Often drug reaction patterns are subtly different from the classic lesion or there is a combination of reaction patterns that would not normally occur together, or the reaction pattern varies from area to area within the biopsy. For example, what are often (and incorrectly) called "sarcoid-like" drug reactions[11] to agents such as anti–tumor necrosis factor (TNF) agents such as adalimumab (Humira) are in fact collections of noncaseating granulomas that do not actually show the

Table 18.2
Drug reactions in relation to underlying anatomy

Parenchyma—many patterns mimic ILD
  Interstitial inflammation
  Interstitial fibrosis
  Granulomas, occasionally necrotizing
  Organizing pneumonia
  Diffuse alveolar damage (AIP/ARDS)
  Mimicking NSIP
  Mimicking hypersensitivity pneumonitis
  Mimicking UIP
  Lymphoid hyperplasia and lymphocytic interstitial pneumonia
  Pulmonary alveolar proteinosis
  Eosinophilic pneumonias (acute and chronic)
  Diffuse alveolar hemorrhage
Parenchyma—nodular lesions, occasionally necrotizing
Airways (bronchiolitis, constrictive bronchiolitis [bronchiolitis obliterans], bronchiectasis, asthma)
Vascular (vasculitis, hemorrhage, veno-occlusive disease, pulmonary hypertensive changes)
Pleura (pleural fibrosis, eosinophilic pleuritis)

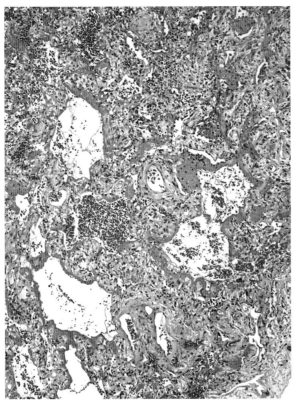

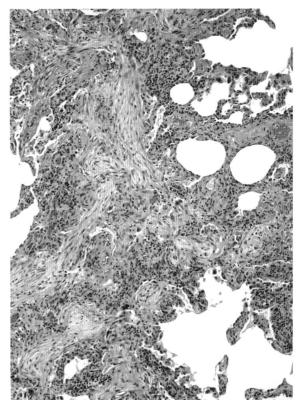

18.4   18.5

FIGURES 18.4 to 18.7. See figure legend 18.7.

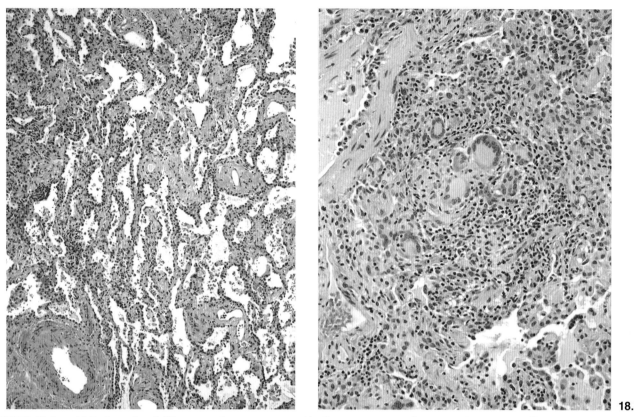

FIGURES 18.4 to 18.7. Examples of different reaction patterns caused by the same agent, methotrexate. **Figure 18.4:** Diffuse alveolar damage; **Figure 18.5:** OP; **Figure 18.6:** Fibrotic NSIP; **Figure 18.7:** Granulomas. Note that **Figures 18.5** and **18.6** are from the same case.

characteristic lymphangitic distribution of sarcoid in the lung (see Chapter 13). One useful rule of thumb is that when one encounters a strange pattern of ILD, a pattern that does not fit classic descriptions of a specific disease, a drug reaction or an underlying collagen vascular disease should be considered.

Sometimes it is not possible to separate a drug reaction from the underlying disease. For example, penicillamine, a drug used in the past as a treatment for rheumatoid arthritis (RA), appears to produce diffuse alveolar damage, OP, constrictive bronchiolitis, and follicular bronchiolitis, but all of these lesions are seen in patients with RA who have not been treated with penicillamine, and it is still unclear whether penicillamine itself is really producing adverse effects. Another example of this problem in a patient with RA treated with leflunomide (Arava) is illustrated in Case Study 4 below. Many drugs produce immunosuppression, and such patients are at risk of infections that may mimic drug reactions (see Case Study 5).

Amiodarone, and to a much lesser extent, statins, bear special mention because they will produce coarsely foamy alveolar macrophages in anyone who has accumulated a sufficient dose.[1,12] By themselves foamy macrophages are not a cause of a clinical drug reaction unless they are present in enormous numbers and produce a desquamative interstitial pneumonia (DIP)-like pattern (Figs. 18.8 and 18.9).

Cytotoxic drugs are another problem because many can produce very atypical appearing nuclei (see Fig. 7.26) that in some cases mimic viral inclusions and in others make one worry about a neoplasm. However, cytotoxic drugs do not produce the pattern of lepidic growth seen in adenocarcinoma in situ.

New categories of drugs can produce new reaction patterns. Florid granulomatous responses to anti-TNF agents such as adalimumab (Humira) (see Case Study 1) are well known[11]; and granulomatous reactions are also seen with interferons and antiretroviral therapy. It is our impression that granulomatous responses seem to be a frequent form of toxicity with a variety of other humanized antibodies.

Immune checkpoint inhibitors are now widely used for treating malignancies and such agents can produce toxicity in various organs including the lung; in a series of 915 patients treated with anti-PD1/PDL-1 therapy, what was called clinically "pneumonitis" was seen in 5% of patients.[13] Only a few biopsies were performed and the pathologic findings included diffuse alveolar damage, OP, cellular NSIP, eosinophilic infiltrates, and granulomas. Recent reports suggest that, as with other antibodies, granulomatous reactions, frequently systemic, are particularly common with antibodies against immune checkpoint inhibitors.[11,13,14]

Recreational drugs can cause adverse reactions in the lung, either because the drug itself is toxic or because it has been cut with a toxic agent that may be another drug, a soluble filler, or an insoluble particulate. Crack cocaine may produce diffuse alveolar hemorrhage as well diffuse alveolar damage and OP.[15] A hint to a crack-induced drug reaction is the presence of numerous alveolar macrophages completely filled with black pigment (Figs. 18.10 and 18.11).

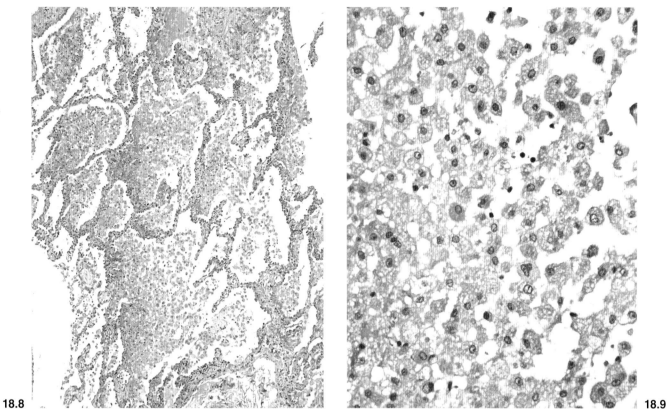

FIGURES 18.8 and 18.9. Marked macrophage reaction to amiodarone. Amiodarone induces small numbers of coarsely foamy macrophages in everyone who takes the drug, and these are useful for identifying exposure to amiodarone but by themselves do not indicate a pathologic reaction. However, the extensive filling of airspaces by such macrophages in this example (corresponding to radiologic ground-glass opacities) is indicative of drug toxicity. This is only one of the numerous patterns of toxicity seen with amiodarone.

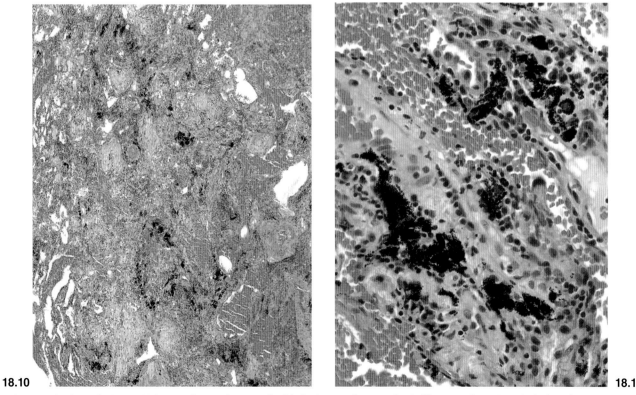

FIGURES 18.10 and 18.11. OP in a crack user. The extensive black pigment that completely fills macrophages is typical of crack use.

The effects of marijuana are surprisingly poorly defined, but chronic marijuana use can mimic some of the effects of cigarette smoke including Langerhans cell histiocytosis and DIP (see Chapter 8, Figs. 8.20 and 8.21).

Sometimes the "drug" in question may be any of a wide variety of chemical compounds and this makes adverse reactions even more unpredictable. So-called synthetic marijuana (synthetic cannabinoids) is a good example[16,17] (see Case Study 7).

Intravenous (IV) drug users not uncommonly develop pulmonary disease because the tablets of drugs intended for oral consumption contain a variety of insoluble particulate fillers. IV injection of ground up tablets can lead to vascular obstruction, vascular and interstitial granulomas, various forms of diffuse interstitial fibrosis, and emphysema[18]; this topic is discussed in Chapter 22.

EXAMPLES OF SPECIFIC CASES ILLUSTRATING THE APPROACH TO DRUG REACTIONS

Case studies 1 to 9 provide examples of how to apply the principles set out in Table 18.1 to specific cases.

Case study 1: Granulomatous Lung Disease Caused By An Anti-TNF Agent

A 48-year-old woman with a long history of RA, treated with methotrexate, developed increasingly severe joint disease. Humira (anti-TNF agent) was started in September 2008. By October 2008, she had diffuse opacities on imaging (Fig. 18.12) and was in respiratory failure. A biopsy was performed and showed a granulomatous interstitial pneumonia (Figs. 18.14 and 18.15). Special stains and cultures of the biopsy for organisms were negative. Humira was discontinued. Her symptoms rapidly disappeared and

there was considerable clearing of her radiologic abnormalities by January 2009 (Fig. 18.13).

Analysis of Case Study 1

- The temporal sequence is correct: disease appeared shortly after starting Humira.
- The pathologic reaction pattern is correct: anti-TNF agents are known to produce granulomatous interstitial pneumonias[19] (pneumotox.com). Note that the pattern of disease does not correspond exactly to any ordinary ILD and in particular does not mimic the distribution of sarcoid granulomas. Strange ILD-like patterns are a common finding with drug reactions and sometimes an important clue to the diagnosis.
- The process was not infectious by special stains and cultures.
- The temporal sequence suggests that Humira rather than methotrexate is the offending agent.
- Conclusion at the time of biopsy: granulomatous interstitial pneumonia consistent with reaction to Humira (i.e., probable drug reaction).
- Conclusion after drug discontinued and patient improved: definite drug reaction to Humira.

Case Study 2: Pulmonary Alveolar Proteinosis Caused by Smoking Fentanyl Patches

A 50-year-old woman presented with a 1-month history of cough and shortness of breath. She was afebrile. She had smoked about half pack of cigarettes per day for 35 years. She had been prescribed Fentanyl patches for chronic pain related to old burn scars, but smoked the patches instead of applying them to the skin. An initial chest radiograph showed diffuse parenchymal opacities and a CT scan demonstrated innumerable ground-glass centrilobular

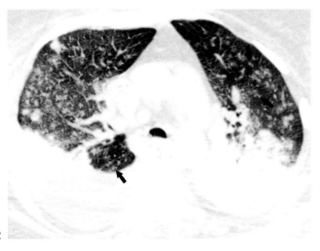

18.12

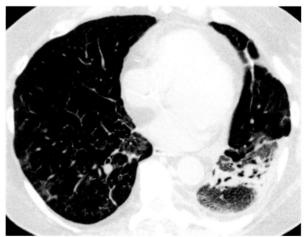

◄ 18.13

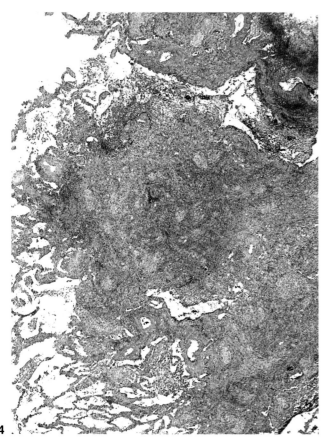

18.14

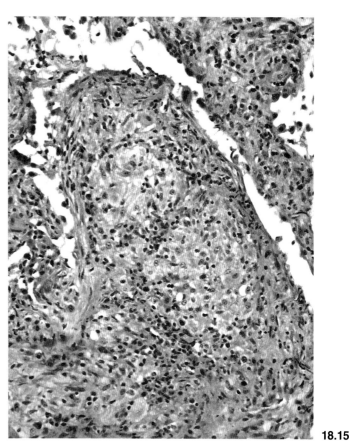

18.15

FIGURES 18.12 to 18.15. Case Study 1: Humira toxicity. **Figure 18.12:** CT image shows extensive bilateral consolidation, patchy ground-glass opacities, and several small nodules (*arrows*). The patient also had bilateral pleural effusions. **Figures 18.14:** Low-power view of the biopsy shows masses of aggregated, somewhat ill-defined, granulomas, seen better at higher power in **Figure 18.15.** A granulomatous response somewhat mimicking sarcoid is well described with anti-TNF agents. **Figure 18.13:** CT performed 3 months after Figure 18.10 shows marked improvement. The findings now consist of patchy bilateral ground-glass opacities, left lower lobe consolidation and volume loss, and residual left pleural effusion and thickening.

nodules (Fig. 18.16). A biopsy was performed and showed pulmonary alveolar proteinosis but with some degree of interstitial fibrosis and interstitial eosinophils (Figs. 18.17 and 18.18). Post biopsy, she discontinued smoking the Fentanyl patches and her symptoms and radiologic abnormalities rapidly cleared.

Analysis of Case Study 2

- The temporal sequence supports a reaction to Fentanyl patch smoke.
- The imaging studies are typical of an inhalation injury.
- Pulmonary alveolar proteinosis is occasionally seen as a drug reaction, but there is nothing in the literature on Fentanyl patch smoke.
- Conclusion post biopsy: pulmonary alveolar proteinosis consistent with reaction to Fentanyl patch smoke (probable drug reaction).
- Conclusion after drug discontinued and disease disappeared: definite reaction to Fentanyl patch smoke.

Case Study 3: Eosinophilic Pneumonia as a Late Complication of Asacol (Mesalamine) Use

A 45-year-old woman had used Asacol (mesalamine) for ulcerative colitis since 1998 with a good response. In November 2005, she developed cough and night sweats, and was found to have an elevated sedimentation rate. In January 2006, iritis and abnormal chest imaging with migratory peripheral consolidation (Fig. 18.19) were seen, and she was found to have a peripheral eosinophilia. A transbronchial biopsy (Figs. 18.20 and 18.21) showed an eosinophilic pneumonia, in this instance appearing largely as OP, a common pathologic pattern in chronic eosinophilic pneumonia (see Chapter 15).

Analysis of Case Study 3

- The peripheral eosinophilia, imaging, and biopsy are characteristic of eosinophilic pneumonias and eosinophilic pneumonias are a common form of drug reaction.

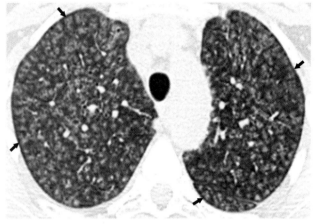

18.16

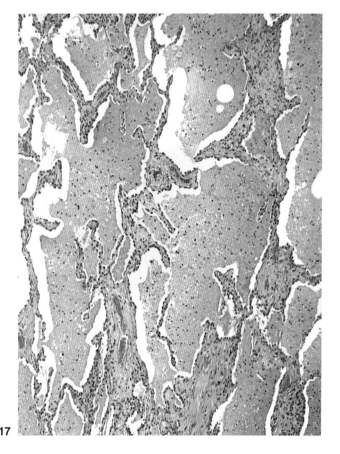

18.17

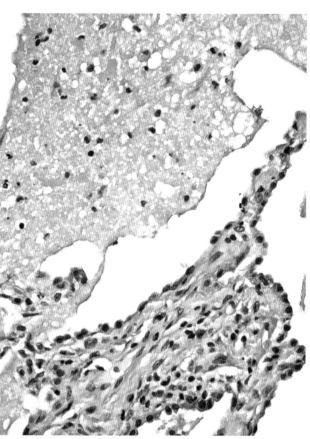

18.18

FIGURES 18.16 to 18.18. Case Study 2: Pulmonary alveolar proteinosis caused by smoking Fentanyl patches. **Figure 18.16:** HRCT demonstrates bilateral centrilobular ground-glass nodules (*arrows*) and mild patchy ground-glass opacities. The centrilobular distribution is consistent with an inhalational injury. **Figures 18.17** and **18.18:** Alveolar filling by proteinosis material and a modest degree of interstitial fibrosis, and eosinophils. Fibrosis is uncommon in PAP and eosinophils are very rare; the combination of findings suggests a drug reaction.

- The development of eosinophilic pneumonias after Asacol use is well established in the literature.[2]
- The temporal sequence is somewhat unusual because of the 7-year hiatus between beginning drug use and the appearance of an adverse reaction; however, cases of this type with long temporal gaps as a reaction to Asacol have been published.[2]
- There is no other obvious cause for an eosinophilic pneumonia.
- Conclusion at the time of biopsy: Eosinophilic pneumonia consistent with reaction to Asacol (probable drug reaction).
- Comment: No follow-up information was available, but disappearance of her pulmonary disease after drug cessation would put this case into the category of definite drug reaction.

Case Study 4: Constrictive Bronchiolitis Possibly Caused by Leflunomide in a Patient with Rheumatoid Arthritis

A 40-year-old woman presented with progressive shortness of breath. She had a 10-year history of RA, treated with steroids. Because of increasingly severe disease, leflunomide (Arava) was started a few months before she became short of breath. Pulmonary function testing showed airflow obstruction not responsive to bronchodilators. Imaging demonstrated extensive air-trapping (Fig. 18.22). Lung biopsy showed constrictive bronchiolitis (bronchiolitis obliterans) (Figs. 18.23 to 18.25, and see Chapter 20 for detailed descriptions of constrictive bronchiolitis).

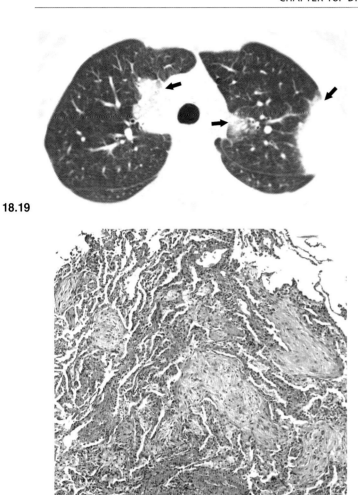

18.19

18.20

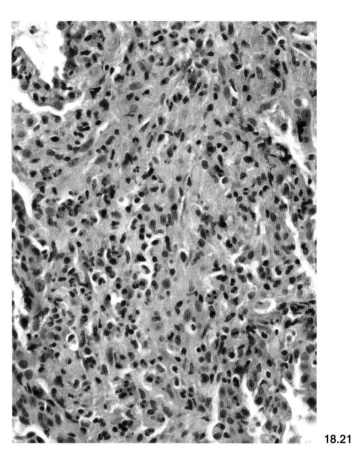

18.21

FIGURES 18.19 to 18.21. Case Study 3: Eosinophilic pneumonia induced by Asacol. **Figure 18.19:** CT image shows bilateral peripheral areas of consolidation (*arrows*) in both lung apices. The pattern and distribution are characteristic of eosinophilic pneumonia. **Figures 18.20 and 18.21:** Transbronchial biopsy shows a pattern of OP, but the high-power view demonstrates numerous eosinophils. Chronic eosinophilic pneumonia frequently mimics OP. Eosinophilic pneumonias are a very common drug reaction pattern.

Analysis of Case Study 4

- The temporal sequence is correct for a drug reaction.
- Leflunomide is known to cause a variety of forms of pulmonary toxicity including eosinophilic pneumonias, NSIP-like reactions, granulomas, and pulmonary alveolar proteinosis (see www.pneumotox.com), but has not been reported to cause constrictive bronchiolitis.
- RA itself is an established cause of constrictive bronchiolitis.[20]
- Conclusion: Possible drug reaction. Sign out the biopsy as "Surgical lung biopsy showing constrictive bronchiolitis. This might be a reaction to leflunomide but might also be caused by underlying RA."
- Comment: if follow-up showed that discontinuing leflunomide stabilized her pulmonary function, then this would be evidence for a definite drug reaction.

Case Study 5: Organizing Pneumonia as a Possible Reaction to Cyclophosphamide

A 71-year-old woman was treated with steroids and cyclophosphamide for glomerulonephritis. A few weeks after treatment was begun, she developed shortness of breath. HRCT showed peripheral consolidation. A video-assisted thoracoscopic (VATS) biopsy was performed and showed OP (Fig. 18.26). Special stains and cultures of the biopsy were negative.

Analysis of Case Study 5

- The temporal sequence is correct for a drug reaction
- The negative stains and cultures of the biopsy suggest that this is not OP on the basis of an *overt* infection

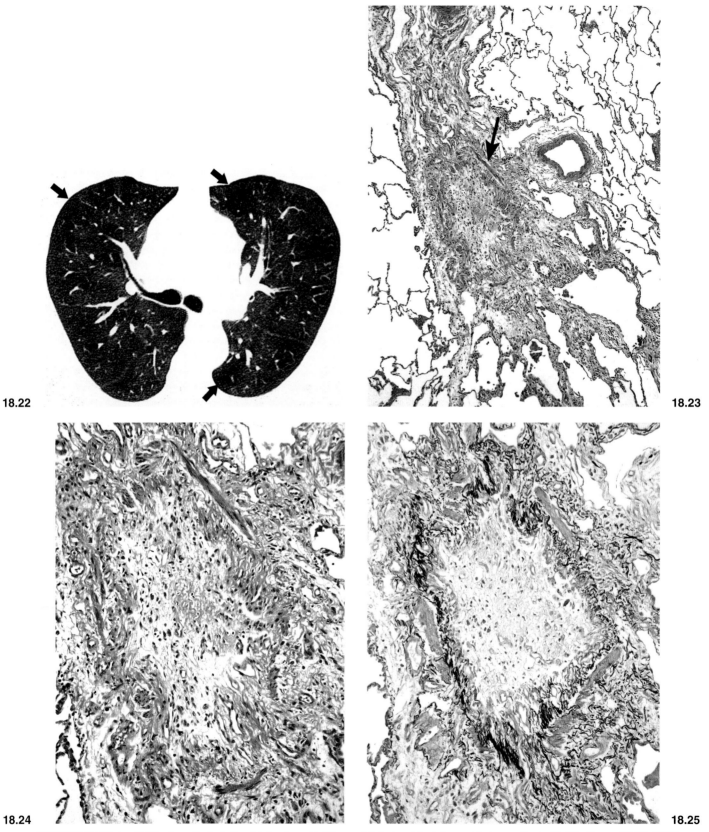

FIGURES 18.22 to 18.25. Case Study 4: Constrictive bronchiolitis possibly induced by leflunomide in a patient with RA. **Figure 18.22:** HRCT demonstrates bilateral areas of decreased attenuation and vascularity (*arrows*). Redistribution of blood flow to relatively normal lung results in areas of increased attenuation and vascularity. The findings are characteristic of constrictive bronchiolitis (bronchiolitis obliterans). **Figure 18.23:** Low-power view of the biopsy shows what at first appears to be a scar (*arrow*) next to a pulmonary artery branch. At higher power (**Fig. 18.24**) there is remnant muscle in the scar and elastic stain (**Fig. 18.25**) confirms that this is completely fibrosed bronchiole. In this case it was impossible to determine whether the disease was caused by the drug or the underlying disease.

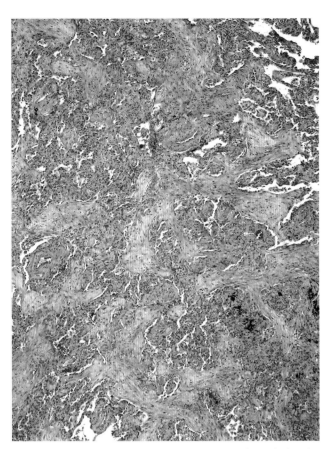

FIGURES 18.26. Case study 5: OP possibly induced by cyclophosphamide. The biopsy shows a typical pattern of OP. Cyclophosphamide is known to produce OP. However, OP is a very common finding in lung biopsies, particularly in immunocompromised patients, and the biopsy at best can be labeled a "possible" drug reaction.

- OP is well described as a reaction to cyclophosphamide (pneumotox.com), but OP is a very common and fairly nonspecific finding in lung biopsies from immunocompromised patients.
- Biopsy should be signed out as "Surgical lung biopsy showing OP. OP can be caused by cyclophosphamide, but is a common finding in immunocompromised patients. Infection needs to be ruled out."
- As it stands, this is a possible drug reaction. If the clinical and imaging picture improved after discontinuing cyclophosphamide, then this would be a probable to definite drug reaction.

Case Study 6: Mixed Pattern of ILD Caused By Chemotherapeutic And Anti-Estrogen Agents

A 75-year-old woman presented with shortness of breath. She had been treated for the preceding 2 years with Taxol (Paclitaxel), Carboplatin, Taxotere (Docetaxel), and Topotecan for Stage IV ovarian cancer. Imaging (Fig. 18.27) showed mild peripheral reticulation (indicative of underlying fibrosis) and some ground-glass opacities. VATS bi-

opsy showed a fibrosing interstitial pneumonia, OP (not illustrated), and fibrotic damage to small airways, including fibrosis between the bronchiolar epithelium and the muscle, the latter raising a question of constrictive bronchiolitis (Figs. 18.28 and 18.29).

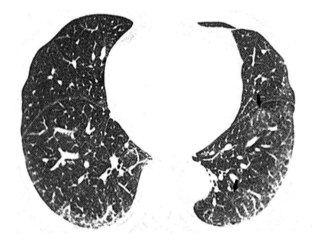

18.27

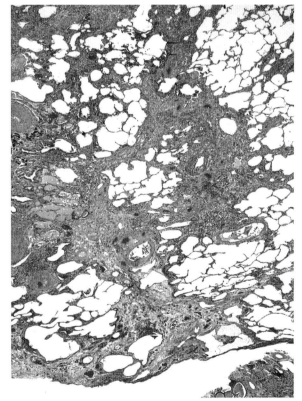

18.28

FIGURES 18.27 to 18.29. Case Study 6: Unusual pattern of interstitial fibrosis probably caused by chemotherapeutic agents for ovarian cancer. **Figure 18.27:** HRCT demonstrates mild peripheral reticulation mainly in the dorsal lung regions and small patchy areas of ground-glass attenuation (*arrows*). The findings are consistent with interstitial fibrosis but are otherwise nonspecific. **Figure 18.28:** Low-power view of the biopsy shows a pattern of patchy fibrosis that somewhat mimics UIP but has more centrilobular disease and less subpleural disease than is typical of UIP. At high power (**Fig. 18.29**) there is also fibrosis extending into the wall of a bronchiole. In other areas of the biopsy OP was present (not shown). Drug reactions can sometimes produce peculiar combinations of ILD patterns, and this is a useful clue to the diagnosis.

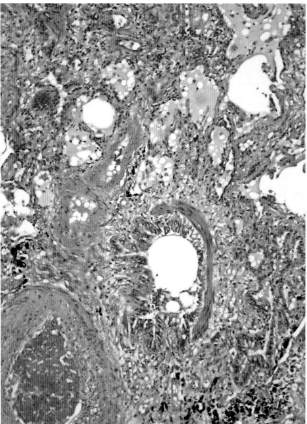

18.29

FIGURES 18.27 to 18.29. (*continued*)

respiratory failure within 24 hours of admission, requiring intubation. All cultures, serologic testing, HIV testing, and vasculitis workup were negative. The patient was a heavy daily smoker of synthetic marijuana, which he obtained from different sources. He had occasionally smoked tobacco, but not in recent months. Imaging (Fig. 18.30) showed centrilobular ground-glass nodules. The clinical impression was hypersensitivity pneumonitis vs. "something caused by synthetic marijuana." A VATS biopsy was performed and demonstrated granulation tissue,

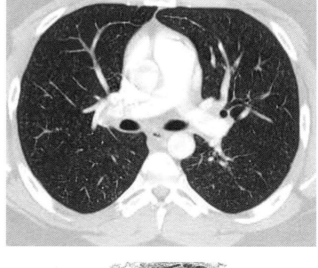

18.30

Analysis of Case Study 6

• Temporal sequence fits for a drug reaction.
• Many chemotherapeutic agents produce fibrotic reactions in the lung and these may take several years to develop.[3] OP is also a common reaction to chemotherapeutic agents. Most fibrosing interstitial pneumonias do not produce bronchiolar fibrosis.
• An argument could be made that the patient actually has UIP (common in this age group) but the pattern is not quite correct for UIP and the OP and bronchiolar damage do not go along with UIP.
• The combination of a set of ILD-like reactions that do not normally occur together suggests a drug reaction.
• Conclusion: Probable drug reaction caused by chemotherapeutic agents.

Case Study 7: Peribronchiolar (Centrilobular) Inflammation Caused by Inhalation of Synthetic Marijuana (Synthetic Cannabinoids) (Case Courtesy Dr. Brandon Larsen)

An 18-year-old male with no prior medical history presented with several days of progressive respiratory distress, fatigue, and a dry cough. This progressed to acute

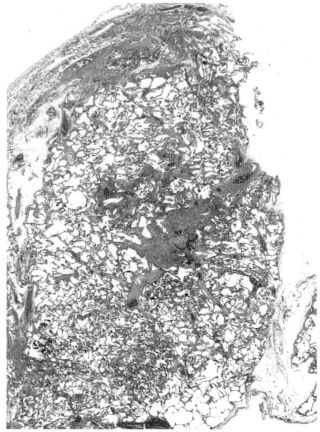

18.31

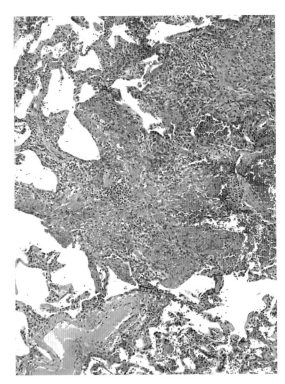

18.32

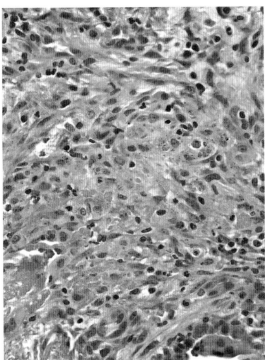

18.33

FIGURES 18.30 to 18.33. Case Study 7: Reaction to synthetic marijuana (Case Courtesy Dr. Brandon Larsen). **Figure 18.30:** HRCT shows innumerable centrilobular ground-glass nodules. **Figures 18.31** and **18.32:** Low- and medium-power views showing a collection of inflammatory cells and developing fibrosis confined to the centrilobular region of the lung. Both the imaging and the location of the lesion on biopsy strongly suggest a reaction to an inhaled agent, although the morphology does not fit any specific pathologic pattern. **Figure 18.33:** High-power view showing numerous golden-brown dots that presumably represent the residue of the inhaled material.

macrophages, and fibrin confined to the peribronchiolar regions; the macrophages contained numerous pale brown particles (Figs. 18.31 to 18.33). Cultures of the biopsy were negative.

Analysis of Case Study 7

- Temporal sequence fits for a drug reaction.
- The patient gives a history of heavy exposure to synthetic marijuana, a generic name for a variety of synthetic cannabinoids,[16,17] many of them believed to be more potent and potentially more toxic than marijuana itself.
- The imaging finding of centrilobular ground-glass nodules is strongly suggestive of an inhalation injury, either hypersensitivity pneumonitis or, in this case, a reaction to synthetic marijuana.
- An inflammatory reaction in/around bronchioles also fits with an inhalation injury, although the pattern is not specific. This is not the morphologic picture of hypersensitivity pneumonitis (see Chapter 12).
- Conclusion: There is little in the literature on pathologic reactions to synthetic marijuana, but the imaging and pathologic findings are entirely consistent with a reaction to an inhaled agent. The numerous brown particles probably are residua of the actual inhaled material. Sign out as probable drug reaction.
- Improvement if the patient stops using synthetic marijuana would be confirmatory.

CASE STUDY 8

A 30-year-old man with a history of hepatitis B infection was found to have an unresectable hepatocellular carcinoma. Treatment with sorafenib was started and 2 weeks later the patient became progressively more short of breath and developed respiratory failure, eventually requiring intubation. Imaging showed extensive bilateral ground-glass opacities and consolidation in dependent lung regions, consistent with diffuse alveolar damage/ARDS (Fig. 18.34). A VATS biopsy showed diffuse alveolar damage (Fig. 18.35). Cultures of the biopsy were negative.

Analysis of Case Study 8

- Temporal sequence fits for a reaction to sorafenib. Sorafenib has been reported to produce diffuse alveolar damage, which is in fact the most common pulmonary reaction to this agent[21] (pneumotox.com). Development of pulmonary disease within as little as 2 weeks is frequent.[21]
- The imaging and VATS biopsy results, although not at all specific, are consistent with a drug reaction.
- Cultures of the biopsy were negative and there is no good competing cause for this patient's lung disease
- Conclusion: sign out as to definite reaction to sorafenib.

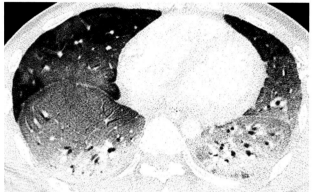

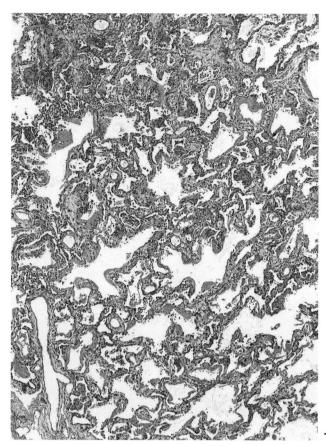

FIGURES 18.34 and 18.35. Diffuse alveolar damage/ARDS caused by sorafenib. **Figure 18.34:** HRCT shows extensive bilateral ground-glass opacities with relative sparing of the tips of the right middle lobe and lingula and areas of consolidation in the dependent regions of the lower lobes. **Figure 18.35:** Medium-power view showing diffuse alveolar damage. Rapid onset diffuse alveolar damage/ARDS is a common reaction to sorafenib.

CASE STUDY 9

A 45-year-old woman presented with Grave disease. She was treated with radioiodine and propylthiouracil (PTU). Several months after starting PTU she developed hemoptysis. PTU was stopped but she continued to have hemoptysis. Imaging showed ground-glass opacities throughout both lungs consistent with diffuse alveolar hemorrhage (Fig. 18.36). Antineutrophil cytoplasmic antibodies (ANCA) were initially negative but then became positive. The working impression was PTU-induced alveolar hemorrhage vs. vasculitis. PTU was discontinued, but ANCA remained positive. Rheumatologic workup was negative. Because of continuing intermittent hemoptysis, a VATS biopsy was performed 5 years after starting PTU and showed numerous hemosiderin-laden macrophages as well as very fine focal interstitial fibrosis associated with hemosiderin (Figs. 18.37 and 18.38). There was no evidence of vasculitis in the biopsy.

Analysis of Case Study 9

- The temporal sequence fits for a reaction to PTU.
- PTU-induced alveolar hemorrhage is well established in the literature and some cases of PTU pulmonary toxicity are associated with the presence of ANCA[22,23] (pneumotox.com).

- Extensive workup excluded a systemic vasculitis or any other cause of pulmonary hemorrhage.
- Conclusion: Definite PTU-induced pulmonary hemorrhage. Sign out as "surgical lung biopsy showing diffuse alveolar hemorrhage consistent with PTU toxicity." Note that this case is somewhat unusual in that there is no evidence of capillaritis at the time of biopsy, although there may have been capillaritis in the past. The fine linear fibrosis with incorporated hemosiderin is a common reaction to long-standing hemorrhage. Persistence of ANCA after discontinuation of PTU has been described.[23]

DIAGNOSTIC MODALITIES

Transbronchial biopsies are occasionally useful in documenting drug reactions when a very specific pattern such as eosinophilic pneumonia (Figs. 18.20 and 18.21) or non-necrotizing granulomas is found. Because many drug reactions produce relatively nonspecific patterns and often produce more than one pattern, VATS biopsy is usually required to obtain an adequately large sample. The potential efficacy of cryobiopsy is not known. The choice and limitations of each type of biopsy depend very much on the drug and the specific lesion identified.

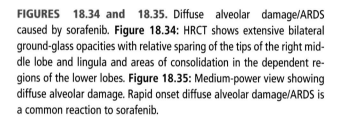

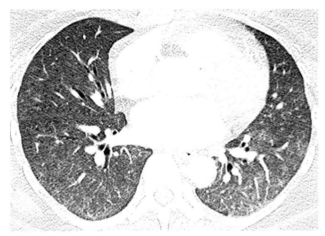

18.36

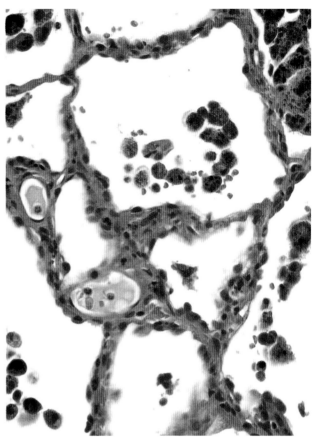

18.38

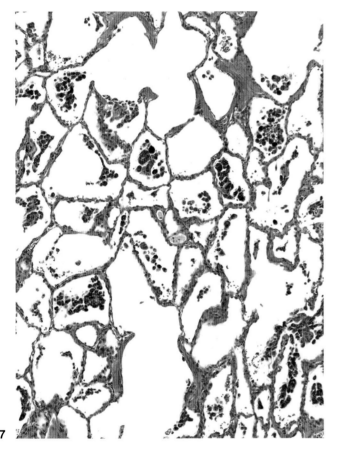

18.37

FIGURES 18.36 to 18.38. Case study 9: PTU-induced chronic hemorrhage. **Figure 18.36:** HRCT demonstrates diffuse bilateral ground-glass opacities slightly denser in the lower lobes. **Figures 18.37** and **18.38:** Low- and high-power views showing evidence of chronic hemorrhage in the form of numerous hemosiderin-laden macrophages and a small amount of interstitial hemosiderin. There is very fine interstitial fibrosis secondary to chronic hemorrhage.

REFERENCES

1. Camus P, Martin WJ 2nd, Rosenow EC 3rd. Amiodarone pulmonary toxicity. *Clin Chest Med.* 2004;25:65–75.
2. Foster RA, Zander DS, Mergo PJ, et al. Mesalamine-related lung disease: clinical, radiographic, and pathologic manifestations. *Inflamm Bowel Dis.* 2003;9:308–315.
3. Twohig KJ, Matthay RA. Pulmonary effects of cytotoxic agents other than bleomycin. *Clin Chest Med.* 1990;11:31–54.
4. Skeoch S, Weatherley N, Swift AJ, et al. Drug-induced interstitial lung disease: a systematic review. *J Clin Med.* 2018;7(10).
5. Silva CI, Müller NL. Drug-induced lung diseases: most common reaction patterns and corresponding high-resolution CT manifestations. *Semin Ultrasound CT MR.* 2006;27:111–116.
6. Torrisi JM, Schwartz LH, Gollub MJ, et al. CT findings of chemotherapy-induced toxicity: what radiologists need to know about the clinical and radiologic manifestations of chemotherapy toxicity. *Radiology.* 2011;258:41–56.
7. Rossi SE, Erasmus JJ, McAdams HP, et al. Pulmonary drug toxicity: radiologic and pathologic manifestations. *Radiographics.* 2000;20:1245–1259.
8. Camus P, Fanton A, Bonniaud P, et al. Interstitial lung disease induced by drugs and radiation. *Respiration.* 2004;71:301–326.
9. Matsuno O. Drug-induced interstitial lung disease: mechanisms and best diagnostic approaches. *Respir Res.* 2012 31;13:39.
10. Roden AC, Camus P. Iatrogenic pulmonary lesions. *Semin Diagn Pathol.* 2018;35:260–271.

11. Chopra A, Nautiyal A, Kalkanis A, et al. Drug-induced sarcoidosis-like reactions. *Chest*. 2018;154:664–677. doi:10.1016/j.chest.2018.03.056.

12. Papiris SA, Triantafillidou C, Kolilekas L, et al. Amiodarone: review of pulmonary effects and toxicity. *Drug Safety*. 2010;33:539–558.

13. Naidoo J, Wang X, Woo KM, et al. Pneumonitis in patients treated with anti-programmed death-1/programmed death ligand 1 therapy. *J Clin Oncol*. 2017;35(7):709–717.

14. Gkiozos I, Kopitopoulou A, Kalkanis A, et al. Sarcoidosis-like reactions induced by checkpoint inhibitors. *J Thorac Oncol*. 2018;13(8):1076–1082.

15. Haim DY, Lippmann ML, Goldberg SK, et al. The pulmonary complications of crack cocaine. A comprehensive review. *Chest*. 1995;107:233–240.

16. Cohen K, Weinstein AM. Synthetic and non-synthetic cannabinoid drugs and their adverse effects-a review from public health prospective. *Front Public Health*. 2018;6:162.

17. Berkowitz EA, Henry TS, Veeraraghavan S, et al. Pulmonary effects of synthetic marijuana: chest radiography and CT findings. *AJR Am J Roentgenol*. 2015;204:750–757.

18. Milroy CM, Parai JL. The histopathology of drugs of abuse. *Histopathology*. 2011;59:579–593.

19. Daïen CI, Monnier A, Claudepierre P, et al; Club Rheumatismes et Inflammation (CRI). Sarcoid-like granulomatosis in patients treated with tumor necrosis factor blockers: 10 cases. *Rheumatology (Oxford)*. 2009;48:883–886.

20. Lynch JP 3rd, Weigt SS, Derhovanessian A, et al. Obliterative (constrictive) bronchiolitis. *Semin Respir Crit Care Med*. 2012;33:509–532.

21. Horiuchi-Yamamoto Y, Gemma A, Taniguchi H, et al. Drug-induced lung injury associated with sorafenib: analysis of all-patient post-marketing surveillance in Japan. *Int J Clin Oncol*. 2013;18:743–739.

22. Cordier JF, Cottin V. Alveolar hemorrhage in vasculitis: primary and secondary. *Semin Respir Crit Care Med*. 2011;32:310–321.

23. Yazisiz V, Ongüt G, Terzioglu E, et al. Clinical importance of antineutrophil cytoplasmic antibody positivity during propylthiouracil treatment. *Int J Clin Pract*. 2010;64(1):19–24.

Lymphoid and Hematopoietic Processes Producing a Pattern of Interstitial Lung Disease

NOMENCLATURE ISSUES

Lymphoid proliferations in the lung go by a variety of names (Table 19.1), some of which (follicular bronchiolitis, lymphocytic interstitial pneumonia [LIP]) are generally viewed as interstitial lung disease (ILD) and some of which are circumscribed processes that are nodular or produce localized consolidation. Nomenclature in this area is confused by numerous terms in the literature (Table 19.1), often not very clearly defined, and by the fact that distinctions among the various entities in Table 19.1, particularly the benign diffuse proliferations, are sometimes arbitrary. Because this book concerns diffuse lung disease, the emphasis in this chapter is on diffuse processes, but localized lymphoid lesions are described and illustrated in the section on differential diagnosis.

Table 19.1

Lymphoid and hematopoietic lesions in the lung

Localized
  Intrapulmonary lymph nodes
  Nodular lymphoid hyperplasia (called in the past, pseudolymphoma)
  Malignant lymphoma (primary or secondary)
  IgG4-related disease
  Castleman disease (unicentric or multicentric)
Diffuse
  Follicular bronchiolitis and bronchitis (synonyms: pulmonary lymphoid hyperplasia, hyperplasia of BALT, hyperplasia of MALT)
  Lymphoid hyperplasia
  LIP (sometimes called diffuse lymphoid hyperplasia)
  IgG4-related disease
  Castleman disease (multicentric)
  Malignant lymphoma (primary or secondary)
  Pulmonary involvement by leukemias

CLINICAL FEATURES

Follicular Bronchitis and Bronchiolitis

The clinical findings in follicular bronchitis and bronchiolitis are very heterogeneous. Most patients present with shortness of breath and/or cough, but they may also have fever and weight loss. In some instances, these lesions are the sequelae of pneumonia or other infections. Follicular bronchitis and bronchiolitis are also seen distal to or around bronchiectatic/bronchioloectatic airway segments, and the clinical features of bronchiectasis, particularly recurrent purulent infections, may predominate. Table 19.2[1-7] lists known associations of follicular bronchiolitis/bronchitis. Pulmonary function tests can show an obstructive or restrictive pattern.

Lymphoid Hyperplasia

Lymphoid hyperplasia as defined here (see section Pathologic Features) frequently occurs as a postinflammatory and particularly postinfectious process, around mass lesions such as tumors, and in patients with bronchiectasis. It is also very common in patients with underlying collagen vascular disease–related ILD/interstitial pneumonia with autoimmune features (IPAF, see Chapter 21), but may be seen in idiopathic usual interstitial pneumonia (UIP; UIP/IPF) or nonspecific interstitial pneumonia (NSIP) not clearly associated with a collagen vascular disease; however, multiple lymphoid aggregates always raise a question of underlying collagen vascular disease/IPAF. Occasionally, lymphoid hyperplasia is seen in otherwise morphologically normal lung. When it is not associated with follicular bronchiolitis, it probably produces no clinical symptoms and is purely a pathologic finding.

Lymphocytic Interstitial Pneumonia

LIP usually presents with cough and shortness of breath but systemic symptoms (fever, weight loss), as well as features of an underlying disease, may be present. In adults, Sjögren syndrome is the single strongest association with LIP, accounting for about 25% of cases, but in children

Table 19.2

Associations of follicular bronchitis and bronchiolitis

Collagen vascular diseases, especially rheumatoid arthritis and Sjögren syndrome

IPAF (see Chapter 21)

Postinfectious, including pneumonias and infectious bronchiolitis

As part of active infections (*Pneumocystis, Legionella*)

Immunodeficiency syndromes, including HIV infection, common variable and selective IgA deficiency, Wiskott–Aldrich syndrome

Distal to or around bronchiectasis and bronchiolectasis

Dust inhalation

Drug reactions (penicillamine)

Associated with systemic eosinophilia

Evans syndrome

Secondary to airway obstruction of any cause

From Romero S, Barroso E, Gil J, et al. Follicular bronchiolitis: clinical and pathologic findings in six patients. *Lung*. 2003;181:309–319; Ryu JH. Classification and approach to bronchiolar diseases. *Curr Opin Pulm Med*. 2006;12:145–151; Nicholson AG. Lymphocytic interstitial pneumonia and other lymphoproliferative disorders in the lung. *Semin Respir Crit Care Med*. 2001;22:409–422; Aerni MR, Vassallo R, Myers JL, et al. Follicular bronchiolitis in surgical lung biopsies: clinical implications in 12 patients. *Respir Med*. 2008;102:307–312; Romero S, Barroso E, Gil J, et al. Follicular bronchiolitis: clinical and pathologic findings in six patients. *Lung*. 2003;181:309–319; Carrillo J, Restrepo CS, Rosado de Christenson M, et al. Lymphoproliferative lung disorders: a radiologic-pathologic overview. Part I: reactive disorders. *Semin Ultrasound CT MR*. 2013;34:525–534; Tashtoush B, Okafor NC, Ramirez JF, et al. Follicular bronchiolitis: a literature review. *J Clin Diagn Res*. 2015;9(9):OE01–OE05; Yousem SA, Colby TV, Carrington CB. Follicular bronchitis/bronchiolitis. *Hum Pathol*. 1985;16:700–706.

Table 19.3

Etiologies/associations of LIP

Collagen vascular diseases, especially Sjögren syndrome

Autoimmune diseases (primary biliary cholangitis, myasthenia gravis, Hashimoto thyroiditis, celiac disease, pernicious anemia, autoimmune hemolytic anemia)

Common variable immunodeficiency and selective IgA deficiency

Infection with HIV (almost always in children), Epstein–Barr virus, HHV-8

Chronic viral hepatitis

Crohn disease

Bone marrow transplantation and graft vs host disease

Drugs (amiodarone, carbamazepine, phenytoin, sirolimus, tryptophan)

Idiopathic LIP

From Nicholson AG. Lymphocytic interstitial pneumonia and other lymphoproliferative disorders in the lung. *Semin Respir Crit Care Med*. 2001;22:409–422; Swigris JJ, Berry GJ, Raffin TA, et al. Lymphoid interstitial pneumonia: a narrative review. *Chest*. 2002;122:2150–2164; Panchabhai TS, Farver C, Highland KB. Lymphocytic Interstitial Pneumonia. *Clin Chest Med*. 2016;37:463–474.

the most common association is with HIV infection. Other associations are listed in Table 19.3.[8,9] Some cases are idiopathic and have been included in descriptions/ classifications of the idiopathic interstitial pneumonias.[10] Dysproteinemias, usually hypergammaglobulinemias but sometimes hypogammaglobulinemias, are present in 80% of cases.[10] The presence of a monoclonal gammopathy suggests that the process is really a lymphoma and not LIP. Pulmonary function tests show a restrictive pattern and a decreased diffusing capacity, typical of diffuse ILD.

IMAGING

High-resolution computed tomography (HRCT) findings of follicular bronchiolitis include bilateral centrilobular and peribronchial nodules and patchy ground-glass opacities.[11,12] Most nodules measure less than 3 mm in diameter, although nodules up to 12 mm in diameter may be seen. The centrilobular nodules may be associated with branching linear opacities resulting in a tree-in-bud pattern

(Fig. 19.1). The findings are nonspecific and resemble those seen in a variety of other acute and chronic conditions.

The HRCT manifestations of LIP include bilateral ground-glass opacities, centrilobular and subpleural nodules, mild interlobular septal thickening, and, in up to 70% of patients, cysts (Fig. 19.2).[12] The cysts are usually peribronchovascular, few in number, and have thin walls.[12,13] The abnormalities may be diffuse but tend to involve mainly the lower lobes. Although the findings are nonspecific, the presence of bilateral ground-glass opacities with associated cysts in a predominantly lower lobe distribution in a patient with Sjögren syndrome is highly suggestive of LIP.

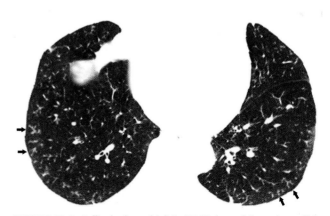

FIGURE 19.1. Follicular bronchiolitis. HRCT shows bilateral centrilobular nodular and branching opacities (*arrows*) in the peripheral lung regions. The patient was a 58-year-old man.

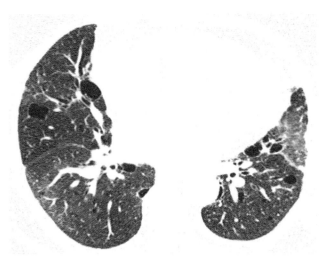

FIGURE 19.2. Lymphocytic interstitial pneumonia. HRCT at the level of the lower lung zones demonstrates patchy bilateral ground-glass opacities and several thin-walled cysts. The patient was a 63-year-old woman with Sjögren syndrome.

PATHOLOGIC FEATURES

Distribution of Lymphoid Tissue in the Normal Lung

In the normal lung, lymphoid tissue, referred to as bronchial-associated lymphoid tissue (BALT) or mucosal-associated lymphoid tissue (MALT), is inconspicuous and appears as occasional small lymphoid nodules, usually without germinal centers, next to small airways (Fig. 19.3).

Pathologic Features of Benign Lymphoid Proliferations

Follicular Bronchitis and Bronchiolitis

Follicular bronchiolitis represents hyperplasia of the normal BALT and is characterized by the formation of numerous lymphoid nodules adjacent to or within the walls of membranous or respiratory bronchioles (Fig. 19.4). When the same process occurs around bronchi, it is termed follicular bronchitis. The lymphoid nodules may or may not contain reactive germinal centers and there can be one nodule or many around any particular airway (Fig. 19.4). The nodules sometimes appear to compress the airway and compromise the airway lumen (Fig. 19.4). Typically, the germinal centers contain B cells that stain for CD20, and the surrounding lymphocytes are T cells that stain for CD3 (Figs. 19.5 and 19.6). Follicular bronchitis/bronchiolitis may also be seen around bronchiectatic and bronchioloectatic airways (Fig. 19.7).

Lymphoid Hyperplasia

We use the term "lymphoid hyperplasia" to refer to the formation of multiple discrete lymphoid aggregates, with or without germinal centers, in alveolar walls, interlobular septa, and the pleura. As opposed to LIP, the aggregates are *discontinuous* spacially separated lesions (Fig. 19.8).

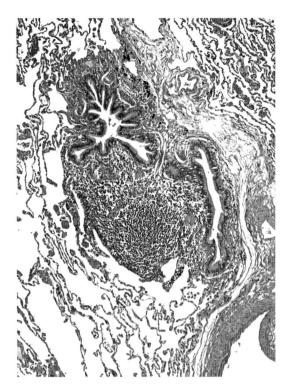

FIGURE 19.3. Normal BALT. Lymphoid aggregates such as this are occasionally seen in normal lung but should be infrequent and scattered; numerous lymphoid aggregates of this type mandate a diagnosis of follicular bronchiolitis (see Fig. 19.4).

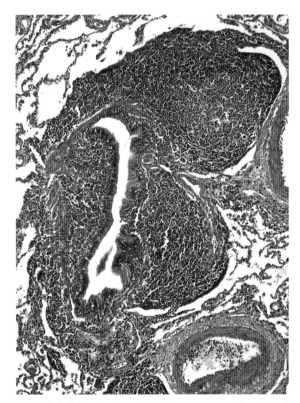

FIGURE 19.4. Follicular bronchiolitis (same case as Fig. 19.1). Lymphoid aggregates surround and compress a bronchiole. Note the presence of a germinal center, a common finding in follicular bronchiolitis. There were many such aggregates in the biopsy.

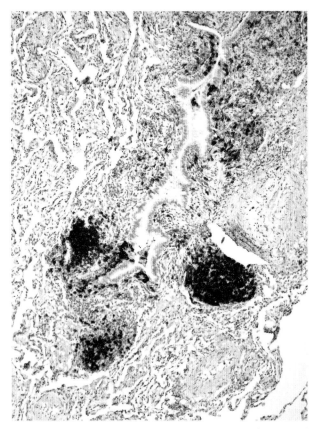

FIGURE 19.5. Same case as Figure 19.4. CD20 stain of a longitudinally cut bronchiole shows B-cell aggregation in follicles.

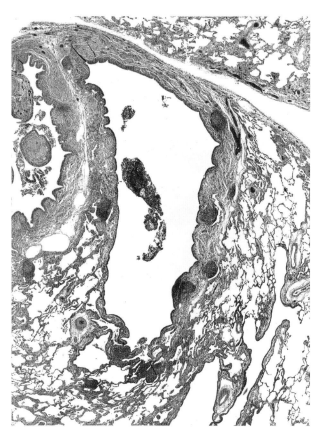

FIGURE 19.7. Follicular bronchitis. Numerous lymphoid nodules are present around a bronchiectactic bronchus.

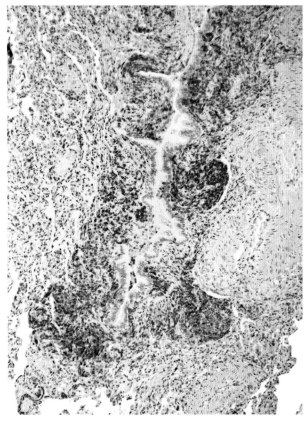

FIGURE 19.6. CD3 stain of the same bronchiole as Figure 19.5 shows a mild diffuse T-cell infiltrate.

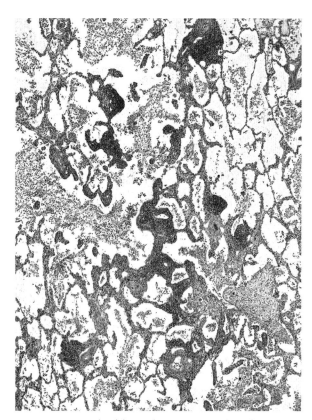

FIGURE 19.8. Lymphoid hyperplasia next to a bronchogenic carcinoma. The lymphoid reaction was localized to the region of lung containing the tumor.

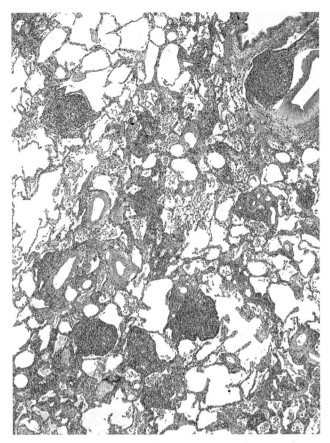

FIGURE 19.9. Lymphoid hyperplasia in a patient taking amiodarone. Some authors would classify this as follicular bronchiolitis, but the lymphoid aggregates don't only associate with bronchioles.

Such cases sometimes have follicular bronchiolitis as well, and some authors view lymphoid hyperplasia as defined here as a variant of follicular bronchiolitis.[14] Lymphoid hyperplasia can be present over large areas of lung, particularly in collagen vascular disease patients or where the process represents a drug reaction (Fig. 19.9), but can occur in a more localized fashion as well (Fig. 19.8). The presence of multiple lymphoid nodules in a biopsy showing an interstitial pneumonia is strongly suggestive of an underlying collagen vascular disease (see Chapter 21).

Lymphocytic Interstitial Pneumonia

In LIP, the lymphoid proliferation is dense and interstitial and involves alveolar walls in a *continuous* fashion over large areas of the lung. Germinal centers may or may not be present, but the defining feature is the marked expansion of alveolar walls by small lymphocytes and plasma cells (Figs. 19.10 to 19.16), sometimes to the point that the airspaces are obliterated and the alveolar walls become contiguous. Small noncaseating granulomas or individual giant cells are common within the lymphoid infiltrates (Fig. 19.14). B cells are found in germinal centers, when these are present, with the remaining lymphocytes usually T cells (Figs. 19.17 and 19.18). By definition, in LIP, the process is polyclonal.

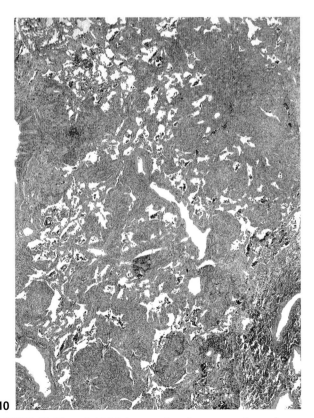

19.10

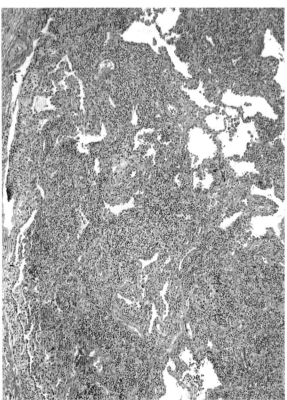

19.11

FIGURES 19.10 and 19.11. Low- and medium-power views of a case of LIP in a patient with IgA deficiency. Note the diffuse lymphoid infiltrate that in this example does not form germinal centers, and the marked widening of the alveolar walls, in some areas to the point of confluence.

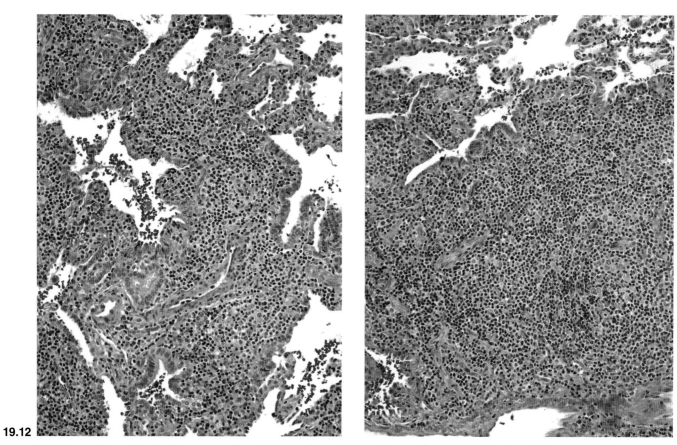

19.12

19.13

FIGURES 19.12 and 19.13. Higher power views of the case shown in Figures 19.10 and 19.11. Note the relatively homogeneous lymphoplasma-cytic infiltrate and the marked widening of the alveolar walls.

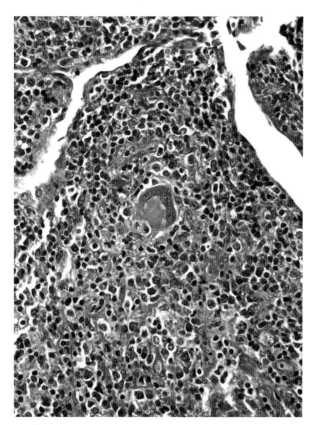

FIGURES 19.14. A giant cell in the midst of lymphocytes and plasma cells in a case of LIP. Interstitial giant cells and small loose granulomas are a common finding in LIP.

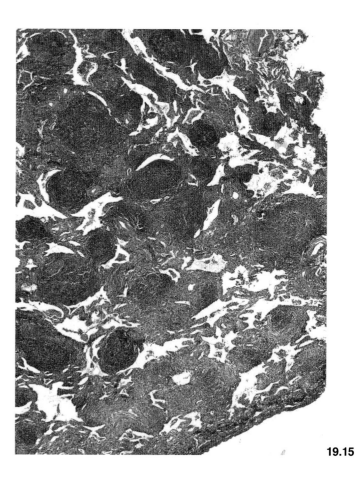

19.15

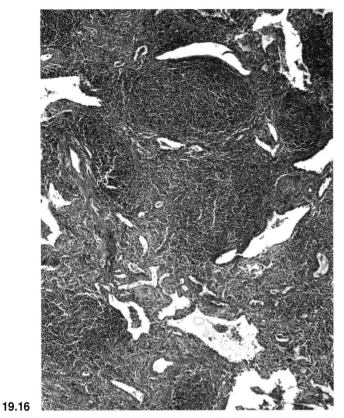

19.16

FIGURES 19.15 and 19.16. Low- and medium-power views of a case of LIP in which there is a suggestion of germinal center formation.

Cysts are common on imaging but are rarely biopsied. It has been suggested that the cysts reflect a check valve effect of bronchioles involved by lymphoid infiltrates.[9] The cysts appear to start immediately distal to bronchioles or represent dilated bronchioles that are partially obstructed by a lymphoid infiltrate (Fig. 19.19); the walls of the cysts contain lymphoid cells, sometimes with a small amount of fibrous tissue. What is not known is whether cysts in the setting of Sjögren syndrome are actually the earliest form of LIP or are a separate process, but we have seen cases in which a process that looks like LIP appears to spread from the cysts into the parenchyma (Figs. 19.20 to 19.22).

In advanced cases of LIP, interstitial fibrosis and honeycombing may be found (Figs. 19.23 and 19.24). Amyloid nodules are sometimes seen, either by themselves or in areas of LIP.

DIFFERENTIAL DIAGNOSIS

Table 19.4 lists the differential diagnosis of LIP. The most important differential diagnosis of all intrapulmonary lymphoid proliferations is malignant lymphoma, and in the lung, this is most commonly a low-grade marginal zone B-cell lymphoma (MALT lymphoma). MALT lymphomas are usually mass lesions and thus the usual distinction is from nodular lymphoid hyperplasia (see below), but they

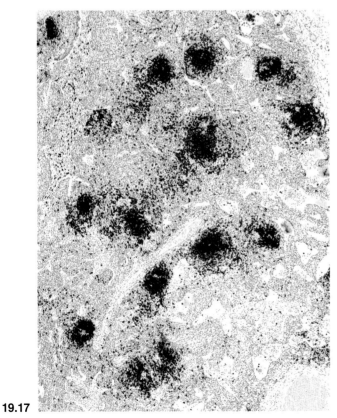

19.17

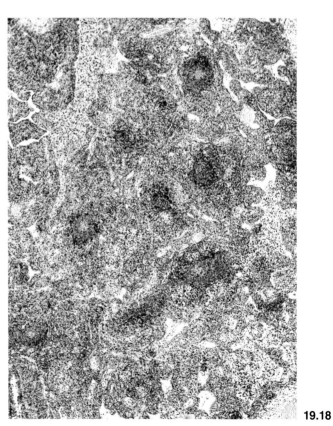

19.18

FIGURES 19.17 and 19.18. CD20 (**Fig. 19.17**) and CD3 (**Fig. 19.18**) stains of a case of LIP showing germinal center–like aggregates of B cells and a diffuse T-cell infiltrate. Not all cases of LIP show formation of germinal centers and in some cases the B-cell infiltrate is more diffuse and raises a question of a lymphoma.

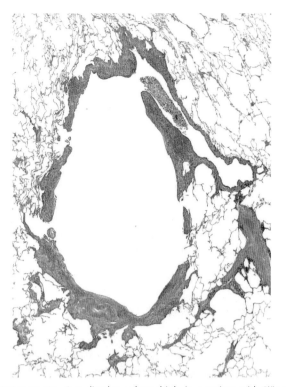

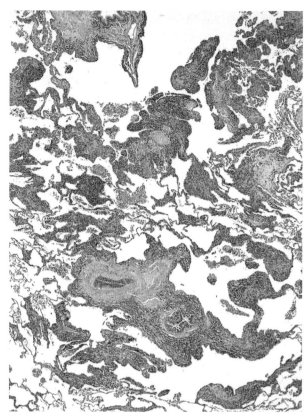

FIGURE 19.19. Cyst distal to a bronchiole in a patient with Sjögren syndrome. The cyst wall is composed of chronic inflammatory cells and fibrous tissue and the same process is present in the bronchiolar wall. Cysts of this type probably develop because of a check valve effect from affected bronchioles. Patient had Sjögren syndrome. Whether cysts of this type progress to LIP is not known.

19.21

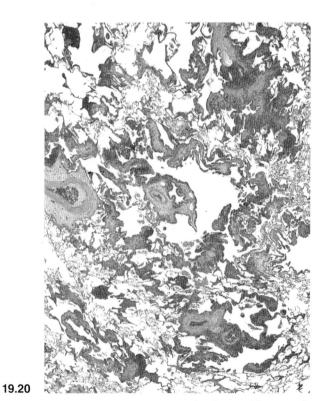

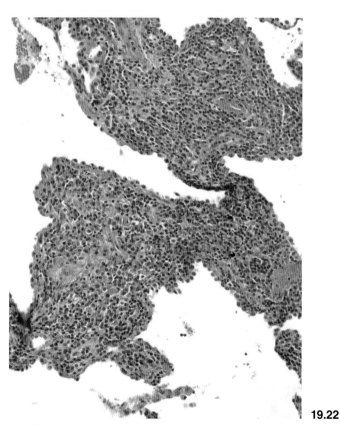

19.20

19.22

FIGURES 19.20 to 19.22. An example of cysts with surrounding interstitial inflammation in a patient with Sjögren syndrome. The lymphoid infiltrate (Figs. 19.20 to 19.22) is locally typical of LIP but occurs in circumscribed areas; this may represent very early LIP. Radiologically, this case was very similar to Figure 19.2.

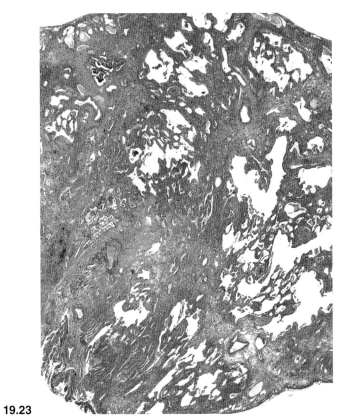
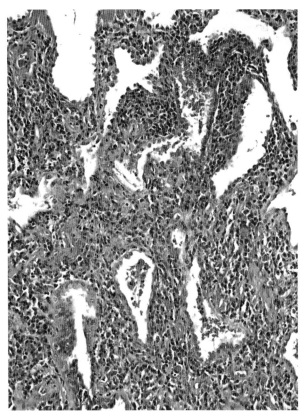

19.23

19.24

FIGURES 19.23 and 19.24. LIP with fibrosis. Some cases of LIP progress to fibrosis and sometimes honeycombing. In this example, LIP-type areas (**Fig. 19.24**) are still present and allow the diagnosis.

Table 19.4

Differential diagnosis of LIP

LIP	NSIP	HP	IgG4 disease	Lymphoma
Marked lymphoid infiltrate widens alveolar walls and may obliterate alveolar spaces	Lymphoid infiltrate usually only a few cells thick (alveolar spaces only obliterated by fibrous tissue not lymphoid cells)	Lymphoid infiltrate is peribronchovascular	Lymphoid infiltrate resembles NSIP but large numbers of IgG4+ plasma cells present (>20/hpf)[a]	Often marked lymphoid infiltrate with widening of alveolar walls and obliteration of alveolar spaces. Lymphoid cells may be monomorphous
Lymphoid infiltrate continuous over large areas	Lymphoid infiltrate continuous over large areas	Alveolar walls often normal away from bronchovascular bundles		Lymphoid infiltrate often continuous over large areas
No vascular infiltration	No vascular infiltration	No vascular infiltration	Vascular infiltration often present	Vascular infiltration often present
Small ill-defined granulomas or giant cells may be present	No granulomas	Granulomas present in areas of lymphoid infiltrate	No granulomas	Small ill-defined granulomas or giant cells may be present
Not clonal	Not clonal	Not clonal	Not clonal	Clonal (often demonstrable by staining for kappa and lambda in MALT lymphoma)

[a]Intrathoracic IgG4 disease may also manifest as hilar lymphadenopathy, pleural nodules, fibrosing pleuritis, sclerosing mediastinitis, peribronchiolar inflammation, OP-like lesions, plasma cell granulomas, eosinophilic infiltrates, phlebitis, arteritis, pulmonary hyalinizing granulomas, and inflammatory pseudotumors (see Travis et al.[14] and Liebow and Carrington[15]).

also can be diffuse and morphologically "interstitial," and at low power closely mimic LIP (see Figs. 24.18 and 24.19). In fact, many of the original cases of LIP described by Liebow and Carrington[15] would now be classified as MALT lymphomas. Other types of lymphomas primary or secondary in the lung can also spread in alveolar walls (see Fig. 24.17). Lymphomas typically do not have cysts, so the finding of cysts favors a diagnosis of LIP.

Distinction of benign from malignant is complicated by the fact that MALT lymphomas frequently contain reactive germinal centers and sometimes small noncaseating granulomas as well, and there may be an admixture of B and T cells by immunohistochemistry. Features that suggest MALT lymphoma are sheets of monomorphous slightly atypical B cells that sometimes have clear cytoplasm (see Figs. 24.18 and 24.19), monoclonal gammopathy, clonality demonstrated by flow cytometry or by immunohistochemical staining of the proliferating cells for only kappa or lambda (see Figs. 24.22 and 24.23) (demonstrable in the majority of MALT lymphomas but not all cases), infiltration of the airway epithelium by B lymphocytes (lymphoepithelial lesions) (see Fig. 24.19), and plaque-like infiltration of the pleura. Molecular studies to show a gene rearrangement/clonal process may be necessary to confirm the diagnosis.

Occasionally lymphomas involving the lung mimic follicular bronchiolitis because lymphomas tend to follow lymphatic pathways; however, in most instances, lymphomas with this pattern produce a more homogeneous and intense lymphoid infiltrate (see Fig. 24.17) than is seen in follicular bronchiolitis and don't form germinal centers. Typically, such cases are secondary rather than primary lymphomas, but primary MALT lymphomas can also spread in the lung in this fashion.

Leukemias involving the lung usually infiltrate the interstitium, as does intravascular lymphoma (see Fig. 24.24), and produce what at first glance appears to be an interstitial pneumonia. However, careful inspection shows that the infiltrating cells are not mature lymphocytes and plasma cells but rather morphologically atypical cells.

Pneumocystis pneumonia and cytomegalovirus (CMV) pneumonia sometimes morphologically produce a chronic interstitial inflammatory process that can mimic LIP, but generally with a less intense interstitial infiltrate that is morphologically closer to cellular NSIP. Usually with pneumocystis foamy alveolar exudates containing obvious organisms on silver stains are present, whereas with CMV viral inclusions are found.

The distinction of LIP from NSIP can be arbitrary (Chapter 7), but in general in NSIP, the interstitial infiltrate is much less intense than in LIP, the alveolar walls are not widened to the same extent, and where NSIP is severe enough to produce confluence of alveolar walls the area of confluence is fibrotic rather than cellular[16] (see Figs. 7.16 and 7.17). The combination of a lymphoid

Table 19.5
Intrathoracic manifestations of IgG4 disease
Parenchymal masses
ILD (NSIP-like, LIP-like, OP-like, UIP-like)
Airway-associated masses or airway stenoses
Vascular infiltration by inflammatory cells ("vasculitis")
Lymphadenopathy
Sclerosing mediastinitis
Pleural masses or fibrosis
Pleural effusions

From Ryu JH, Yi ES. Immunoglobulin G4-related disease and the lung. *Clin Chest Med.* 2016;37:569–578.

infiltrate and small noncaseating granulomas or giant cells in LIP can also mimic hypersensitivity pneumonitis (HP; Chapter 12), but in HP the interstitial inflammatory infiltrate is again much less intense than in LIP and typically is present in the interstitium away from the bronchovascular bundles.

Immunoglobulin (Ig)G4–related disease (IgG4RD) has a wide variety of manifestations in the thorax (Table 19.5). Although the typical picture of IgG4RD in most organs is that of a fibrotic process with a storiform pattern, vascular obliteration, and high numbers of IgG4-positive plasma cells as well as a high IgG4/IgG plasma cell ratio, in the lung, the appearances of IgG4RD disease can be much more varied. IgG4 fibrotic masses in the lung often do not show a storiform pattern.[17] Sometimes, IgG4RD disease in the lung takes the form of interstitial lymphoplasmacytic infiltrates with or without associated interstitial fibrosis and can resemble NSIP (Chapter 7) or LIP. Examples of organizing pneumonia (OP) and UIP associated with increased numbers of IgG4-positive cells have also been reported. In some cases, the interstitial process is quite diffuse and produces a restrictive pattern of pulmonary function impairment, and in others it is fairly localized (Figs. 19.25 and 19.26). The infiltrating cells can invade vessels and mimic lymphoma[18,19] (Fig. 19.27). Staining for IgG4 shows a high number of positive cells, typically greater than 20 per high-power field (hpf) (Fig. 19.28) with an IgG4/IgG-positive plasma cell ratio of greater than 40%. Many of these patients have extrapulmonary manifestations of IgG4RD disease, particularly autoimmune pancreatitis, and this information can be helpful in determining that the pulmonary process is also IgG4 disease.

Multicentric Castleman disease involving the lung may appear as nodular masses or localized areas of interstitial infiltrates of plasma cells and lymphocytes.[20] Fibrosis is generally not a feature. The process is usually localized but there are a few reports of diffuse ILD.[21] Germinal centers and increased numbers of IgG4-positive plasma cells

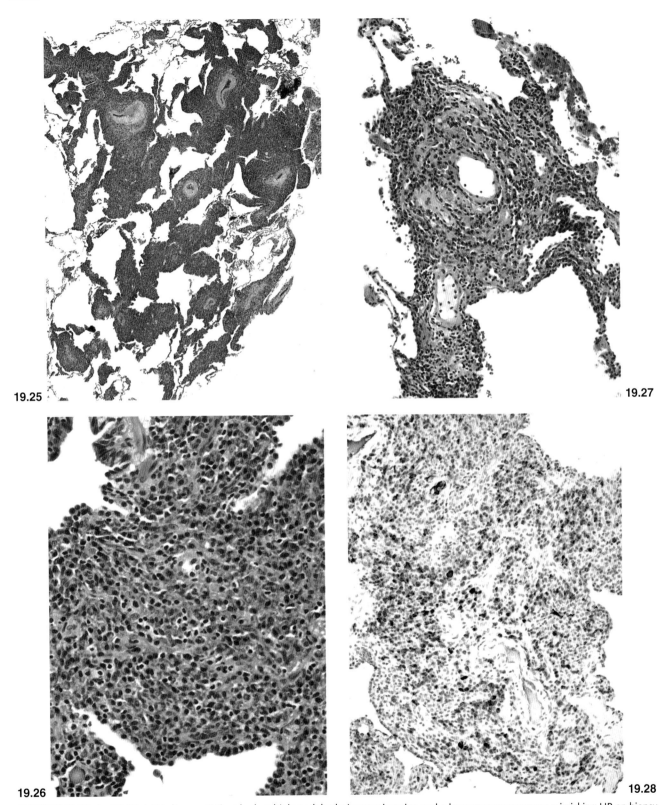

FIGURES 19.25 to 19.28. IgG4 disease. Patient had multiple nodular lesions on imaging and a low-power appearance mimicking LIP on biopsy (**Fig. 19.25**), but the individual areas of interstitial infiltration were localized. At high power (**Fig. 19.26**), there is a marked plasmacellular infiltrate, and the plasma cells and lymphocytes infiltrate vessels (**Fig. 19.27**). IgG4 stain (**Fig. 19.28**) demonstrates very large numbers of staining cells.

are commonly found, but not in the numbers and with the high IgG4/IgG-positive cell ratios seen in IgG4RD. Some cases of multicentric Castleman disease stain for human herpesvirus (HHV)-8. Serum interleukin 6 levels are typically elevated.

Nodular Lymphoid Hyperplasia

Nodular lymphoid hyperplasia consists of nodular or mass-like or occasionally more diffuse but still circumscribed lesions composed of contiguous lymphoid tissue with numerous germinal centers and, usually, some degree of localized interstitial fibrosis (Figs. 19.29 and 19.30). Small noncaseating granulomas may be present. Most cases have only one lesion but occasionally several are found. Microscopically nodular lymphoid hyperplasia and LIP can be identical in a given field, and the distinction is based on the diffuseness or circumscription of the process on biopsy or imaging. Most cases of nodular lymphoid hyperplasia appear to be reactions to previous inflammatory processes, but the disease is also associated with Sjögren syndrome.[22] Of interest, it has also been reported that some cases of nodular lymphoid hyperplasia have increased IgG4-positive plasma cells and an increased IgG4/IgG-positive plasma cell ratio,[23] suggesting that these might be variants of IgG4RD.

Intrapulmonary Lymph Nodes

Intrapulmonary lymph nodes are subpleural single or multiple nodular lymphoid lesions. As opposed to nodular lymphoid hyperplasia, they usually have the sharp circumscription and microscopic structure of a lymph node including a capsule and subcapsular sinus (Fig. 19.31), but sometimes the capsule is missing and the distinction from nodular lymphoid hyperplasia becomes arbitrary. Intrapulmonary lymph nodes accumulate atmospheric carbon pigment in the same fashion as hilar and mediastinal lymph nodes. Occupational dust exposure appears to predispose to the formation of intrapulmonary lymph nodes and such nodes may contain large quantities of the inhaled dust.

DIAGNOSTIC MODALITIES

As a rule, the diagnosis of most lymphoid lesions requires a large biopsy because low-power architecture is important, and areas diagnostic of lymphomas, particularly MALT lymphomas, may be scattered. If transbronchial biopsies are used, they need to be backed up by appropriate immunohistochemical and molecular testing to rule out a low-grade lymphoma. Cryobiopsies presumably would have the same limitations as transbronchial forceps biopsies.

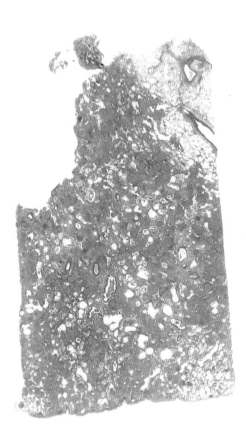

19.29

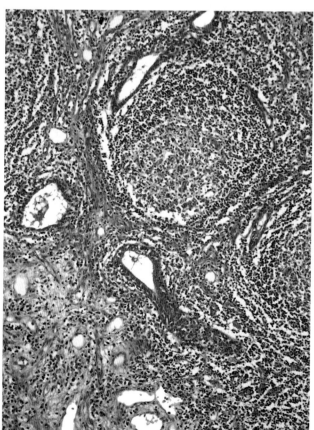

19.30

FIGURES 19.29 and 19.30. Nodular lymphoid hyperplasia. Patient had several discrete nodules on HRCT. The edge of one such nodule is shown in **Figure 19.29** and a high-power view in **Figure 19.30.** Note that the process stops abruptly and is surrounded by normal lung, the typical finding in nodular lymphoid hyperplasia.

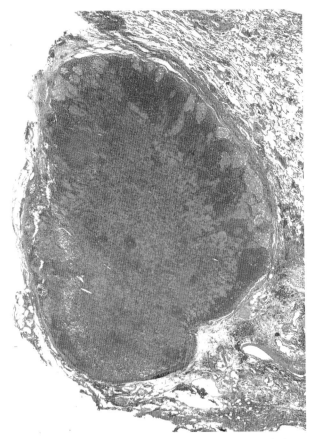

FIGURE 19.31. An intrapulmonary lymph node. This example has a capsule and prominent nodal sinuses.

PROGNOSIS

The prognosis of follicular bronchiolitis when it is the only lesion appears to be good, with stabilization or improvement on steroid therapy[4,1]; however, if it is present in a patient with a collagen vascular disease who has NSIP or UIP, then the latter determines prognosis. Lymphoid hyperplasia by itself probably produces no adverse effects, but is often seen in collagen vascular disease patients who have UIP or NSIP and is a helpful clue to correct diagnosis. The prognosis of LIP is highly variable. Overall survival is said to be 50% to 70% at 5 years, but this number may be biased by inclusion of HIV-positive patients. Some patients improve with steroid therapy, whereas others progress to end-stage fibrosis. Transplantation has been reported in a few cases without recurrence of LIP in the transplanted lung.[9] The proportion of patients with LIP that develop lymphomas is controversial, but probably small (on the order of 5%).[9] There are claims that LIP complicating AIDS improves survival but also reports that it makes survival worse.[8]

REFERENCES

1. Romero S, Barroso E, Gil J, et al. Follicular bronchiolitis: clinical and pathologic findings in six patients. *Lung.* 2003;181:309–319.
2. Ryu JH. Classification and approach to bronchiolar diseases. *Curr Opin Pulm Med.* 2006;12:145–151.
3. Nicholson AG. Lymphocytic interstitial pneumonia and other lymphoproliferative disorders in the lung. *Semin Respir Crit Care Med.* 2001;22:409–422.
4. Aerni MR, Vassallo R, Myers JL, et al. Follicular bronchiolitis in surgical lung biopsies: clinical implications in 12 patients. *Respir Med.* 2008;102:307–312.
5. Carrillo J, Restrepo CS, Rosado de Christenson M, et al. Lymphoproliferative lung disorders: a radiologic-pathologic overview. Part I: reactive disorders. *Semin Ultrasound CT MR.* 2013;34:525–534.
6. Tashtoush B, Okafor NC, Ramirez JF, et al. Follicular bronchiolitis: a literature review. *J Clin Diagn Res.* 2015;9(9):OE01–OE05.
7. Yousem SA, Colby TV, Carrington CB. Follicular bronchitis/bronchiolitis. *Hum Pathol.* 1985;16:700–706.
8. Swigris JJ, Berry GJ, Raffin TA, et al. Lymphoid interstitial pneumonia: a narrative review. *Chest.* 2002;122:2150–2164.
9. Panchabhai TS, Farver C, Highland KB. Lymphocytic interstitial pneumonia. *Clin Chest Med.* 2016;37:463–474.
10. Travis WD, Costabel U, Hansell DM, et al.; ATS/ERS Committee on Idiopathic Interstitial Pneumonias. An official American Thoracic Society/European Respiratory Society statement: update of the international multidisciplinary classification of the idiopathic interstitial pneumonias. *Am J Respir Crit Care Med.* 2013;188:733–748.
11. Howling SJ, Hansell DM, Wells AU, et al. Follicular bronchiolitis: thin-section CT and histologic findings. *Radiology.* 1999;212:637–642.
12. Sirajuddin A, Raparia K, Lewis VA, et al. Primary pulmonary lymphoid lesions: radiologic and pathologic findings. *Radiographics.* 2016;36:53–70.
13. Johkoh T, Müller NL, Pickford HA, et al. Lymphocytic interstitial pneumonia: thin-section CT findings in 22 patients. *Radiology.* 1999;212:567–572.
14. Travis WD, Colby TV, Koss MN, et al. *Non-Neoplastic Disorders of the Lower Respiratory Tract.* Washington, DC: American Registry of Pathology; 2002:266–276.
15. Liebow AA, Carrington CB. Diffuse pulmonary lymphoreticular infiltrations associated with dysproteinemia. *Med Clin North Am.* 1973;57:809–843.
16. Churg A, Bilawich A. Confluent fibrosis and fibroblast foci in fibrotic non-specific interstitial pneumonia. *Histopathology.* 2016;69:128–135.
17. Ryu JH, Yi ES. Immunoglobulin G4-related disease and the lung. *Clin Chest Med.* 2016;37:569–578.
18. Guinee DG Jr. Update on nonneoplastic pulmonary lymphoproliferative disorders and related entities. *Arch Pathol Lab Med.* 2010;134:691–701.
19. Yi ES, Sekiguchi H, Peikert T, et al. Pathologic manifestations of Immunoglobulin(Ig)G4-related lung disease. *Semin Diagn Pathol.* 2012;29:219–225.

20. Terasaki Y, Ikushima S, Matsui S, et al.; Tokyo Diffuse Lung Diseases Study Group. Comparison of clinical and pathological features of lung lesions of systemic IgG4-related disease and idiopathic multicentric Castleman's disease. *Histopathology*. 2017;70:1114–1124.

21. Huang H, Feng R, Li J, et al. Castleman disease-associated diffuse parenchymal lung disease: a STROBE-compliant retrospective observational analysis of 22 cases in a tertiary Chinese hospital. *Medicine (Baltimore)*. 2017;96:e8173.

22. Song MK, Seol YM, Park YE, et al. Pulmonary nodular lymphoid hyperplasia associated with Sjögren's syndrome. *Korean J Intern Med*. 2007;22:192–196.

23. Guinee DG Jr, Franks TJ, Gerbino AJ, et al. Pulmonary nodular lymphoid hyperplasia (pulmonary pseudolymphoma): the significance of increased numbers of IgG4-positive plasma cells. *Am J Surg Pathol*. 2013;37:699–709.

Bronchiolitis

CLINICAL FEATURES AND NOMENCLATURE ISSUES

Bronchiolar disorders are a complicated problem in that there are numerous, frequently overlapping, pathologic patterns with no universally agreed on names for many of them, considerably fewer patterns on imaging, and a variety of clinical and pulmonary functional associations that often don't correspond to any single morphologic entity.[1] As well, bronchiolar abnormalities may be isolated to the bronchioles but may also be part of more proximal airway disease, as in asthma or bronchiectasis (including cystic fibrosis), or of diffuse distal disease involving large portions of the lobule such as Langerhans cell histiocytosis (Chapter 10) and hypersensitivity pneumonitis

---

Table 20.1

Etiologic/clinical associations of bronchiolitis

Idiopathic
Infectious
Smoking related
Asthma
Distal to bronchiectasis
Collagen vascular disease related
Primary biliary cholangitis (primary biliary cirrhosis)
Inhalation of mineral dusts
Inhalation of toxic gases and fumes
Inhalation of hard metal (tungsten carbide, see
    Chapter 22)
Drug related (see Chapter 18)
Aspiration
Inflammatory bowel disease
Lung transplant rejection
Bone marrow transplantation (GVHD)
Bronchiolitis obliterans (pathologic constrictive
    bronchiolitis)
Diffuse panbronchiolitis
Granulomatosis with polyangiitis (Wegener
    granulomatosis)

(Chapter 12). Table 20.1 shows a general listing of etiologic/clinical associations of bronchiolitis and Tables 20.2 to 20.4 break down bronchiolitis by pathologic pattern.

The clinical features of bronchiolitis are extremely varied and often reflect another underlying systemic disease; for example, cystic fibrosis, collagen vascular disease, or inflammatory bowel disease. Although some forms of morphologic bronchiolitis, especially acute infectious bronchiolitis, fibrosing bronchiolitis,[2] constrictive bronchiolitis (bronchiolitis obliterans),[3-5] and diffuse panbronchiolitis,[6] produce signs and symptoms such as shortness of breath, others such as smoker's respiratory bronchiolitis usually do not, and the significance of bronchiolitis found in biopsies can only be determined by consultation with the radiologist and clinician.

In North America, acute infectious bronchiolitis in infants is usually caused by respiratory syncytial virus (RSV), which accounts for 50% to 80% of cases,[7] and less frequently by adenovirus, metapneumovirus, varicella, influenza, parainfluenza, or measles virus; and is associated with pneumonia-like symptoms, wheezing, and often hypercapnea.[7,8] Acute diffuse infectious bronchiolitis in adults is relatively rare, at least compared to pneumonia; etiologies include mycoplasma, influenza, *Streptococcus pneumoniae*, *Haemophilus influenzae*, RSV, and rhinovirus.[9]

Table 20.2

Etiologies of acute bronchiolitis (with or without epithelial ulceration/necrosis, with or without chronic inflammation)

Infection (may have epithelial necrosis/ulceration)
Aspiration (may have granulomas and foreign material)
Distal to bronchiectasis
Inflammatory bowel disease (may have granulomas in
    Crohn disease)
Inhaled fumes and gases (nitrogen dioxide, sulfur
    dioxide, chlorine, ammonia, phosgene)
Diffuse panbronchiolitis
Granulomatosis with polyangiitis (Wegener
    granulomatosis)

Table 20.3
Etiologies of chronic bronchiolitis (with or without airway wall fibrosis but without acute inflammation)

Infection
Cigarette smoke–induced "small airways disease" ("small airway remodeling")
Smoker's respiratory bronchiolitis (Chapter 8)
Aspiration (may have granulomas and foreign material)
Distal to bronchiectasis
Inflammatory bowel disease (may have granulomas, Chapter 14)
Inhalation of mineral dusts (may have inhaled dust, asbestos bodies)
Hard metal disease (Chapter 22)
Collagen vascular disease (follicular bronchiolitis) (Chapter 19)
Inhaled fumes and gases (nitrogen dioxide, sulfur dioxide, chlorine, ammonia, phosgene)
Drugs
Asthma
Hypersensitivity pneumonitis (may have granulomas) (Chapter 12)
Lung transplant rejection
Bone marrow transplantation (GVHD)
Diffuse panbronchiolitis
Lymphoma
Granulomatosis with polyangiitis (Wegener granulomatosis)
Idiopathic

Table 20.4
Etiologies of constrictive bronchiolitis (bronchiolitis obliterans)

Asthma (rare)
Postinfectious (viral [adenovirus, RSV, influenza, parainfluenza, measles, varicella, coronavirus, Epstein–Barr virus], mycoplasma), usually in very young children[4,26]
Inhaled gases and fumes (fire smoke, nitrogen dioxide, hydrogen sulfide, sulfur dioxide, chlorine gas, ammonia, phosgene gas, fly ash, nylon flock, sulfur mustard, polyamide-amine dyes, polyester resins used in fiberglass boat manufacturing, thionyl chloride, flavoring agents [2,3-pentanedione, diacetyl])[5,27]
Drugs (Aurothiopropanosulfonite, busulfan, CCNU, penicillamine,[a] tiopronin, sulfasalazine, rituximab)
Inflammatory bowel disease
DIPNECH
Lung transplantation and bone marrow transplantation
Distal to bronchiectasis (e.g., in cystic fibrosis)
Idiopathic

[a]It is not clear whether penicillamine itself causes constrictive bronchiolitis or the process is actually related to underlying rheumatoid arthritis.

In infants, acute infectious bronchiolitis may lead to postinfectious constrictive bronchiolitis, generally called bronchiolitis obliterans in the clinical literature. If one lung is affected much more than the other, unilateral hyperlucent lung (Swyer–James–MacLeod syndrome) may develop. Worldwide, adenovirus is the most common cause of postinfectious constrictive bronchiolitis in children, but some cases are associated with influenza, parainfluenza, varicella, mycoplasma, and RSV.[10,11] Postinfectious constrictive bronchiolitis also occurs in adults but is uncommon and is typically caused by mycoplasma infection. Constrictive bronchiolitis is usually associated with progressive shortness of breath, nonproductive cough and sometimes wheezing, and an obstructive pulmonary functional pattern that is not improved with bronchodilators.[1,3,4]

In lung transplant recipients, the clinical diagnosis of bronchiolitis obliterans syndrome (BOS, so named because pathologic constrictive bronchiolitis is histologically patchy and often cannot be demonstrated on transbronchial biopsy) requires a reduced FEV₁ for more than 3 weeks and the exclusion of acute rejection, infection, anastomotic complications, or other diseases affecting pulmonary function.[12] BOS also develops in a small percentage of bone marrow patients, in whom it is believed to represent a form of chronic graft-versus-host disease (GVHD) and is strongly associated with chronic GVHD elsewhere in the body.[13–15]

Diffuse panbronchiolitis is largely seen in Japan or persons of Japanese heritage and to a lesser extent in other areas of East Asia; it is rare in Western populations. Patients present with shortness of breath, productive cough, and airflow obstruction on pulmonary function testing. Most (>80%) also have signs and symptoms of chronic sinusitis. Cold agglutinins are persistently elevated in the face of negative mycoplasma antibody titers, and rheumatoid factor may be positive.[6]

IMAGING

High-resonance computed tomography (HRCT) manifestations of bronchiolitis can be classified into three main types: solid centrilobular nodules and tree-in-bud pattern, ill-defined (ground-glass) centrilobular nodules, and areas of decreased attenuation and vascularity resulting in a mosaic attenuation pattern.[16] The tree-in-bud pattern consists of well-defined (solid) centrilobular nodules attached to branching linear or tubular opacities. Centrilobular opacities can be recognized on HRCT by their distribution a few millimeters away from the periphery of the secondary

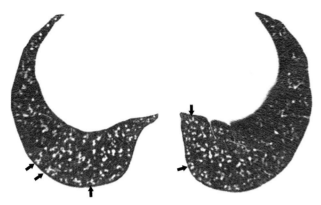

FIGURE 20.1. Infectious bronchiolitis. HRCT demonstrates well-defined small bilateral nodules that are clustered a few millimeters away from the pleura and the interlobular septa (arrows) characterizing a centrilobular distribution. Many of the nodules are attached to branching tubular opacities resulting in a pattern that resembles a tree-in-bud. The patient was a 20-year-old woman with infectious bronchiolitis.

lobule, that is, from the interlobular septa, pleura, and large pulmonary vessels.

The tree-in-bud pattern usually reflects the presence of bronchiolar wall thickening and accumulation of intraluminal material (secretions, inflammatory cells, granulation tissue, etc.) and is a characteristic feature of infectious bronchiolitis (Fig. 20.1).[16] In infectious bronchiolitis, the abnormalities usually have a patchy unilateral or asymmetric bilateral distribution. Similar findings may be seen in endobronchial spread of tuberculosis, atypical mycobacterial infection, and bronchiolar mucus impaction associated with bronchiectasis or allergic bronchopulmonary aspergillosis. In aspiration bronchiolitis, the tree-in-bud pattern may be diffuse or involve mainly the dependent lung regions. Diffuse panbronchiolitis is characterized by the presence of extensive bilateral tree-in-bud pattern,

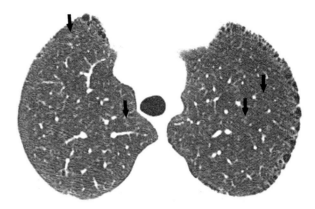

FIGURE 20.3. Respiratory bronchiolitis. HRCT shows bilateral poorly defined centrilobular ground-glass nodules (*arrows*) and mild emphysema. The patient was a 45-year-old smoker.

bronchiolectasis, bronchiectasis, and, commonly, areas of decreased attenuation and vascularity, resulting in a mosaic pattern of attenuation (Fig. 20.2).[17]

Ill-defined centrilobular ground-glass nodules are seen most commonly in patients with respiratory bronchiolitis (typically in the upper lobes in smokers) and in hypersensitivity pneumonitis (usually diffuse or with a lower lobe predominance) (Fig. 20.3). Centrilobular ground-glass nodules can also occur in a large number of other less common conditions including follicular bronchiolitis and mineral dust exposure.[16]

Areas of decreased attenuation and vascularity resulting in a heterogeneous appearance (mosaic attenuation) on inspiratory HRCT and associated with air-trapping on HRCT scans obtained at end-expiration are a characteristic manifestation of constrictive bronchiolitis (Fig. 20.4).[16] Ancillary findings include bronchiectasis and bronchial wall thickening. A mosaic attenuation pattern is a nonspecific finding seen on HRCT in a number of conditions.

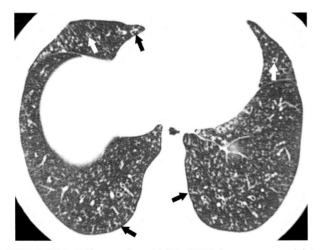

FIGURE 20.2. Diffuse panbronchiolitis. HRCT shows numerous bilateral well-defined centrilobular nodules and branching tubular structures resulting in a tree-in-bud pattern (*black arrows*). Also noted is mild bronchiectasis (*white arrows*). The patient was a 34-year-old woman with diffuse panbronchiolitis.

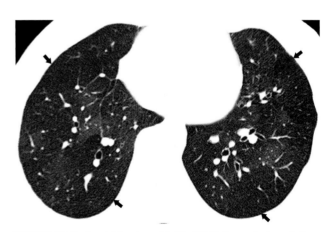

FIGURE 20.4. Constrictive bronchiolitis. HRCT demonstrates a heterogeneous appearance of the lungs (mosaic attenuation) caused by the presence of extensive bilateral areas of decreased attenuation and vascularity (*arrows*). The patient was a 23-year-old woman with constrictive bronchiolitis and severe airflow obstruction secondary to chronic GVHD.

However, mosaic attenuation as the predominant or only abnormality and associated with decreased vascularity usually is due to constrictive bronchiolitis, asthma, hypersensitivity pneumonitis, or chronic pulmonary thromboembolism.[16]

NORMAL ANATOMY

Bronchioles are conducting airways that lack cartilage in their walls. They are divided into more proximal membranous bronchioles, which have a completely muscularized wall (Figs. 20.5 and 20.6), and more distal respiratory bronchioles, which have a partially muscularized and partially alveolated wall (Fig. 20.5). Both types of bronchiole normally have a predominantly ciliated epithelium with interspersed Clara (club) cells, identified by apical snouts. Small numbers of mucus-secreting cells are found in the normal membranous bronchioles but are rare in normal respiratory bronchioles. Most forms of bronchiolitis affect predominantly membranous bronchioles.

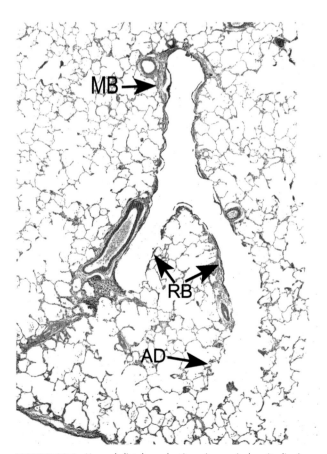

FIGURE 20.5. Normal distal conducting airways in longitudinal section. Membranous bronchioles (MB) have a continuous muscular wall. Respiratory bronchioles (RB) have a partially muscular and partially alveolated wall, whereas alveolar ducts (AD) have a completely alveolated wall.

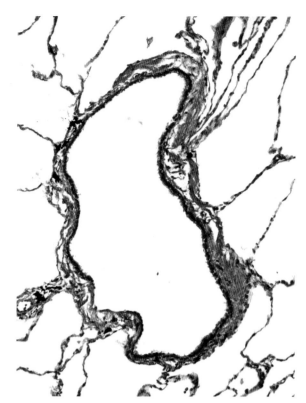

FIGURE 20.6. Higher power view of a normal membranous bronchiole in cross section. There is at most a small space between the muscular layer and the epithelium.

PATHOLOGIC FEATURES

Acute Bronchiolitis

Bronchiolitis with acute inflammation is most commonly infectious but can be seen in a variety of other conditions (Table 20.2). In immunocompetent patients, infections caused by viruses and mycoplasma frequently show a combination of neutrophils in the lumen and lymphocytes in the wall (Figs. 20.7 to 20.10), something that is less common in most of the other conditions listed in Table 20.2. Diffuse panbronchiolitis (Figs. 20.11 and 20.12, and see below) can demonstrate the same combination, but with interstitial foamy macrophages as well. The airway epithelium in viral and mycoplasma infections is often hyperplastic, disordered, and sometimes cytologically atypical (Fig. 20.8 to 20.10), useful clues to the underlying etiology. In severe cases, the epithelium may be ulcerated or even obliterated by inflammation.

In the immunocompromised patient, acute bronchiolitis is often much more severe with destruction of the airway wall, extensive acute inflammation, and large amounts of karyorrhexis (Figs. 20.13 and 20.14), producing a low-power view of necrotizing airway-centered nodules. This picture can be caused by viruses (usually adenovirus, herpes, or cytomegalovirus), fungi, and toxoplasma.

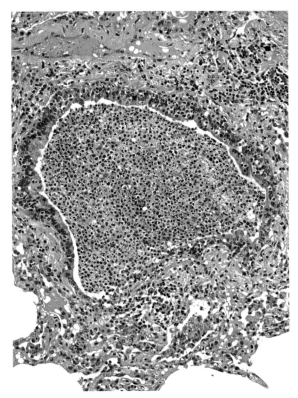

FIGURE 20.7. Acute bronchiolitis caused by mycoplasma. The lumen is filled with neutrophils, whereas the surrounding tissue contains chronic inflammatory cells. The epithelium is inflamed but otherwise normal.

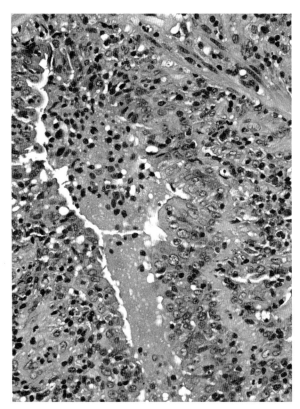

FIGURE 20.10. Acute bronchiolitis caused by mycoplasma. In this example, the airway epithelium is disorganized and cytologically atypical.

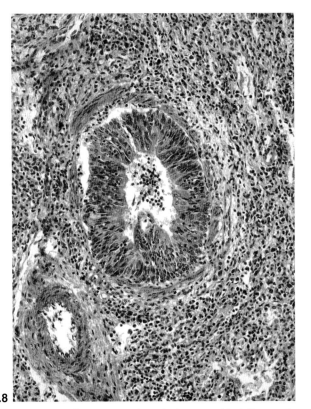

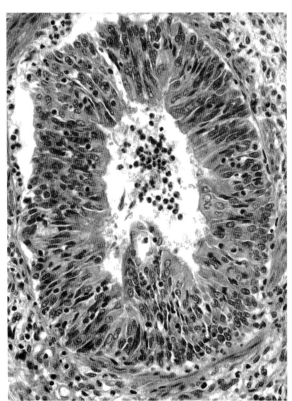

20.8   20.9

FIGURES 20.8 and 20.9. Acute bronchiolitis caused by influenza. The same pattern of luminal neutrophils and surrounding chronic inflammatory cells as seen in Figure 20.7 is present, but the epithelium is markedly hyperplastic.

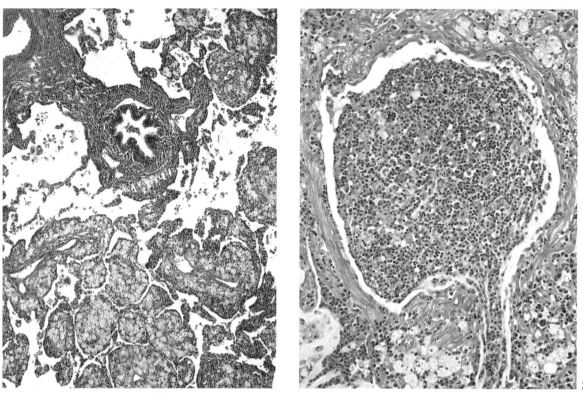

20.11

20.12

FIGURES 20.11 and 20.12. Diffuse panbronchiolitis. In **Figure 20.11** there are a few neutrophils in the lumen and surrounding chronic inflammation, similar to the findings in many forms of acute infectious bronchiolitis (Figs. 20.7 to 20.10). However, the presence of foamy macrophages in the interstitium is strongly suggestive of diffuse panbronchiolitis. **Figure 20.12.** An example of diffuse panbronchiolitis with a marked luminal neutrophil infiltrate and foamy macrophages in the bronchiolar wall.

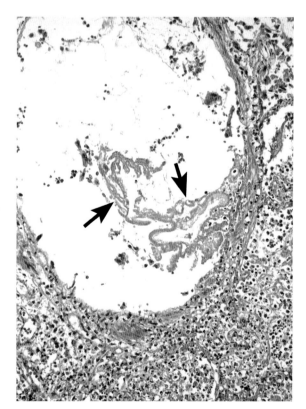

FIGURE 20.13. Herpes bronchiolitis in an immunocompromised patient. The airway epithelium (*arrows*) is completely necrotic. The surrounding tissue contains numerous karyorrhectic fragments.

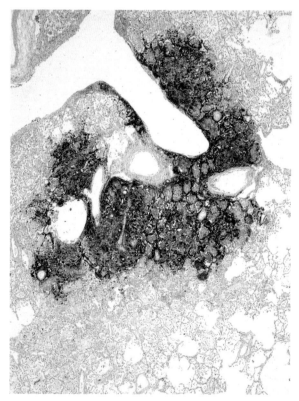

FIGURE 20.14. Herpes bronchiolitis. Immunostain for herpes shows extensive viral infection in the tissue surrounding the airway.

Inflammatory bowel disease can produce a picture of an acute or chronic bronchiolitis; in most cases, lung involvement occurs in patients already known to have Crohn disease or ulcerative colitis, but occasionally the initial presentation is in the lung. Biopsies from Crohn disease patients frequently, but not invariably, show granulomas (see Chapter 14).

Granulomatosis with polyangiitis (Wegener granulomatosis), although a vasculitis, often involves the trachea and large airways and occasionally the bronchioles as well and can produce ulceration with acute and chronic inflammation. Unless vasculitis is also present, the morphologic features of the bronchiolitis are not specific.

Diffuse panbronchiolitis has distinctive clinical features (see above) and also reasonably distinctive pathologic findings including some combination of acute and chronic inflammation involving membranous and respiratory bronchioles and sometimes also small bronchi and, by definition, foamy macrophages present in the bronchiolar walls, walls of alveolar ducts, and sometimes alveoli (Figs. 20.11 and 20.12). However, the diagnosis of diffuse panbronchiolitis requires these findings in conjunction with typical clinical features, because, rarely, interstitial foamy macrophages can be found in the walls of alveolar ducts (and even more uncommonly in the walls of membranous bronchioles) in constrictive and follicular bronchiolitis, cystic fibrosis, aspiration, hypersensitivity pneumonitis, granulomatosis with polyangiitis (Wegener granulomatosis), collagen vascular diseases, and lymphomas.[18]

Chronic Bronchiolitis

Bronchiolitis characterized by chronic inflammation in the wall without a significant neutrophil component is much less specific and has a wide range of etiologies (Table 20.3). There are three fundamental patterns: disorganized infiltration of the bronchiolar wall by lymphocytes and plasma cells; follicular bronchiolitis (see Chapter 19) in which one or more discrete lymphoid nodules, frequently with germinal centers, expand the bronchiolar wall and narrow the lumen (see Fig. 19.4); and fibrosis of the airway wall with or without chronic inflammation. The latter pattern overlaps into constrictive bronchiolitis.

Chronic bronchiolitis may be found in many of the same conditions that cause acute bronchiolitis, including infectious bronchiolitis (Figs. 20.15 to 20.17), but statistically the most common morphologic cause of chronic bronchiolitis is cigarette smoking, which produces both smoker's respiratory bronchiolitis (Chapter 8) and small airways disease (small airway remodeling) in the membranous bronchioles.

Smoker's respiratory bronchiolitis (Chapter 8) is characterized by accumulation of pale golden or pale brown macrophages in the bronchiolar lumen (see Figs. 8.5 to 8.9) and a variable amount of fibrosis in the bronchiolar wall, sometimes with interstitial extension of the fibrosis into the distal parenchyma.

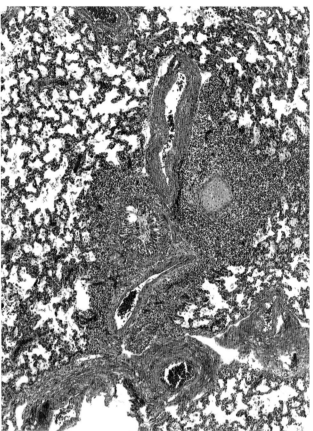

20.15

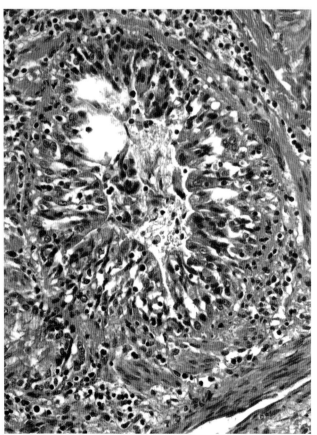

20.16

FIGURES 20.15 to 20.17. See figure legend 20.17.

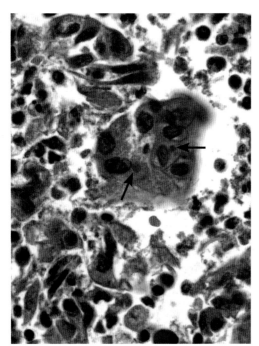

20.17

FIGURES 20.15 to 20.17. Chronic bronchiolitis, in this case caused by RSV infection in a child. **Figure 20.15:** Low-power view shows an intense chronic inflammatory infiltrate surrounding the airways. **Figure 20.16:** Marked chronic inflammatory infiltration of the airway wall and epithelium with epithelial hyperplasia. **Figure 20.17:** Eosinophilic RSV inclusions (*arrows*). (Case Courtesy Dr. Michael Graham)

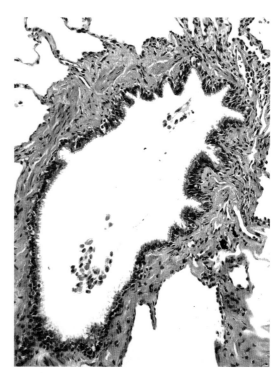

FIGURE 20.18. Cigarette smoke–induced chronic bronchiolitis. This process is referred to as "small airways disease" or "small airway remodeling." The bronchiolar wall is thickened by fibrous tissue and some degree of chronic inflammation.

In cigarette smoke–induced small airways disease (Fig. 20.18), the bronchiolar wall is thickened by fibrous tissue and the lumen narrowed, and there is an associated chronic inflammatory infiltrate, sometimes with lymphoid follicles. Small numbers of neutrophils may be present. There is often extensive mucus metaplasia of the airway epithelium and mucus plugs may obstruct the airway lumen. By convention, the process is not referred to, diagnostically, as "bronchiolitis" but rather as cigarette smoke–induced small airways disease or small airway remodeling; however, functionally and morphologically, it is really a variant of constrictive bronchiolitis. Recent data suggest that many such bronchioles end up as fibrous scars.[19]

Bronchiolitis caused by inhalation of mineral dusts (asbestos, iron oxide, aluminum oxide, talc, mice, silicates)[20] is morphologically similar to cigarette smoke–induced small airways disease, but statistically there is more fibrosis of the airway wall and less chronic inflammation (Fig. 20.19); however, individual membranous bronchioles with changes caused by cigarette smoke and mineral dusts are often not distinguishable unless the mineral dust is pigmented or birefringent. With mineral dust exposure, the fibrosis sometimes extends into the respiratory bronchioles, often with considerable accompanying pigmented dust (Figs. 20.19 and 20.20), and this is much less common with cigarette smoking.

Hard metal disease is a pneumoconiosis caused by exposure to tungsten carbide. The bronchiolar walls are

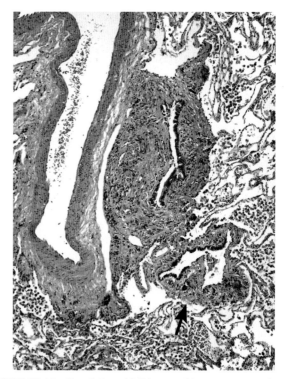

FIGURE 20.19. Chronic bronchiolitis caused by exposure to asbestos. The changes in the membranous bronchiole are similar to those caused by cigarette smoke, but the process also markedly thickens the wall of the adjacent respiratory bronchiole (*arrow*), something not usually seen with cigarette smoke exposure.

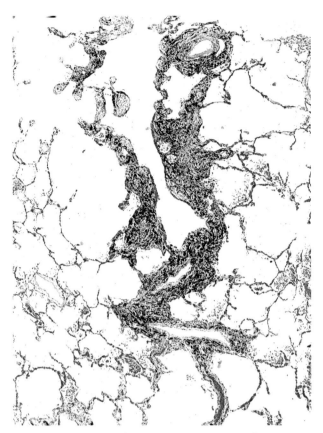

FIGURE 20.20. Marked fibrosis and pigmentation of a respiratory bronchiole in a patient with heavy exposure to silica plus another pigmented dust of uncertain nature.

chronically inflamed and markedly thickened and distorted by fibrous tissue, and the bronchiolar lumens contain macrophages and giant cells (see Figs. 22.26 and 22.27).

"Bronchiolitis" characterized by chronic inflammatory cells in bronchiolar walls may also be seen in hypersensitivity pneumonitis (see Fig. 12.13). By convention, the term "bronchiolitis" is not used when diagnosing hypersensitivity pneumonitis, but patients with hypersensitivity pneumonitis may have some degree of airflow obstruction, indicating that the bronchiolitis is functionally important.

Asthma is another condition in which a bronchiolitis is often present but is not named as such pathologically. The findings in asthma are very variable and can include goblet cell metaplasia of the epithelium, luminal mucus plugs, a markedly thickened basement membrane (uniformly present in the large airways, sometimes present in bronchioles), increased smooth muscle, eosinophils and chronic inflammatory cells, and, rarely, fibrosis of the airway wall.

Acute or chronic bronchiolitis with granulomas or foreign body giant cells (Figs. 20.21 and 20.22) should raise a question of aspiration; if aspirated food particles are not evident on routine stains, digested periodic acid–Schiff (PAS) stain can be helpful because the walls of vegetable particles are strongly PAS positive. Polarization may also be useful to demonstrate foreign material. The combination of organizing pneumonia (OP, Chapter 5) with giant cells or granulomas with or without acute inflammation is also strongly suggestive of aspiration (see Figs. 5.29 and 5.30).

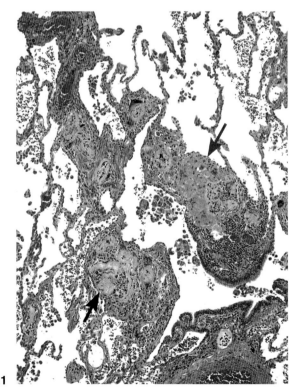

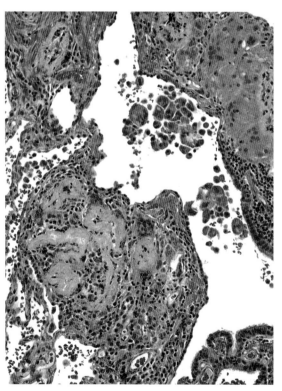

20.21   20.22

FIGURES 20.21 and 20.22. Chronic bronchiolitis caused by aspiration. **Figure 20.21:** The bronchiolar wall contains chronic inflammatory cells, a foreign body granuloma (*red arrow*), and a partially degraded aspirated vegetable particle (*black arrow*), seen better in the high-power view (**Fig. 20.22**).

In addition to aspiration, granulomas associated with bronchioles can be found in sarcoid (see Figs. 13.15 and 13.16), Crohn disease, and tuberculosis and fungal infections (usually necrotizing), and in the latter situation, a diagnosis of tuberculous or fungal bronchiolitis is appropriate.

Lymphomas often show a lymphangitic distribution in the lung and hence can produce a morphologic picture resembling chronic bronchiolitis (see Fig. 24.17).

Constrictive Bronchiolitis

Historically, the term "bronchiolitis obliterans" was used by pathologists both for bronchiolitis with intraluminal granulation tissue polyps and for fibrous narrowing/obliteration of the bronchiolar lumen. Luminal granulation tissue polyps are now regarded as either part of OP (also called bronchiolitis obliterans with OP and cryptogenic OP, see Chapter 5) if the granulation tissue is also present in alveolar ducts; or if confined to the bronchiolar lumens, as fibrosing bronchiolitis (see below). Constrictive bronchiolitis is the name applied to processes in which the bronchiolar lumen is narrowed or obliterated by scar tissue. The distinction is important because OP is generally a treatable disease with a good prognosis, and fibrosing bronchiolitis also improves

with treatment, whereas constrictive bronchiolitis may lead to respiratory failure.

The newer term "constrictive bronchiolitis" has been extensively adopted by pathologists, but clinicians generally use the older name bronchiolitis obliterans or obliterative bronchiolitis for the clinical syndrome[4,15] and may not understand "constrictive bronchiolitis," so it is advisable to use both names in the diagnosis. However, in lung transplant rejection biopsies and in patients with bone marrow transplants, the pathologic term "bronchiolitis obliterans" is still used; in these two settings, the clinical scenario is referred to as BOS.[13,14]

In the normal bronchiolar wall, there is almost no space between the epithelium and the muscular layer (Fig. 20.6). In constrictive bronchiolitis, fibrous tissue, which may be accompanied early on by acute or chronic inflammatory cells and epithelial ulceration, is deposited between the epithelium and the muscle, so that the lumen is narrowed or completely obliterated (Figs. 20.23 to 20.31).

Constrictive bronchiolitis may be very patchy and is easy to overlook. In the normal lung, there should be a bronchiole next to a pulmonary artery branch, and the airway and vessel should be of approximately the same diameter. A scarred bronchiole with an internal diameter much smaller than the artery represents constrictive bronchiolitis (Fig. 20.25). The presence of what at first

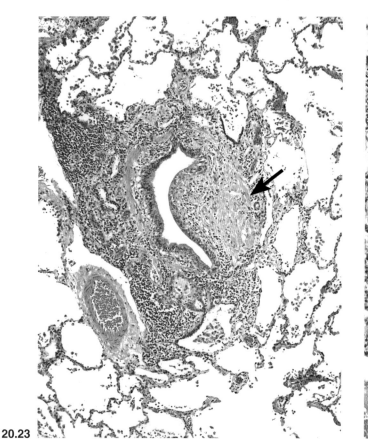
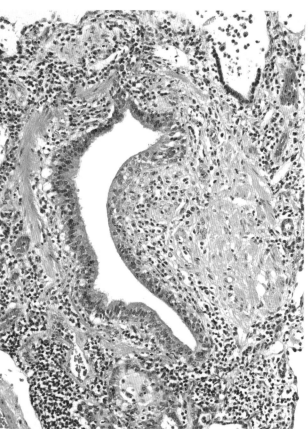

20.23

20.24

FIGURES 20.23 and 20.24. Early constrictive bronchiolitis in a patient with cystic fibrosis. There is a chronic inflammatory infiltrate in the bronchiolar wall along with a nodular scar (*arrow*) internal to the muscle layer. The process narrows the lumen.

glance appears to be a scar next to a pulmonary artery branch (see Figs. 18.23 to 18.25) should always raise a suspicion of constrictive bronchiolitis. Elastic stains are extremely helpful in finding old constrictive bronchiolitis because the normal bronchiole has an elastic layer and elastic stains outline the obliterated lumen in completely scarred constrictive bronchiolitis (Figs. 20.27 to 20.29 and see Fig. 18.25); however, if the inflammatory process that has caused the bronchiolitis is severe enough, most of the elastica of the bronchiole may be lost, with only a few fragments left to indicate the correct diagnosis (Figs. 20.30 and 20.31).

Most etiologies of constrictive bronchiolitis (Table 20.4) are morphologically indistinguishable. One exception is diffuse idiopathic neuroendocrine cell hyperplasia (DIPNECH) where minute carcinoid tumors (tumorlets) in bronchiolar lumens or neuroendocrine cell hyperplasia in the bronchiolar epithelium evoke a fibrotic reaction that obliterates the lumen (Fig. 20.32). This process is believed to be mediated through production of gastrin-releasing peptide by the neuroendocrine cells.

It should be noted that the morphologic presence of constrictive bronchiolitis in such cases may be misleading, because only about 30% of the patients reported in the literature as DIPNECH actually have airflow obstruction and air-trapping on imaging or pulmonary function testing.[21] Rossi et al.[22] have suggested that only patients with airflow obstruction should be labeled as "DIPNECH syndrome";

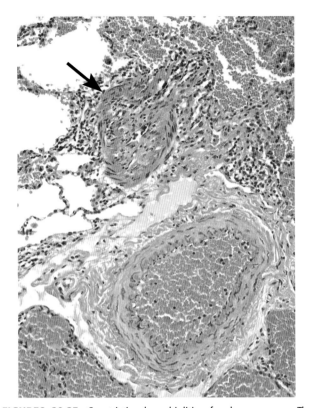

FIGURES 20.25. Constrictive bronchiolitis of unknown cause. The bronchiole (*arrow*) is much smaller than the accompanying pulmonary artery and the lumen is almost completely obstructed by organizing granulation tissue.

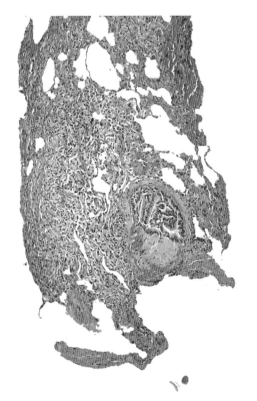

20.26

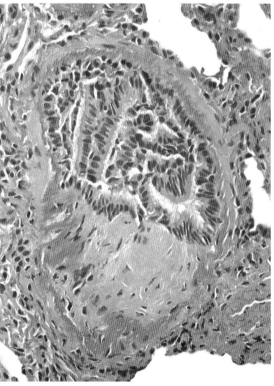

20.27

FIGURES 20.26 and 20.27. Constrictive bronchiolitis in a transbronchial biopsy from a lung transplant patient. A dense scar internal to the bronchiolar elastica narrows the lumen. The bronchiolar elastica is bright red (hematoxylin and aqueous eosin stain).

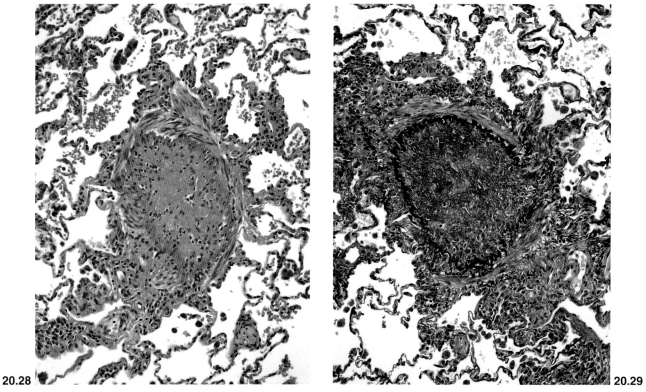

20.28 **20.29**

FIGURES 20.28 and 20.29. Constrictive bronchiolitis of unknown cause (same case as Fig. 20.25). **Figure 20.28:** On hematoxylin and eosin, the obliterated bronchiole appears as a scar with surrounding muscle. **Figure 20.29:** Elastic stain confirms that the apparent scar is really an obliterated bronchiole.

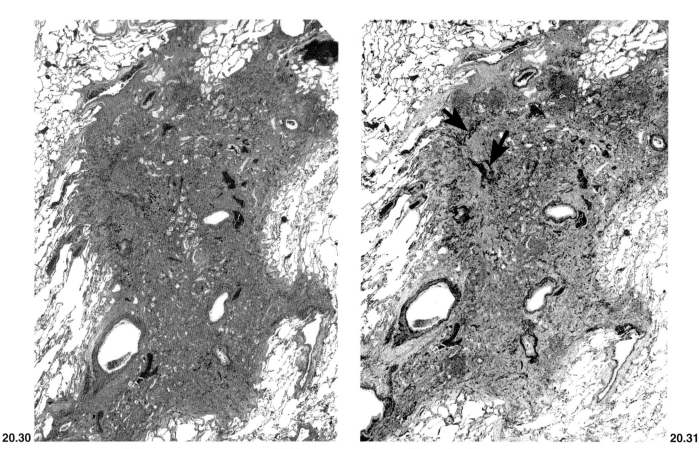

20.30 **20.31**

FIGURES 20.30 and 20.31. Severe constrictive bronchiolitis in a patient with cystic fibrosis. The inflammatory process has completely destroyed the bronchiole, and only a few fragments of elastic tissue (*arrows*) are seen in the elastic stain (Fig. 20.29). Location of scar next to a pulmonary artery branch is an important clue to the diagnosis.

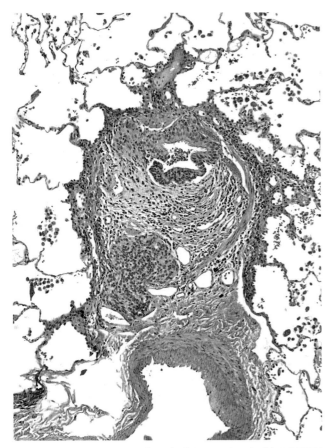

FIGURE 20.32. Constrictive bronchiolitis associated with DIPNECH. The image shows both a tumorlet and neuroendocrine hyperplasia in the residual bronchiolar epithelium. The bronchiolar lumen is narrowed by surrounding fibrous tissue.

in the remaining cases, neuroendocrine cell hyperplasia is mostly associated with the presence of macroscopic carcinoid tumors.

Fibrosing Bronchiolitis

Fibrosing bronchiolitis (Figs. 20.33 to 20.36) is an uncommon and somewhat poorly defined entity in which there are granulation tissue polyps in the lumens of bronchioles with no or minimal extension outside the bronchioles and normal parenchyma away from the bronchioles. The polyps organize to dense fibrous tissue and become epithelialized with narrowing and distortion of the bronchiolar lumens (Figs. 20.34 and 20.35). Morphologically, there is an overlap with OP, but OP covers relatively large areas of parenchyma and has granulation tissue plugs in alveolar ducts, a feature not seen in fibrosing bronchiolitis. There is also an overlap with constrictive bronchiolitis, but the usual case of constrictive bronchiolitis shows fibrosis in the airway wall rather than luminal granulation tissue polyps.

Lesions of this type have been referred to in the literature as constrictive bronchiolitis, proliferative bronchiolitis, and fibrosing bronchiolitis.[2] On imaging, there are centrilobular nodules or tree-in-bud opacities (Fig. 20.33 and 20.34), but no air-trapping as would be seen in constrictive bronchiolitis (Fig. 20.4), nor the peribronchovascular consolidation typical of OP.[2] Clinically, the process appears to be caused by (unidentified) infectious agents or inhaled fumes/toxins.[2]

We believe that these lesions represent early constrictive bronchiolitis at a stage when the process can be stopped and potentially reversed. In our experience, patients with fibrosing bronchiolitis respond reasonably well to high-dose immunosuppressive agents with at least partial recovery of pulmonary function,[2] so separation from established constrictive bronchiolitis, which typically does not respond well to therapy, is important.

DIAGNOSTIC MODALITIES

Accurate assessment of bronchiolitis generally requires one or preferably more whole bronchioles, and as a rule transbronchial biopsy does not provide adequate sampling. However, lung transplant rejection is one exception in which there are agreed upon rules for grading the inflammatory response even in partially sampled bronchioles in transbronchial biopsies.[23] Another exception is diffuse panbronchiolitis where a transbronchial biopsy

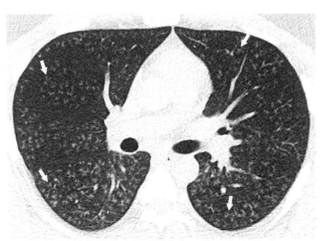

20.33

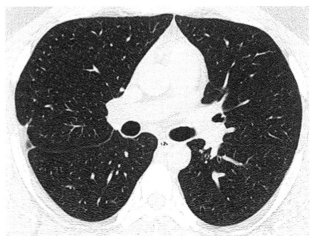

20.34

FIGURES 20.33 to 20.36. See figure legend 20.36.

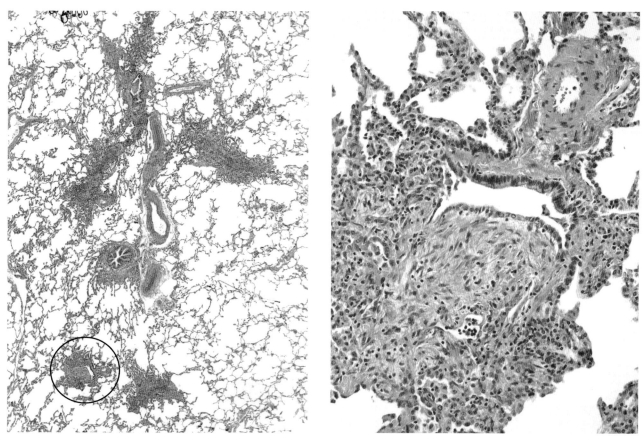

20.35   20.36

FIGURES 20.33 to 20.36. Fibrosing bronchiolitis, probably postinfectious. **Figure 20.33:** HRCT demonstrates numerous well-defined bilateral centrilobular nodules and tree-in-bud pattern (*arrows*). **Figure 20.34:** HRCT 3 months later is normal except for small area of subpleural scarring in the right lung at the site of the surgical lung biopsy. **Figure 20.35:** Low-power view showing inflammatory lesions confined to the bronchioles with normal intervening parenchyma. **Figure 20.36:** High-power view of the bronchiole circled in **Figure 20.35**. A re-epithelialized granulation tissue plug narrows the bronchiolar lumen and there is surrounding chronic inflammation. Morphologically, this process is similar to early constrictive bronchiolitis, but the imaging is completely different, as is the improvement with treatment. (Reprinted with permission of the American Thoracic Society. Copyright 2019 American Thoracic Society from Ryerson CJ, Olsen SR, Carlsten C, et al. Fibrosing bronchiolitis evolving from infectious or inhalational acute bronchiolitis. A reversible lesion. *Ann Am Thorac Soc.* 2015;12:1323–1327. *The American Journal of Respiratory* and *Critical Care Medicine* is an official journal of the American Thoracic Society.)

may sample an inflamed bronchiole and show the characteristic foamy macrophages. The utility of cryobiopsy in this setting is unclear; despite having larger pieces, Roden et al.[24] did not find a higher incidence of bronchiolitis obliterans in lung transplant patients in a series of cryobiopsies compared to conventional forceps biopsies.

PROGNOSIS

For many types of bronchiolitis, pathologic features do not provide a good guide to prognosis, and an underlying systemic disease, if present, may be the major determinant of outcome. However, cigarette smoke–induced small airways disease is now recognized as a major contributor to airflow obstruction in most patients with COPD.[19] Acute

adenovirus bronchiolitis in infants is associated with a mortality rate up to 20%.[8] The prognosis of constrictive bronchiolitis depends on the clinical setting. Postinfectious constrictive bronchiolitis in infants is associated with low mortality but considerable morbidity including recurrent respiratory infections.[8]

In adults, constrictive bronchiolitis often causes progressive fixed (i.e., unresponsive to bronchodilators) airflow obstruction and may lead to respiratory failure, but some patients appear to stabilize, albeit with residual functional impairment.[1,4] Constrictive bronchiolitis develops in about 50% of lung transplant recipients by 5 years and is the major cause of graft failure and mortality in long-term lung transplant survivors.[25,26] The 2-year survival of BOS in patients with bone marrow transplant has been reported as 70% to 80%, but some of those patients end up needing lung transplants.[14]

Untreated, diffuse panbronchiolitis is slowly progressive, with a 10-year survival of about 30% and may be complicated by colonization of the airways with infectious organisms, especially *Pseudomonas*, and by the development of bronchiectasis.[6] Treatment with macrolides (clarithromycin, roxithromycin, or azithromycin) dramatically improves survival.[6,15,27]

Somatostatin analogs (octreotide, lanreotide) have sometimes been reported to improve airflow in some patients with DIPNECH, but most patients do not improve on this regime.[15]

REFERENCES

1. Ryu JH. Classification and approach to bronchiolar diseases. *Curr Opin Pulm Med.* 2006;12:145–151.
2. Ryerson CJ, Olsen SR, Carlsten C, et al. Fibrosing bronchiolitis evolving from infectious or inhalational acute bronchiolitis. A reversible lesion. *Ann Am Thorac Soc.* 2015;12:1323–1327.
3. Markopoulo KD, Cool CD, Elliot TL, et al. Obliterative bronchiolitis: varying presentations and clinicopathological correlation. *Eur Respir J.* 2002;19:20–30.
4. Lynch JP 3rd, Weigt SS, DerHovanessian A, et al. Obliterative (constrictive) bronchiolitis. *Semin Respir Crit Care Med.* 2012;33:509–532.
5. Barker AF, Bergeron A, Rom WN, et al. Obliterative bronchiolitis. *N Engl J Med.* 2014;370:1820–1828.
6. Poletti V, Chilosi M, Casoni G, et al. Diffuse panbronchiolitis. *Sarcoidosis Vasc Diffuse Lung Dis.* 2004;21:94–104.
7. Meissner HC. Viral bronchiolitis in children. *N Engl J Med.* 2016;374:62–72.
8. Fischer GB, Sarria EE, Mattiello R, et al. Post infectious bronchiolitis obliterans in children. *Paediatr Respir Rev.* 2010;11:233–239.
9. Ryu K, Takayanagi N, Ishiguro T, et al. Etiology and outcome of diffuse acute infectious bronchiolitis in adults. *Ann Am Thorac Soc.* 2015;12:1781–1787.
10. Li YN, Liu L, Qiao HM, et al. Post-infectious bronchiolitis obliterans in children: a review of 42 cases. *BMC Pediatr.* 2014;14:238–243.
11. Castro-Rodriguez JA, Giubergia V, Fischer GB, et al. Postinfectious bronchiolitis obliterans in children: the South American contribution. *Acta Paediatr.* 2014;103:913–921.
12. Hayes D Jr. A review of bronchiolitis obliterans syndrome and therapeutic strategies. *J Cardiothorac Surg.* 2011;18;6:92.
13. Chien JW, Duncan S, Williams KM, et al. Bronchiolitis obliterans syndrome after allogeneic hematopoietic stem cell transplantation-an increasingly recognized manifestation of chronic graft-versus-host disease. *Biol Blood Marrow Transplant.* 2010;16(1 Suppl.):S106–S114.
14. Bergeron A, Cheng GS. Bronchiolitis obliterans syndrome and other late pulmonary complications after allogeneic hematopoietic stem cell transplantation. *Clin Chest Med.* 2017;38:607–621.
15. Cordier JF, Cottin V, Lazor R, et al. Many faces of bronchiolitis and organizing pneumonia. *Semin Respir Crit Care Med.* 2016;37:421–440.
16. Winningham PJ, Martínez-Jiménez S, Rosado-de-Christenson ML, et al. Bronchiolitis: a practical approach for the general radiologist. *Radiographics.* 2017;37:777–794.
17. Nishimura K, Kitaichi M, Izumi T, et al. Diffuse panbronchiolitis: correlation of high-resolution CT and pathologic findings. *Radiology.* 1992;184:779–785.
18. Iwata M, Colby TV, Kitaichi M. Diffuse panbronchiolitis: diagnosis and distinction from various pulmonary diseases with centrilobular interstitial foam cell accumulations. *Hum Pathol.* 1994;25:357–363.
19. McDonough JE, Yuan R, Suzuki M, et al. Small-airway obstruction and emphysema in chronic obstructive pulmonary disease. *N Engl J Med.* 2011;365:1567–1575.
20. Churg A, Green FHY. *Pathology of Occupational Lung Disease.* 2nd ed. Baltimore, MA: Williams and Wilkins; 1998.
21. Marchevsky AM, Walts AE. Diffuse idiopathic pulmonary neuroendocrine cell hyperplasia (DIPNECH). *Semin Diagn Pathol.* 2015;32:438–444.
22. Rossi G, Cavazza A, Spagnolo P, et al. Diffuse idiopathic pulmonary neuroendocrine cell hyperplasia syndrome. *Eur Respir J.* 2016;47:1829–1841.
23. Stewart S, Fishbein MC, Snell GI, et al. Revision of the 1996 working formulation for the standardization of nomenclature in the diagnosis of lung rejection. *J Heart Lung Transplant.* 2007;26:1229–1242.
24. Roden AC, Kern RM, Aubry MC, et al. Transbronchial cryobiopsies in the evaluation of lung allografts: do the benefits outweigh the risks? *Arch Pathol Lab Med.* 2016;140:303–311.
25. Aguilar PR, Michelson AP, Isakow W. Obliterative bronchiolitis. *Transplantation.* 2016;100:272–283.
26. Todd JL, Palmer SM. Bronchiolitis obliterans syndrome: the final frontier for lung transplantation. *Chest.* 2011;140:502–508.
27. Friedlander AL, Albert RK. Chronic macrolide therapy in inflammatory airways diseases. *Chest.* 2010;138:1202–1212.

Interstitial Lung Disease in Patients with Collagen Vascular Diseases and Interstitial Pneumonias with Autoimmune Features

NOMENCLATURE AND CONCEPTUAL ISSUES

Interstitial lung disease (ILD) is common in patients with diagnosed collagen vascular disease (CVD); however, ILD can also be seen in patients who have some clinical, serologic, radiologic, or pathologic features suggestive of a CVD but do not meet the rheumatologic criteria for a defined CVD. Various names have been proposed for such patients including "undifferentiated connective tissue disease-associated ILD," "lung dominant connective tissue disease," or "autoimmune featured ILD"; the definitions of each are only partially overlapping and there is variability in how these definitions are applied in the literature.

In this chapter, we will use the more recent term "interstitial pneumonia with autoimmune features" (IPAF),[1] largely because of the comprehensive and detailed criteria set out for this designation[1] (see details below). Strictly speaking, IPAF is not a specific diagnosis, but from the point of view of pathology, IPAF incorporates a set of biopsy findings that can be identical to those in patients with overt CVD.[2–4] Hence, in a patient not known to have a CVD, reporting a biopsy as having features of IPAF alerts the clinician to the possibility that the process in question has an autoimmune basis.

Patients with CVDs and IPAF may have not only ILD but disease involving the pleura, the pulmonary vasculature, and several other lesions (Tables 21.1 and 21.2). In the past, there was a tendency to simply lump such conditions together into "rheumatoid lung" or "lupus lung," etc., but this approach provides no useful information to clinicians because the prognosis, and to a certain extent the treatment, varies by pathologic pattern. For example, a diagnosis of "rheumatoid lung" could in theory be applied to usual interstitial pneumonia (UIP) or to cellular nonspecific interstitial pneumonia (NSIP) developing in

a patient with underlying rheumatoid arthritis, or even to rheumatoid nodules, but the former probably behaves just as badly as idiopathic UIP (see section Treatment and Prognosis), whereas cellular NSIP appears to have a very good prognosis, and rheumatoid nodules generally do not require any treatment once their nature is established.

Table 21.1

Intrathoracic lesions in patients with CVD

Chronic pleural or pericardial effusion/pleural or pericardial fibrosis
Diffuse alveolar damage/ARDS
Usual interstitial pneumonia
Nonspecific interstitial pneumonia
Organizing pneumonia (BOOP, COP, OP)
Lymphocytic interstitial pneumonia
Chronic bronchiolitis
Follicular bronchiolitis/lymphoid hyperplasia
Lymphocytic interstitial pneumonia
Constrictive bronchiolitis
Xerotrachea (Sjögren syndrome)
Eosinophilic pneumonia
Apical fibrosis
Rheumatoid nodules
Diffuse alveolar hemorrhage with/without capillaritis
Vasculitis
Vasculopathy (in systemic sclerosis)
Vascular thrombosis (typically in patients with lupus and anti-phospholipid antibodies)
Aspiration pneumonia (usually in polymyositis/dermatomyositis or systemic sclerosis)
Lymphoma (most commonly in Sjögren syndrome)

Table 21.2

Criteria for a designation of IPAF

Clinical domain
"Mechanic's Hands" (distal digital fissuring)
Ulceration of digital tips
Inflammatory arthritis or polyarticular morning stiffness lasting more than 60 minutes
Raynaud phenomenon
Palmar telangiectasia
Gottron sign (unexplained fixed rash on the digital extensor surfaces)
Unexplained digital edema

Serologic domain
ANA titer 1:320 or greater with a diffuse, speckled, or homogeneous pattern
ANA of any titer with a centromere or nucleolar pattern
Rheumatoid factor >2× the upper limit of normal
Greater than normal anti-CCP, anti-dsDNA, anti-SSA, anti-SSB, anti-RNP, anti-Smith, anti-Scl 70 (topoisomerase), anti-tRNA synthetase antibodies (most commonly Jo-1, PL-7, PL-12), anti-PM-Scl, anti-MDA-5

Morphologic domain
HRCT pattern of NSIP, OP, NSIP plus OP, LIP
Biopsy pattern of NSIP, OP, NSIP plus OP, LIP, lymphoid aggregates with germinal centers, diffuse interstitial lymphoplasmacytic infiltrates
Other morphologic compartments in addition to interstitial pneumonia:
  a. Unexplained pleural or pericardial effusion or thickening
  b. Unexplained intrinsic airways disease (by pulmonary function testing, imaging, or biopsy)
  c. Unexplained pulmonary vasculopathy

One clue to the diagnosis of CVD/IPAF is the presence of more than one ILD pattern or unusual combinations of ILD patterns in a given biopsy (but see comments about drug reactions, below). We suggest that when dealing with ILD in such patients, the pathologist should attempt to put the biopsy in question into as close a fit as possible to the corresponding idiopathic ILD(s) so that the clinician has some guide to treatment and prognosis. Thus a patient with rheumatoid arthritis and a UIP pattern should be diagnosed as "UIP in a patient with rheumatoid arthritis" or, alternately, if morphologic features suggestive of CVD/IPAF (see below and Table 21.2) are present but the patient is not known to have a CVD, a diagnosis of "UIP with features of CVD/IPAF" would be appropriate. A patient with a mixture of cellular NSIP and organizing pneumonia (OP), a combination that is common in CVDs, should be diagnosed as such: "Surgical lung biopsy showing a mixture of cellular NSIP and OP in a patient with underlying [disease]."

CLINICAL FEATURES

These diseases in general do not have obvious etiologies beyond autoimmunity, but the same MUC5B promoter variant (rs35705950) that confers an increased risk of idiopathic pulmonary fibrosis and chronic hypersensitivity pneumonitis (HP) increases the risk of UIP developing in patients with rheumatoid arthritis.[5] There is also considerable evidence that a large proportion of systemic sclerosis cases in men are associated with silica exposure,[6] probably because silica can act as a hapten. Drugs can induce lupus.[7]

Pleuropulmonary manifestations vary considerably by type of CVD. ILD-type patterns in particular are common in CVD, and it has been estimated that 15% of ILD patients actually have an underlying CVD.[8] ILD is especially frequent in rheumatoid arthritis and systemic sclerosis (in the latter up to 75% of patients in some series).[9–11] Some authors suggest that almost all cases of NSIP represent some form of autoimmune disease[4,12–14]; however, because drug reactions and HP can also have an NSIP morphology (see Chapters 12 and 18), a more accurate view is that NSIP is usually an immunologically mediated process.

The extrapulmonary clinical features of CVD vary with the disease and are beyond the scope of this book. When ILD is present, the basic clinical pulmonary features are no different from idiopathic ILD with the same histologic pattern, although patients with systemic sclerosis also have a high incidence of pulmonary hypertension secondary to vasculopathy.[9] In addition to ILD, recurrent exudative pleural and/or pericardial effusions, sometimes leading to visceral pleural or pericardial fibrosis, as well as ARDS (sometimes labeled "acute lupus pneumonitis" in patients with lupus), diffuse pulmonary hemorrhage, vasculitis, vasculopathy (in systemic sclerosis), and pulmonary hypertension may be found in patients with underlying CVD.

In most CVD patients, pulmonary disease develops after the diagnosis of CVD but sometimes pulmonary disease is the initial manifestation and a defined CVD appears later[15–17]; it appears that some patients who initially meet IPAF criteria fall into this group.[18] Alternatively, overt CVD may never appear and the patient would then remain in the IPAF category.

The detailed criteria[1] for a diagnosis of IPAF are set out in Table 21.2. The a priori requirements include the presence of an interstitial pneumonia on high-resolution computed tomography (HRCT) or biopsy, exclusion of alternative etiologies for the interstitial pneumonia, absence of criteria for a defined CVD, and at least one finding from at least two of the clinical, serologic, and morphologic domains shown in Table 21.2. It should be appreciated than any of the findings listed in Table 21.2 can be found in patients with overt CVD as well.

In reported series, patients with IPAF have tended to be female, often with a positive ANA, Raynaud phenomenon, and most commonly NSIP or UIP on HRCT or biopsy,[18] although strictly speaking a UIP pattern is not an IPAF criterion unless the IPAF clinical and serologic domains are met or a biopsy shows UIP with germinal centers or a considerable number of plasma cells (see below).

IMAGING

Pulmonary abnormalities seen in patients in CVD may be related to the underlying CVD or result from complications of treatment, such as drug toxicity and opportunistic infection. The radiologic manifestations of ILD in patients with CVD are similar to those found in idiopathic interstitial pneumonias.[19] The only difference is that patients with CVD are more likely to have more than one pattern, the most common combination being NSIP and OP.[20]

The most common radiologic patterns of ILD seen in CVD are NSIP, UIP, and OP. NSIP is characterized on HRCT by bilateral symmetric ground-glass opacities, irregular linear (reticular) opacities, and traction bronchiectasis involving mainly the lower lobes (Figs. 21.1 and 21.2). UIP typically manifests with reticulation and honeycombing involving predominantly the subpleural regions and lung bases (Fig. 21.3). The characteristic HRCT of OP consists of patchy bilateral consolidation, which in 60% to 80% of cases has a subpleural and/or peribronchial distribution (Fig. 21.4).

Certain extraparenchymal findings when present can be helpful in suggesting the possibility of CVD on imaging. These include an enlarged pulmonary artery out of proportion to the extent of ILD, pleural effusion or pleural thickening, dilated esophagus (systemic sclerosis), shoulder and acromioclavicular joint abnormalities (rheumatoid arthritis), and soft tissue calcifications (polymyositis/dermatomyositis or scleroderma).[19]

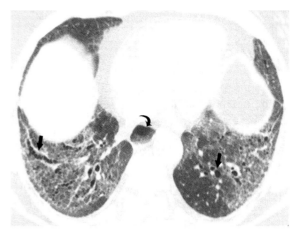

FIGURE 21.2. Same case as Figure 21.1. HRCT at the level of the lung bases demonstrates extensive bilateral ground-glass opacities with superimposed reticulation and traction bronchiectasis (*straight arrows*). The esophagus (*curved arrow*) is dilated and contains air and debris, a common finding in patients with scleroderma. The patient was a 61-year-old woman with NSIP associated with scleroderma.

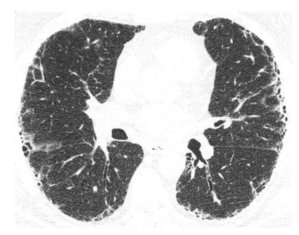

FIGURE 21.3. UIP in rheumatoid arthritis. HRCT demonstrates peripheral reticulation and honeycombing. The patient was a 64-year-old man with UIP associated with rheumatoid arthritis.

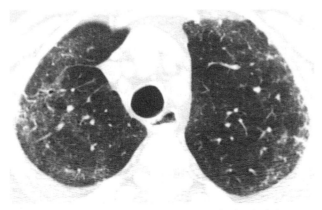

FIGURE 21.1. NSIP in scleroderma. HRCT at the level of the upper lobes shows bilateral ground-glass opacities and mild peripheral reticulation.

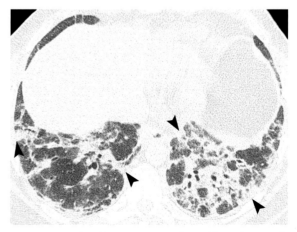

FIGURE 21.4. OP in polymyositis. HRCT shows bilateral areas of consolidation in a predominantly peripheral (*arrowheads*) and peribronchial distribution. The patient was a 44-year-old man with polymyositis.

PATHOLOGIC FEATURES OF COLLAGEN VASCULAR DISEASE–ASSOCIATED ILD AND IPAF

Many of the pathologic features of ILD in CVD/IPAF are identical to those seen in patients without CVD, although there is variation in pattern frequency from CVD to CVD; for example, UIP is relatively common in patients with rheumatoid arthritis[21,22] and uncommon in patients with lupus, whereas fibrotic NSIP is the most common ILD in systemic sclerosis[21,23] and polymyositis/dermatomyositis.[24] If one takes all forms of CVD, an NSIP pattern is the most frequent.[22] However, these statistical differences are not diagnostically useful in an individual case.

As opposed to idiopathic forms of ILD, CVD/IPAF biopsies often have mixtures of patterns, sometimes patterns that are easily classified as specific forms of ILD (Figs. 21.5 to 21.7) and sometimes odd patterns that do not fit any ordinary ILD or that mimic other forms of ILD such as isolated foci of centrilobular fibrosis mimicking chronic HP (Fig. 21.8). Very rarely, LE cells similar to those seen in peripheral blood can be found in tissue in biopsies from patients with lupus[25] and electron microscopy may reveal lupus fingerprint-type immune complex deposits.[26]

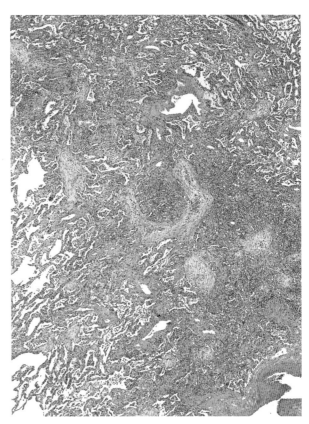

21.6

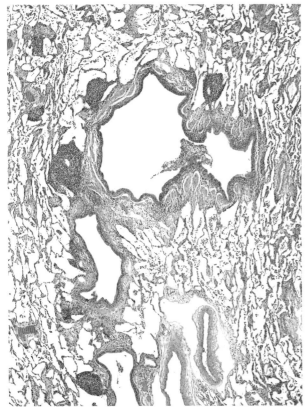

21.5

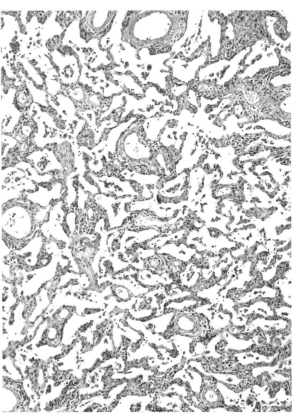

21.7

FIGURES 21.5 to 21.7. Mixture of pathologic patterns in the same biopsy from a patient with rheumatoid arthritis. **Figure 21.5** shows follicular bronchiolitis associated with bronchiolectasis. **Figure 21.6** shows OP. Other areas (**Fig. 21.7**) demonstrate a cellular NSIP pattern. Combinations of ILD patterns are common in patients with CVD.

The finding of follicular bronchiolitis, NSIP, numerous lymphoid aggregates, lymphoid aggregates with germinal centers, a high proportion of plasma cells in the interstitial infiltrate (Fig. 21.9), or lymphocytic interstitial pneumonia (see Chapters 7 and 19 for definitions) should always raise a question of underlying CVD/IPAF. Sometimes follicular bronchiolitis or lymphoid aggregates are the only lesions in a biopsy but frequently they are superimposed on a UIP or NSIP picture[27] (see Fig. 6.34 and 7.10 to 7.12). Idiopathic UIP (IPF) is generally quite paucicellular and the presence of a UIP pattern with germinal centers or increased interstitial lymphocytes and plasma cells (see Fig. 6.35) is suggestive of underlying CVD/IPAF[27]; Lymphocytic interstitial pneumonia is strongly associated with Sjögren syndrome, but occasionally is seen in other CVD as well as in patients with dysgammaglobulinemias (see Chapter 19).

There are no established rules for how many/much of these phenomena one needs to see before suggesting CVD/IPAF. Adegunsoye et al.[28] proposed that three germinal centers per low power field or more than 40 plasma cells per high power field supported a diagnosis of IPAF. However, these criteria are probably too stringent and the finding of any number of lymphoid aggregates with germinal centers should at least raise a question of

CVD/IPAF. Some CVD/IPAF cases are relatively paucicellular, but most of the interstitial inflammatory cells are nonetheless plasma cells. We found that, ignoring lymphoid aggregates, an interstitial plasma cell to lymphocyte ratio of 1:1 or greater was typical of CVD/IPAF;[3] and in a comparison of CVD/IPAF vs. chronic HP cases, the presence of any germinal centers favored a diagnosis of CVD/IPAF by 10:1. In that series, there were no morphologic differences between CVD and IPAF cases and this conclusion has been reported by others.[2]

When any of these features are present but the history of CVD is not known, the possibility that the patient has CVD/IPAF should be indicated in the diagnosis line; for example, "UIP with features of CVD/IPAF" or "UIP with numerous lymphoid aggregates suggestive of underlying CVD/IPAF."

Although the findings just listed point to a diagnosis of underlying CVD/IPAF, they are by no means always present, even in well-established CVD patients. Systemic sclerosis in particular can be very paucicellular (Figs. 21.10 to 21.12), although such biopsies frequently show marked vasculopathy (Fig. 21.12). As noted above, there are those who believe that that almost all NSIP cases are manifestations of autoimmune disease whether or not a biopsy shows features of CVD/IPAF. Conversely, areas of honeycombing

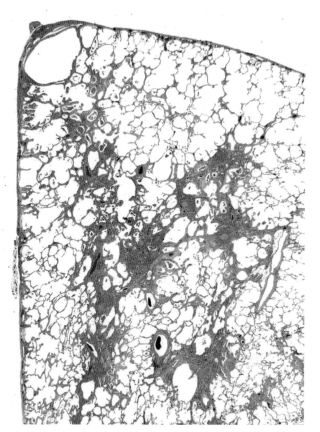

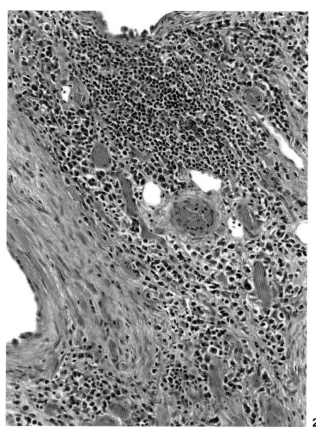

21.8   21.9

FIGURES 21.8 and 21.9. A fibrosing interstitial pneumonia with isolated centrilobular fibrosis and subpleural fibrosis mimicking chronic HP in a patient with CVD. Note the numerous lymphoid aggregates, some with germinal centers and the preponderance of plasma cells away from the lymphoid aggregate at high power; these are typical CVD/IPAF findings.

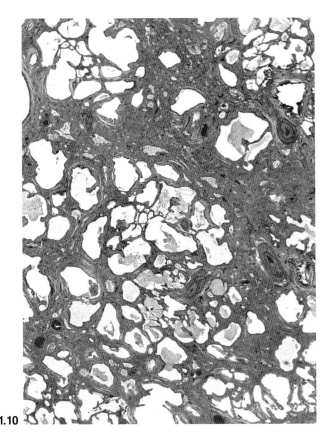
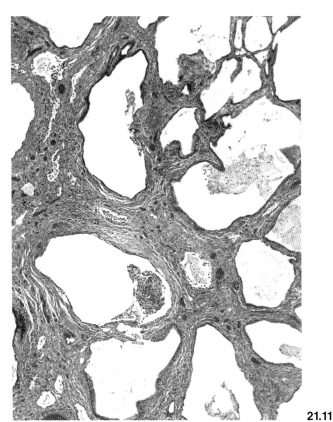

21.10

21.11

FIGURES 21.10 and 21.11. Low and high power views of fibrotic NSIP in a patient with systemic sclerosis. The process is very paucicellular.

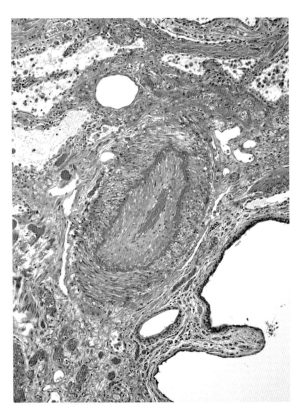

FIGURE 21.12. A pulmonary arterial branch showing marked intimal proliferation and a thickened muscular wall in the same case. Vasculopathy is extremely common in biopsies from patients with systemic sclerosis.

in UIP/IPF often have lymphoid aggregates and a considerable number of interstitial inflammatory cells (see Figs. 6.16 and 6.18), which by themselves are nonspecific findings. However, if the honeycombed foci contain germinal centers or a high proportion of plasma cells, the question of underlying CVD/IPAF should be raised.

Small noncaseating granulomas or giant cells are commonly viewed as features of chronic HP (see Chapter 12). However, we[3] found granulomas/giant cells in one-third of well worked up cases of CVD/IPAF (Figs. 21.13 and 21.14) versus roughly one half of chronic HP cases. Increased interstitial inflammatory cells, including some number of plasma cells, can also be seen in chronic HP, but typically plasma cells are not the majority of inflammatory cells in chronic HP.[3]

Small numbers of eosinophils are common in the interstitial infiltrates of CVD/IPAF[3] but are seen in chronic HP and to a lesser extent in UIP/IPF, and offer little help in diagnosis.

PATHOLOGIC CONFOUNDERS/ DIFFERENTIAL DIAGNOSIS

Patients with CVD/IPAF may be immunosuppressed because they have been treated with steroids and/or other immunosuppressive agents, and biopsy may demonstrate an infectious agent with or without pathologic features of CVD/IPAF.

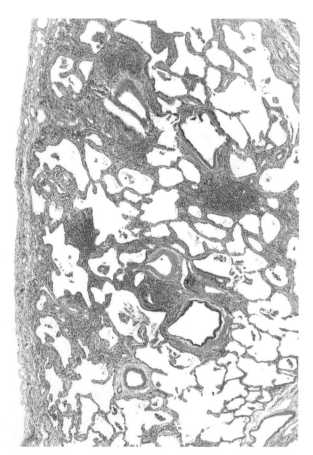

FIGURE 21.13. NSIP pattern in a patient meeting IPAF criteria. Note the numerous lymphoid aggregates.

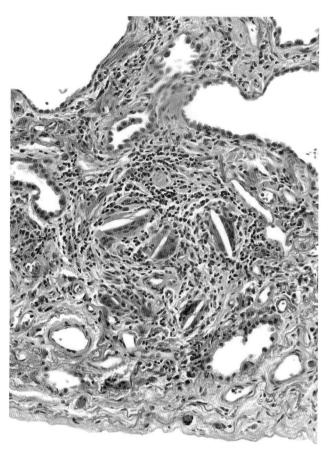

FIGURE 21.14. Higher power view of the same case showing giant cells. Although giant cells are common markers of chronic HP, they can be found in CVD/IPAF cases as well.

Patients with systemic sclerosis and dermatomyositis are at risk of aspiration pneumonias because of esophageal dysfunction (see Chapters 5 and 20 for a discussion of pathologic patterns of aspiration).

Drug reactions represent a more complex problem. For one thing drug reactions can produce strange combinations of ILD-like patterns, the same phenomenon that is seen in CVD/IPAF. For example, methotrexate, which is commonly employed in patients with CVD, can cause a whole range of pathologic reactions including NSIP-like and hypersensitivity-like ILD with granulomas as well as eosinophilic pneumonias (see Figs. 18.4 to 18.7). Antitumor necrosis factor agents such as etanercept and infliximab often cause a picture of multiple sarcoid-like granulomas (see Figs. 18.12 and 18.13) and this is a reasonably specific finding in context, but needs to be separated from the effects of methotrexate, because these agents are often used together, and from infections.

Second, drugs can produce pathologic patterns identical to those in untreated CVD. Thus penicillamine, which has been used in the past to treat rheumatoid arthritis, is believed to cause constrictive bronchiolitis, OP, follicular bronchiolitis, diffuse alveolar damage, and eosinophilic pneumonias,[29,30] all processes found in rheumatoid

arthritis absent drug therapy, and there is controversy about whether these lesions are really penicillamine reactions or underlying disease.[31] Figures 18.21 to 18.23 illustrate the same problem in a patient with rheumatoid arthritis treated with leflunomide who developed constrictive bronchiolitis.

The general principles set forth in Chapter 18 for evaluating potential drug reactions should be followed in such cases; in particular, the development of new disease shortly after starting drug therapy, and unusual new systemic findings such as fever or rash after starting drug therapy,[32] support a drug reaction, but in most instances morphology cannot sort out the problem and such cases should be signed out to indicate that the drug or the underlying disease could cause the picture in question.

DIAGNOSTIC MODALITIES

As a rule, transbronchial forceps biopsy is not suitable for the diagnosis of ILD-like manifestations of CVD and video-assisted thoracoscopic biopsy is required, although cryobiopsy may be satisfactory in some cases.[33] Core needle biopsy is potentially useful for diagnosing rheumatoid nodules.

TREATMENT AND PROGNOSIS

As a general rule, patients with overt CVD and ILD are treated with some form of immunosuppression which may be steroids, azathioprine, mycophenolate, rituximab, cyclosporin, or tacrolimus, and sometimes cyclophosphamide in systemic sclerosis.[34,35] Hematopoietic stem cell transplant has also been used for systemic sclerosis.[34,35] Patients with progressive disease may receive lung transplants.

Treatment for patients who meet IPAF but not CVD criteria is more varied in the literature and is complicated by a variety of case definitions as well as by the fact that all of the studies to date are retrospective and therapies that were applied may not have taken an autoimmune component into consideration. Typically, immunosuppressives have been used in most patients, but antifibrotics (pirfenidone, nintedanib) have been employed for some patients with a UIP pattern (e.g., Yoshimura et al.[12]). Cyclophosphamide has been used in some cases.[36]

The prognosis of ILD-type lesions in patients with CVD is difficult to evaluate, in part because the literature often is based on radiologic rather than pathologic diagnoses,[37] and in part because it is unclear whether there are differences among different CVD with the same pathologic pattern. Patients with OP or cellular NSIP do relatively well.[23] Overall, patients with systemic sclerosis and ILD tend to fare worse than patients with other CVD,[23] but that conclusion appears to reflect the greater prevalence of fibrotic ILD in systemic sclerosis[23,37] and the frequent development of pulmonary hypertension.

The prognosis of UIP in the setting of CVD is controversial, with some reports claiming a considerably better outcome than is seen in idiopathic UIP[38,39]; and others finding no difference, at least for patients with rheumatoid arthritis and a UIP pattern.[22,40–42] In systemic sclerosis, pulmonary involvement is the leading cause of death[35] and some reports suggest that there is no difference between fibrotic NSIP and UIP patterns.[23]

The prognosis for patients with IPAF varies considerably in different reports and again is confounded by purely retrospective studies, but seems to relate in some part to the underlying histologic or radiologic pattern. Some authors find that IPAF patients with a UIP pattern have the same prognosis as idiopathic UIP; however, others describe a better prognosis.[12] In general, patients with other IPAF histologic patterns fare considerably better[43,44] (see Nascimento et al.[2] for other reports).

REFERENCES

1. Fischer A, Antoniou KM, Brown KK, et al. "ERS/ATS Task Force on Undifferentiated Forms of CTD-ILD." An official European Respiratory Society/American Thoracic Society research statement: interstitial pneumonia with autoimmune features. *Eur Respir J*. 2015;46:976–987.
2. Nascimento ECTD, Baldi BG, Sawamura MVY, et al. Morphologic aspects of interstitial pneumonia with autoimmune features. *Arch Pathol Lab Med*. 2018;142:1080–1089.
3. Churg A, Wright JL, Ryerson CJ. Pathologic Separation of chronic hypersensitivity pneumonitis from fibrotic connective tissue disease-associated interstitial lung disease. *Am J Surg Pathol*. 2017;41:1403–1409.
4. Nicholson AG, Colby TV, Wells AU. Histopathological approach to patterns of interstitial pneumonia in patient with connective tissue disorders. *Sarcoidosis Vasc Diffuse Lung Dis*. 2002;19:10–17.
5. Juge PA, Lee JS, Ebstein E, et al. MUC5B promoter variant and rheumatoid arthritis with interstitial lung disease. *N Engl J Med*. 2018;379:2209–2219.
6. Freire M, Alonso M, Rivera A, et al. Clinical peculiarities of patients with scleroderma exposed to silica: a systematic review of the literature. *Semin Arthritis Rheum*. 2015;45:294–300.
7. He Y, Sawalha AH. Drug-induced lupus erythematosus: an update on drugs and mechanisms. *Curr Opin Rheumatol*. 2018;30(5):490–497.
8. Antin-Ozerkis D, Rubinowitz A, Evans J, et al. Interstitial lung disease in the connective tissue diseases. *Clin Chest Med*. 2012;33:123–149.
9. Steele R, Hudson M, Lo E, et al.; Canadian Scleroderma Research Group (CSRG). A clinical decision rule to predict the presence of interstitial lung disease in systemic sclerosis. *Arthritis Care Res (Hoboken)*. 2012;64:519–524.
10. Bussone G, Mouthon L. Interstitial lung disease in systemic sclerosis. *Autoimmun Rev*. 2011;10:248–255.
11. Mira-Avendano I, Abril A, Burger CD, et al. Interstitial lung disease and other pulmonary manifestations in connective tissue diseases. *Mayo Clin Proc*. 2019;94:309–325. doi:10.1016/j.mayocp.2018.09.002.
12. Yoshimura K, Kono M, Enomoto Y, et al. Distinctive characteristics and prognostic significance of interstitial pneumonia with autoimmune features in patients with chronic fibrosing interstitial pneumonia. *Respir Med*. 2018;137:167–175.
13. Fujita J, Ohtsuki Y, Yoshinouchi T, et al. Idiopathic non-specific interstitial pneumonia: as an "autoimmune interstitial pneumonia." *Respir Med*. 2005;99(2):234–240.
14. Kinder BW, Collard HR, Koth L, et al. Idiopathic nonspecific interstitial pneumonia: lung manifestation of undifferentiated connective tissue disease? *Am J Respir Crit Care Med*. 2007;176:691–697.
15. Fischer A, Solomon JJ, du Bois RM, et al. Lung disease with anti-CCP antibodies but not rheumatoid arthritis or connective tissue disease. *Respir Med*. 2012;106:1040–1047.
16. Bauer PR, Schiavo DN, Osborn TG, et al. Influence of interstitial lung disease on outcome in systemic sclerosis: a population-based historical cohort study. *Chest*. 2013;144:571–577.
17. Kono M, Nakamura Y, Enomoto N, et al. Usual interstitial pneumonia preceding collagen vascular disease: a retrospective case control study of patients initially diagnosed with idiopathic pulmonary fibrosis. *PLoS One*. 2014;9(4):e94775.
18. Sambataro G, Sambataro D, Torrisi SE, et al. State of the art in interstitial pneumonia with autoimmune features: a systematic review on retrospective studies and suggestions for further advances. *Eur Respir Rev*. 2018;27: pii: 170139.

19. Henry TS, Little BP, Veeraraghavan S, et al. The spectrum of interstitial lung disease in connective tissue disease. *J Thorac Imaging*. 2016;31:65–77.

20. Tansey D, Wells AU, Colby TV, et al. Variations in histological patterns of interstitial pneumonia between connective tissue disorders and their relationship to prognosis. *Histopathology*. 2004;44:585–596.

21. Kocheril SV, Appleton BE, Somers EC, et al. Comparison of disease progression and mortality of connective tissue disease-related interstitial lung disease and idiopathic interstitial pneumonia. *Arthritis Rheum*. 2005;53:549–557.

22. Kim EJ, Collard HR, King TE Jr. Rheumatoid arthritis-associated interstitial lung disease: the relevance of histopathologic and radiographic pattern. *Chest*. 2009;136:1397–1405.

23. Bouros D, Wells AU, Nicholson AG, et al. Histopathologic subsets of fibrosing alveolitis in patients with systemic sclerosis and their relationship to outcome. *Am J Respir Crit Care Med*. 2002;165:1581–1586.

24. Douglas WW, Tazelaar HD, Hartman TE, et al. Polymyositis-dermatomyositis-associated interstitial lung disease. *Am J Respir Crit Care Med*. 2001;164:1182–1185.

25. Haupt HM, Moore GW, Hutchins GM. The lung in systemic lupus erythematosus. Analysis of the pathologic changes in 120 patients. *Am J Med*. 1981;71:791–798.

26. Churg A, Franklin W, Chan KL, et al. Pulmonary hemorrhage and immune complex deposition in the lung in a patient with systemic lupus erythematosus. *Arch Pathol Lab Med*. 1980;l04:388–39l.

27. Song JW, Do KH, Kim MY, et al. Pathologic and radiologic differences between idiopathic and collagen vascular disease-related usual interstitial pneumonia. *Chest*. 2009;136:23–30.

28. Adegunsoye A, Oldham JM, Valenzi E, et al. Interstitial pneumonia with autoimmune features: value of histopathology. *Arch Pathol Lab Med*. 2017;141(7):960–969.

29. Smith DH, Scott DL, Zaphiropoulos GC. Eosinophilia in D-penicillamine therapy. *Ann Rheum Dis*. 1983;42:408–410.

30. Stein HB, Patterson AC, Offer RC, et al. Adverse effects of D-penicillamine in rheumatoid arthritis. *Ann Intern Med*. 1980;92:24–29.

31. Dawes PT, Smith DH, Scott DL. Massive eosinophilia in rheumatoid arthritis: report of four cases. *Clin Rheumatol*. 1986;5:62–65.

32. Tomioka R, King TE Jr. Gold-induced pulmonary disease: clinical features, outcome, and differentiation from rheumatoid lung disease. *Am J Respir Crit Care Med*. 1997;155:1011–1120.

33. Ussavarungsi K, Kern RM, Roden AC, et al. Transbronchial cryobiopsy in diffuse parenchymal lung disease: retrospective Analysis of 74 cases. *Chest*. 2017;151:400–408.

34. Cottin V, Brown KK. Interstitial lung disease associated with systemic sclerosis (SSc-ILD). *Respir Res*. 2019;20(1):13.

35. Suzuki A, Kondoh Y, Fischer A. Recent advances in connective tissue disease related interstitial lung disease. *Expert Rev Respir Med*. 2017;11:591–603.

36. Wiertz IA, van Moorsel CHM, Vorselaars ADM, et al. Cyclophosphamide in steroid refractory unclassifiable idiopathic interstitial pneumonia and interstitial pneumonia with autoimmune features (IPAF). *Eur Respir J*. 2018;51:1702519.

37. Tan A, Denton CP, Mikhailidis DP, et al. Recent advances in the diagnosis and treatment of interstitial lung disease in systemic sclerosis (scleroderma): a review. *Clin Exp Rheumatol*. 2011;29(2 Suppl. 65):S66–S74.

38. Flaherty KR, Colby TV, Travis WD, et al. Fibroblastic foci in usual interstitial pneumonia: idiopathic versus collagen vascular disease. *Am J Respir Crit Care Med*. 2003;167:1410–1415.

39. Park JH, Kim DS, Park IN, et al. Prognosis of fibrotic interstitial pneumonia: idiopathic versus collagen vascular disease-related subtypes. *Am J Respir Crit Care Med*. 2007;175:705–711.

40. Hubbard R, Venn A. The impact of coexisting connective tissue disease on survival in patients with fibrosing alveolitis. *Rheumatology (Oxford)*. 2002;41:676–679.

41. Solomon JJ, Ryu JH, Tazelaar HD, et al. Fibrosing interstitial pneumonia predicts survival in patients with rheumatoid arthritis-associated interstitial lung disease (RA-ILD). *Respir Med*. 2013;107:1247–1252.

42. Moua T, Zamora Martinez A, Baqir M, et al. Predictors of diagnosis and survival in idiopathic pulmonary fibrosis and connective tissue disease-related usual interstitial pneumonia. *Respir Res*. 2014;15:154.

43. Luppi F, Wells A. Interstitial pneumonia with autoimmune features (IPAF): a work in progress. *Eur Respir J*. 2016;47:1622–1624.

44. Ahmad K, Barba T, Gamondes D, et al. Interstitial pneumonia with autoimmune features: clinical, radiologic, and histological characteristics and outcome in a series of 57 patients. *Respir Med*. 2017;123:56–62.

Pneumoconioses Producing a Pattern of Interstitial Lung Disease

NOMENCLATURE ISSUES

Pneumoconioses are lung diseases caused by the inhalation of dusts. Although generally viewed as a distinctive set of entities, many pneumoconioses are very similar in terms of pulmonary function, imaging, and pathologic changes to interstitial lung disease (ILD), and occasionally the distinction between pneumoconiosis and non–dust-related ILD can be difficult.

Pneumoconioses are usually separated into those characterized by macular/nodular lesions around the bronchovascular bundles in the centers of the lobules (see definitions under Pathologic Features), and those that appear as diffuse

Table 22.1

Types of macular/nodular pneumoconioses

Size of lesion	Terminology
Up to 1 cm	Simple pneumoconiosis
>1 cm	Complicated pneumoconiosis, also called PMF

interstitial disease, but this distinction is somewhat artificial because most dust-related diseases start in or around the bronchioles, and many of the dusts that usually produce bronchiolocentric macular/nodular lesions can occasionally cause diffuse interstitial inflammation/fibrosis; for example, coal dust and silica (see below). Conversely, some of the diseases that typically cause diffuse interstitial fibrosis start as peribronchovascular lesions; for example, asbestosis.

Pneumoconioses characterized by nodular lesions on imaging and nodular or macular lesions on pathologic examination are subclassified into "simple" pneumoconioses, meaning the lesions measure up to 1 cm on imaging or pathology, or "complicated" pneumoconioses (also called "progressive massive fibrosis" [PMF]), meaning the nodules or mass-like lesions are larger than 1 cm[1] (Tables 22.1 and 22.2). This terminology only applies to nodular/macular lesions and is not used for diseases that appear as interstitial fibrosis.

CLINICAL FEATURES

The clinical features of the pneumoconioses vary enormously. Many dusts that produce macules on pathologic examination and nodules on imaging have no or minimal functional

Table 22.2

Summary of disease patterns by agent

Agent/disease	Simple pneumoconiosis[a]	Complicated pneumoconiosis[a]	Diffuse interstitial inflammation/fibrosis	Mineral dust–induced bronchiolitis	PAP[b]
Coal dust (CWP)	Yes	Yes	Uncommon	Yes	No
Silica/silicosis and mixed dust fibrosis	Yes	Yes	Uncommon	Yes	Yes
Silicates (e.g., talc/talcosis)	Yes	Yes	Yes	Yes	No
Asbestos/asbestosis	No[c]	No	Yes	Yes	No
Hard metal/hard metal disease	No[c]	No	Yes[d]	Yes	No

[a]Simple pneumoconiosis = dust macules or nodules measuring up to 1 cm. Complicated pneumoconiosis = nodules or masses larger than 1 cm.
[b]PAP = pulmonary alveolar proteinosis. PAP has also been reported with aluminum, indium, and titanium dioxide exposure.
[c]Early asbestosis and hard metal disease appear as centrilobular fibrotic lesions involving the walls of bronchioles, but by convention are not referred to as simple pneumoconiosis.
[d]Diffuse lesions of hard metal disease may mimic DIP or be similar to UIP.

effects (typically some degree of airflow obstruction if any-thing) and are usually picked up on imaging. Examples are siderosis ("welder's pneumoconiosis") caused by exposure to iron dust or fumes and stannosis caused by exposure to tin dust or fumes. However, simple coal worker's pneumoconi-osis (CWP) is associated with shortness of breath and signif-icant airflow obstruction in some patients.[2] Simple silicosis may produce no functional abnormality and no symptoms, or may cause airflow obstruction, or, if the nodules are pres-ent in great profusion, some degree of restriction.

When the same dusts produce large lesions of PMF, pa-tients are often short of breath and pulmonary function tests can show an obstructive or restrictive or combined abnor-mality. Pulmonary hypertension may also be present if the mass lesions have destroyed many small arterial branches.

In contrast, dusts that produce diffuse interstitial in-flammation/fibrosis, for example asbestos (asbestosis), result in a restrictive pulmonary function profile and de-creased diffusing capacity when the disease is advanced and this is accompanied by shortness of breath. However, mild forms of asbestosis may produce minimal functional changes and may not be symptomatic.

Silica exposure can produce ILD in forms that would not ordinarily be considered pneumoconioses. There is good evidence for an association of silica exposure and sclero-derma, at least in men, and some evidence of an association with rheumatoid arthritis and lupus as well. Latency (time from first exposure to disease) is long, typically decades.[3] Almost 80% of the reported scleroderma patients with silica exposure have ILD (reviewed in Freire et al.[4]), but what that translates to pathologically is not clear. There are suggestive but less strong data to support an association of silica expo-sure and the development of microscopic polyangiitis and Wegener granulomatosis (granulomatosis with polyangii-tis).[5] Both of these forms of vasculitis can also can produce pulmonary hemorrhage that sometimes leads to interstitial fibrosis in patients without silica exposure (see Chapter 24), and presumably could do the same in silica-exposed patients.

IMAGING

For many years, the chest radiograph has been a key compo-nent in the detection and characterization of pneumoconio-sis. The presence, pattern, and severity of abnormalities are assessed objectively by comparing the findings with those of the International Labour Organization (ILO) classification of pneumoconiosis standard radiographs and following the ILO guidelines.[6] The radiograph, however, has limited sen-sitivity and specificity. A number of studies have shown that high-resolution computed tomography (HRCT) is superior to the radiograph in detecting the presence of pneumoco-niosis and in characterizing parenchymal abnormalities.[7,8] Although the imaging workup of pneumoconiosis typi-cally starts with chest radiography, HRCT provides a more accurate detection and characterization of the pulmonary abnormalities and it is recommended that both imaging mo-dalities be performed in the evaluation of these patients.[8]

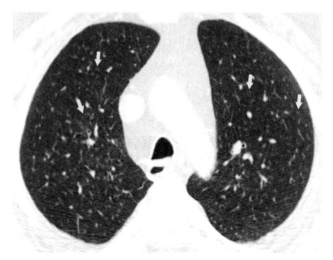

FIGURE 22.1. Coal worker's pneumoconiosis. HRCT image at the level of the upper lobes shows bilateral poorly defined (ground-glass) nod-ules (*arrows*). The patient was a 64-year-old man with CWP.

The parenchymal manifestations of pneumoconiosis on imaging consist mainly of: (a) small nodular opacities which relate to the presence of peribronchiolar dust accu-mulation with or without associated fibrosis; (b) aggrega-tion of small nodular opacities into large nodules (>1 cm) or masses; or (c) findings of ILD consisting mainly of ir-regular linear opacities (reticulation) on the radiograph and ground-glass opacities, reticulation, and, in advanced stage fibrosis, honeycombing, on HRCT.

Pneumoconioses typically presenting with small nod-ular opacities, usually with an upper lobe predominance (on radiograph and HRCT), and predominantly centrilob-ular distribution (HRCT) include CWP (Fig. 22.1), sili-cosis, and siderosis.[8] The nodules may be poorly defined (ground-glass) or well defined. Aggregation of small nod-ules into large nodules and masses (PMF) is seen most commonly in silicosis (Fig. 22.2) and CWP, but may also

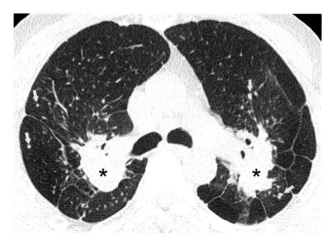

FIGURE 22.2. PMF in silicosis. HRCT image at the level of the main bronchi demonstrates bilateral perihilar conglomerate masses (*). Also noted are architectural distortion caused by the fibrosis and a few well-defined silicotic nodules (*arrows*). The patient was a 65-year-old man with long-standing silicosis.

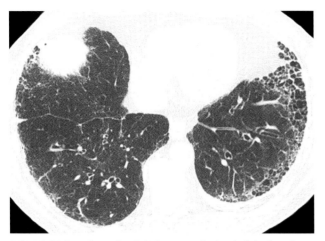

FIGURE 22.3. Asbestosis. HRCT image at the level of the lung bases shows subpleural reticulation in the right lower and middle lobes and honeycombing in the left lower lobe and lingula.

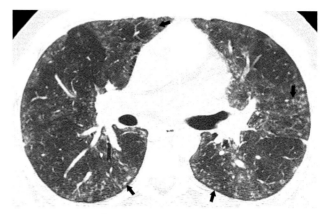

FIGURE 22.5. Hard metal pneumoconiosis. HRCT image demonstrates extensive bilateral ground-glass opacities and several centrilobular nodules (*arrows*). The patient was a 34-year-old man with a 15-year history of exposure to tungsten carbide dust as a machinist sharpening tungsten carbide blades. He had hard metal disease on surgical lung biopsy.

occur in other conditions including mixed dust pneumoconiosis, berylliosis, and talcosis whether inhaled or injected.[9] Findings of diffuse ILD are seen most commonly in asbestosis (Figs. 22.3 and 22.4), hard metal pneumoconiosis (Fig. 22.5), berylliosis, and acute silicosis (silicoproteinosis) but may occasionally occur in many other pneumoconiosis including CWP and silicosis.[9]

The diagnosis of pneumoconiosis is usually based on a history of exposure and consistent radiologic findings. It is important to emphasize, however, that the radiographic and HRCT findings of pneumoconiosis are nonspecific. For example, early CWP and siderosis may be indistinguishable from respiratory bronchiolitis or hypersensitivity pneumonitis on HRCT. Also, although the presence of bilateral pleural plaques is highly suggestive of asbestos exposure, interstitial fibrosis in patients with asbestos exposure may result from other causes or represent idiopathic pulmonary fibrosis rather than asbestosis.[10]

PATHOLOGIC FEATURES

Dust Deposition and Disease Patterns

Most dusts encountered in the workplace or the environment are preferentially deposited in the membranous and respiratory bronchioles. As a consequence, most dust diseases start in or around the bronchioles. Even diffuse fibrosing disease tends to spread from bronchiole to bronchiole and then into the surrounding parenchyma, and when this occurs the typical pattern resembles either fibrotic nonspecific interstitial pneumonia (NSIP; Chapter 7) or usual interstitial pneumonia (UIP; Chapter 6). However, the mimicry is usually not exact, because dust macules or nodules of pigmented or birefringent dust may be mixed with the more diffuse fibrosis (see below).

Macules and Nodules

Macules are defined as nonpalpable, nonfibrotic, collections of dust, usually pigmented, located around the respiratory bronchioles and accompanying pulmonary artery branches. Despite the definition, in practice, many types of macule show some degree of fibrosis. Macules are found with fairly inert dusts such as iron (Fig. 22.6) or tin, silicate minerals such as talc and mica, mixed dust fibrosis (i.e., combinations of silica with another dust) and with coal dust exposure (CWP). In CWP, the macular fibrosis can be locally quite marked with severe distortion of the respiratory bronchiole (Fig. 22.7), and the abnormal bronchiole is frequently surrounded by enlarged airspaces termed "focal emphysema" (Fig. 22.7), a process that is morphologically very similar to centrilobular emphysema found in smokers.

Nodules are rounded or stellate solid lesions that typically start next to respiratory bronchioles. Silicotic nodules have a more or less rounded contour and contain dense whorled collagen (Figs. 22.8 and 22.9) and, if the patient

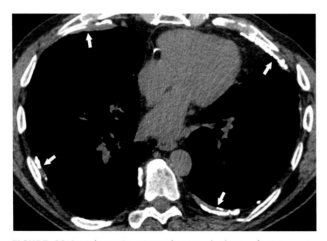

FIGURE 22.4. Asbestosis. HRCT photographed at soft tissue windows shows bilateral calcified pleural plaques (*arrows*). Same case as Figure 22.3. The patient was a 72-year-old man with asbestosis.

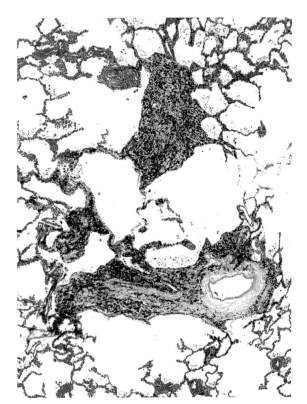

FIGURE 22.6. A dust macule. Dust macules are composed of dust, free and in macrophages, around the bronchovascular bundles. Like many dust macules, this one shows some degree of fibrosis. Patient was a hematite (iron ore) miner.

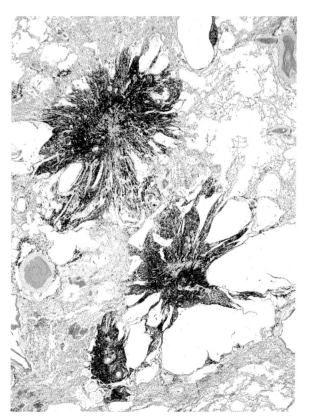

FIGURE 22.7. Simple CWP. The figure illustrates two coal dust macules with associated focal emphysema. The fibrotic portions of the macules are derived from greatly distorted and scarred respiratory bronchioles.

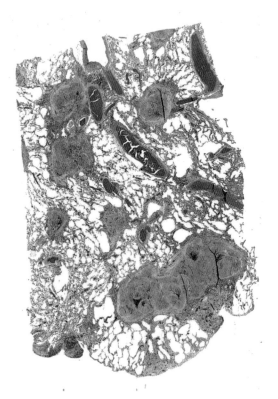

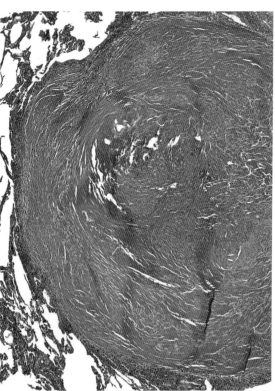

22.8

22.9

FIGURES 22.8 and 22.9. Simple silicosis. The lesions consist of discrete nodules composed of dense whorled collagen. In patients whose silica exposure is fairly remote, the nodules have little or no surrounding macrophage infiltrate, as here.

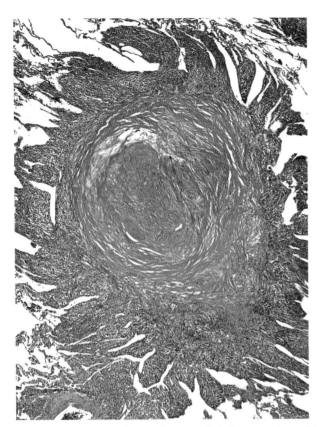

FIGURE 22.10. Simple silicosis. This example is from a patient with current or recent dust exposure and the silicotic nodule is surrounded by a macrophage and chronic inflammatory infiltrate. Nodules of this appearance can raise differential diagnoses of Langerhans cell histiocytosis (which should not have whorled collagenous centers) and sarcoidosis (which should have definite granulomas).

is currently or recently exposed to silica, dust-laden macrophages accumulate around the periphery of the nodules (Fig. 22.10). Although the difference between nodules and macules is usually evident on microscopic examination, both appear as nodules on imaging.

Most macular and nodular lesions are distinctive and do not cause confusion with ILD, but lesions such as that shown in Figure 22.10 could raise a question of Langerhans cell histiocytosis (Chapter 10) because of the appearance of a stellate cellular nodule. However, Langerhans cell histiocytosis produces irregular scars and never nodular scars, and old Langerhans cell histiocytosis scars do not contain whorled collagen (see Figs. 10.22 to 10.24).

Complicated Pneumoconioses (PMF)

PMF is seen with many dusts (Table 22.2) including coal, silica, silicates, and mixed dust fibrosis. PMF consists of masses of heavily collagenized tissue with large amounts of dust; by definition, the lesions are greater than 1 cm in size. PMF almost always develops on a background of simple pneumoconiosis. In silicosis and silicate pneumoconioses, PMF forms by conglomeration of simple silicotic/

silicate nodules/macules, but in CWP, PMF appears to form as a reaction to large amounts of coal dust without agglomeration of macules. PMF lesions can be very large and can occasionally occupy an entire lobe.

Mineral Dust–Induced Bronchiolitis

Mineral dust–induced bronchiolitis, also called mineral dust small airway's disease, consists of fibrosis of the walls of membranous and respiratory bronchioles (see Figs. 20.19 and 20.20), often accompanied by pigmented dust or asbestos bodies. Mineral dust–induced bronchiolitis can be seen with exposure to silica, iron oxide, aluminum oxide, and asbestos.[11,12] Cigarette smoke can produce similar abnormalities, particularly in the membranous bronchioles (see Fig. 20.18), but extension of process down the respiratory bronchioles is more characteristic of dust exposures (see Fig. 20.20).

Granulomatous Reactions

Berylliosis produces noncaseating granulomas that are morphologically indistinguishable from those seen in sarcoid (see Fig. 13.37). As is true of sarcoid granulomas, granulomas in berylliosis can aggregate to form nodules that become hyalinized (see Fig. 13.37). Granulomas may also be seen in organs other than the lung.

Granulomatous responses to silicate minerals such as talc and mica do not produce the well-defined granulomas of sarcoid or berylliosis. These reactions are described and illustrated below.

Diffuse Interstitial Inflammation and Fibrosis

Diffuse interstitial fibrosis is the area in which separation of pneumoconioses from non–dust-induced ILD can be problematic, and, except for asbestosis, the problem is compounded by scanty pathologic descriptions, most of which predate current ILD classifications. Features that are helpful in deciding that diffuse interstitial inflammation/fibrosis is caused by dust exposure are: (1) the presence of large amounts of visible/pigmented and/or birefringent dust in the affected parenchyma; (2) the presence of ferruginous bodies formed on the dust in question; (3) the presence of macular or nodular lesions mixed with the areas of inflammation/fibrosis. History is also crucial, because some dusts that cause fibrosis, notably hard metal, are not visible by light microscopy, and others (asbestos/asbestos bodies) are easily overlooked unless there is a reason to search for them.

Asbestosis

Asbestosis is defined as diffuse interstitial fibrosis caused by asbestos exposure. Disease is always predominantly lower zonal. Advanced asbestosis is grossly very similar to UIP, but asbestosis cases often have asbestos-induced visceral pleural fibrosis and frequently also plaques on the parietal pleura or diaphragm (Fig. 22.4), useful clues to the diagnosis.

The early microscopic lesions of asbestosis consist of small foci of interstitial fibrosis in the alveolar interstitium around membranous and respiratory bronchioles[13] (Figs. 22.11 and 22.12). The type of peribronchiolar scarring shown in Figure 22.11 raises a differential diagnosis of old burnt out Langerhans cell histiocytosis (compare Figs. 10.22 to 10.24), burnt out sarcoid (see Fig. 13.27), or chronic hypersensitivity pneumonitis (see Fig. 12.29). Early asbestosis will have asbestos bodies present (Fig. 22.12) and history is again important in arriving at the correct diagnosis.

As asbestosis progresses, fibrosis spreads interstitially to link bronchioles, and then more diffusely in the parenchyma. Sometimes the disease in advanced asbestosis resembles fibrotic NSIP but more commonly it mimics UIP (Fig. 22.13). The interstitial process in asbestosis is generally more paucicellular than in idiopathic UIP (idiopathic pulmonary fibrosis [IPF]), and fibroblast foci are less common than in UIP,[13] but some cases of asbestosis are morphologically indistinguishable from UIP, aside from the presence of asbestos bodies (Fig. 22.14). A grading scheme for asbestosis[13] is shown in Table 22.3.

By definition, the diagnosis of asbestosis requires the finding of two or more asbestos bodies/cm^2 of lung parenchyma in addition to a proper pathologic pattern.[13] Counting of asbestos bodies should be carried out on iron-stained 5 μm thick sections (Fig. 22.14). Some individuals appear to form asbestos bodies poorly and in such cases electron microscopic analysis to determine total asbestos fiber burden may be helpful; however, cases of this type are quite rare, and in most instances, iron stains provide an excellent way of separating asbestosis from idiopathic ILD.[14]

An unusual differential diagnosis of asbestosis that has emerged in recent years is interstitial fibrosis induced by cigarette smoking, a process that goes under various names including respiratory bronchiolitis with fibrosis (RBF), smoking-related interstitial fibrosis, and airspace enlargement with fibrosis, among others (see Chapter 8 for further discussion). As opposed to asbestosis, which, even in its early stages is a diffuse process, RBF appears as distinctly localized, usually subpleural, patches of very paucicellular hyaline fibrosis mixed with emphysema; the airspaces typically contain smoker's macrophages (see Figs. 8.9 to 8.13).

Although at first glance there does not appear to be much similarity in the appearance of asbestosis and RBF, Bledsoe et al.[15] reported 24 cases that were thought to be asbestosis on the basis of chest radiographs, but on biopsy, 18/24 were actually RBF. Terra-Filho et al.[16] compared chest radiographs to HRCT images in 1,418 miners and millers who had worked at different times with increasingly

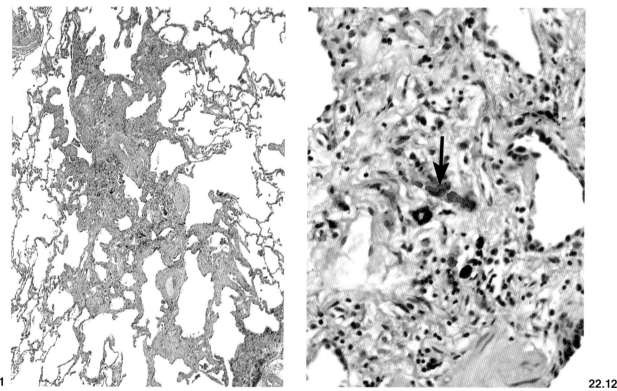

22.11   **22.12**

FIGURES 22.11 and 22.12. Early asbestosis. **Figure 22.11:** The lesions of early asbestosis consist of interstitial fibrosis around membranous and respiratory bronchioles. The morphologic differential diagnosis includes burnt out Langerhans cell histiocytosis, burnt out sarcoid, and chronic hypersensitivity pneumonitis. **Figure 22.12:** An asbestos body (*arrow*) is present in the fibrous tissue. The presence of asbestos bodies in adequate numbers (2 or more/cm^2, see text) supports a diagnosis of asbestosis. This lesion would be graded as 2 under the current diagnostic criteria (see text).

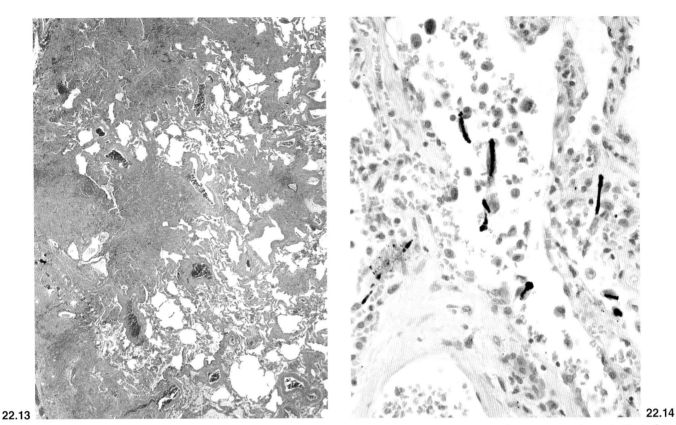

FIGURES 22.13 and 22.14. Advanced asbestosis. This example mimics UIP at low power, but the presence of two or more asbestos bodies/cm² (**Fig. 22.14**, iron stain) allows a diagnosis of asbestosis. This example would be graded as 4 under the current diagnostic criteria (see text).

lower levels of asbestos exposure. Despite considerable differences in exposure levels, chest radiographs showed essentially the same degree of "interstitial" abnormalities in all groups, whereas HRCT demonstrated quite clearly a very marked (down to almost none) drop over time in the number of workers who actually had imaging evidence of

---

Table 22.3

Grading of asbestosis

Grade 0: No interstitial fibrosis or fibrosis confined to bronchiolar walls

Grade 1: Fibrosis confined to the walls of respiratory bronchioles and the first tier of adjacent alveoli

Grade 2: Extension of fibrosis to involve alveolar ducts and/or two or more tiers of alveoli adjacent to the respiratory bronchiole, with sparing of at least some alveoli between adjacent bronchioles

Grade 3: Fibrotic thickening of the walls of all alveoli between two or more adjacent bronchioles

Grade 4: Honeycomb change

From Roggli VL, Gibbs AR, Attanoos R, et al. Pathology of asbestosis—an update of the diagnostic criteria: report of the Asbestosis Committee of the College of American Pathologists and Pulmonary Pathology Society. *Arch Pathol Lab Med.* 2010;134:462–480..

asbestosis. These findings suggest that much of what has been called low ILO reading asbestosis in the past on the basis of chest radiographs may in fact have been related to cigarette smoking.

Diffuse Interstitial Fibrosis with Coal and Silica Exposure

The literature suggests that diffuse interstitial fibrosis is seen in up to 18% of autopsied coal miners,[17] but in our experience the frequency is much lower. Two different patterns of diffuse fibrosis are seen: (1) fibrosis that links macular or nodular lesions of simple CWP, and (2) fibrosis that is more diffuse and resembles fibrotic NSIP or UIP.[17,18] Green[2] has proposed that cases in which there is extensive coal dust mixed with the fibrosis should be regarded as caused by coal exposure (Figs. 22.15 and 22.16), whereas those without much dust should be viewed as idiopathic ILD. The presence or absence of simple CWP on imaging or biopsy may also be a useful guide to etiology.

Diffuse ILD resembling fibrotic NSIP or UIP also occurs in patients with silicosis.[19] We suggest that cases with a mixture of silicotic nodules and diffuse fibrosis should be viewed as caused by dust, whereas in patients with silica exposure but no nodules, the diffuse disease is probably not related to silica exposure.

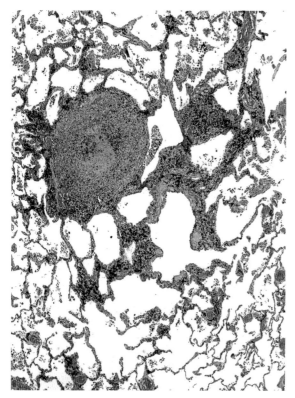

FIGURE 22.15. A silicotic nodule with surrounding early interstitial fibrosis in a coal miner. Note the extensive coal pigment, which indicates that the fibrosis is related to dust exposure.

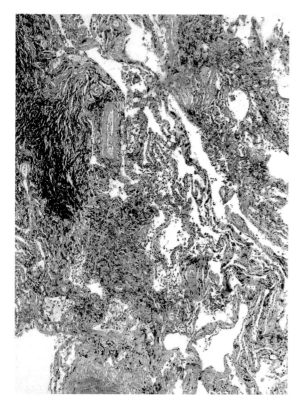

FIGURE 22.16. Diffuse interstitial fibrosis (unclassifiable pattern) in a coal miner. The extensive pigment again indicates that the fibrosis is related to dust exposure.

Diffuse Interstitial Fibrosis with Silicate Exposure

Exposure to silicate minerals (talc, mica, kaolinite, slate, sepiolite, montmorillonite, vermiculite, and wollastonite) causes a variety of pathologic patterns. Most commonly these are macules, but with greater exposure, diffuse interstitial dust collections that are vaguely granulomatous and variably fibrotic may be seen[20–23] (Figs. 22.17 to 22.19). Silicate minerals can also form ferruginous bodies (Fig. 22.18). With heavy exposure, many silicate minerals can produce diffuse fibrosis with or without honeycombing, again in patterns that more or less resemble fibrotic NSIP or UIP but mixed with copious dust (Figs. 22.20 and 22.21). Many, but not all, silicates are brightly birefringent, so polarization is sometimes very helpful in elucidating the cause of fibrosis (Figs. 22.19 and 22.21).

Intravenous Drug Abuse

In intravenous (IV) drug abuse, the drug filler, which is typically insoluble particles of talc or microcrystalline cellulose, is deposited in the lung and can cause interstitial granulomas, diffuse interstitial fibrosis (Figs. 22.22 to 22.25),

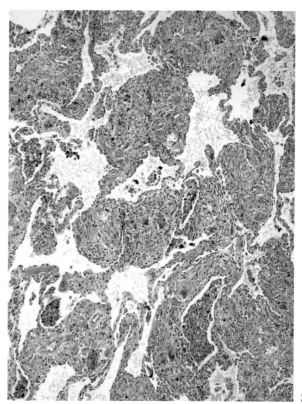

22.17

FIGURES 22.17 to 22.19. Talcosis. This is an example of a sheet silicate (talc) pneumoconiosis mimicking a diffuse ILD. The presence of large amounts of talc, visible as pale staining crystals on H& E (**Fig. 22.18** and brightly birefringent material on polarization **Fig. 22.19**), indicates that this is a pneumoconiosis. Ferruginous bodies (**Fig. 22.18**, *arrow*) also are helpful in diagnosing a pneumoconiosis.

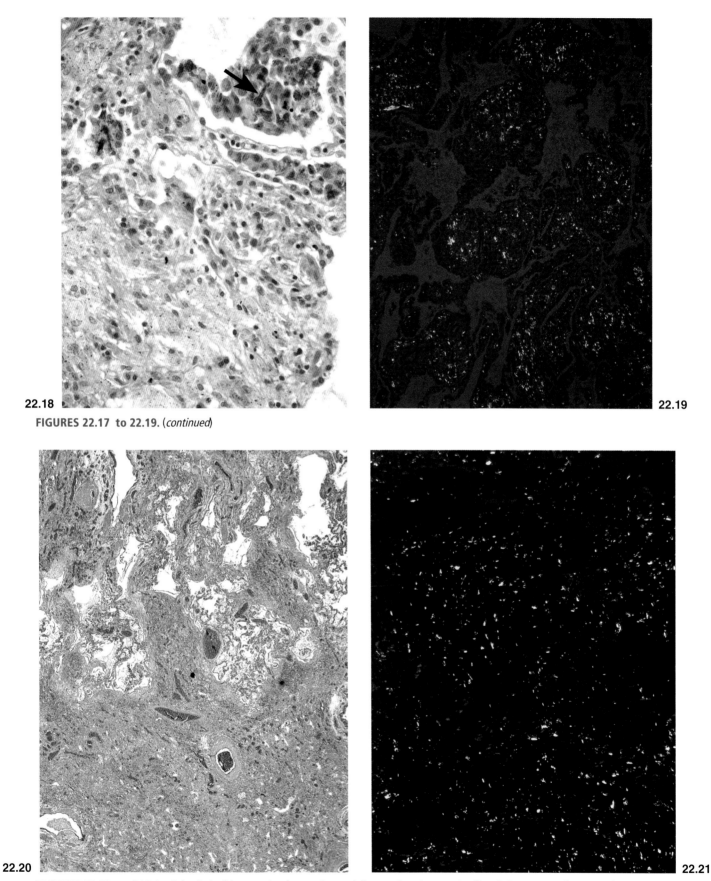

22.18

22.19

FIGURES 22.17 to 22.19. (*continued*)

22.20

22.21

FIGURES 22.20 and 22.21. Talcosis. In this example of very advanced disease, there is extensive fibrosis in a pattern that somewhat mimics UIP. Polarization (**Fig. 22.21**) shows numerous brightly birefringent particles, indicating that this is a pneumoconiosis.

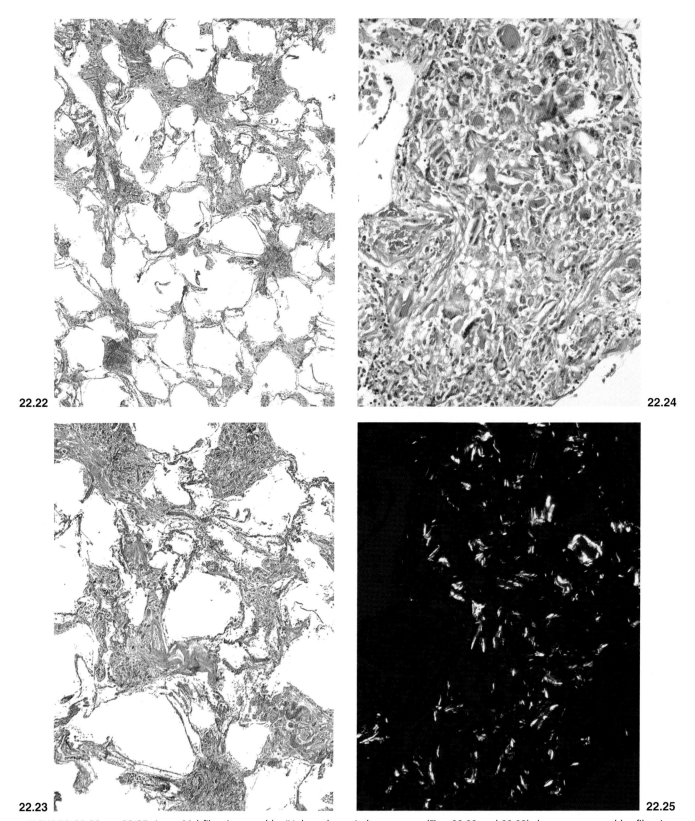

FIGURES 22.22 to 22.25. Interstitial fibrosis caused by IV drug abuse. At lower power (Figs. 22.22 and 22.23) the process resembles fibrotic NSIP, but high-power images show numerous plates of crystalline material (**Fig. 22.24**) that are brightly birefringent on polarized light (**Fig. 22.25**).

PMF, and lesions that resemble macules. IV drug abuse can usually be separated from inhalation particulate exposure because in the former the particles are all interstitial and generally also intravascular, whereas in inhalation injuries dust is usually present in the alveoli as well as the interstitium and is not present in vessels. Talc and microcrystalline cellulose are brightly birefringent (Figs. 22.25), useful clues to the diagnosis.

Pulmonary Alveolar Proteinosis

Pulmonary alveolar proteinosis can be caused by exposure to very large amounts of finely divided dust (see Chapter 16) including silica (quartz), titanium dioxide, aluminum, and indium. Silicoproteinosis, also called acute silicosis, is morphologically very similar to primary (autoimmune) alveolar proteinosis (see Chapter 16), but in our experience always shows a mild interstitial inflammatory reaction, something that is not present in most cases of primary proteinosis (see Fig. 16.10). Numerous poorly birefringent silica particles are usually visible on polarization (see Fig. 16.10), but occasionally the dust may be too small to resolve with the light microscope.

Hard Metal Disease

Hard metal disease or hard metal pneumoconiosis (called in the past "giant cell interstitial pneumonia") is caused by exposure to hard metal (tungsten carbide), either during manufacture of hard metal cutting tools, or during grinding or welding of hard metal tools. Hard metal disease is actually a hypersensitivity reaction to cobalt, which is added as a binder in manufacturing, and exposure to cooling baths that extract cobalt from hard metal blades, for example in sawmills, can cause hard metal disease. Hard metal disease has also been reported in diamond polishers using a cobalt polish but not hard metal[24] and in workers in the bonded diamond tool industry where cobalt is used as the matrix for microdiamonds.[25]

Hard metal disease is pathologically distinctive. In its earliest stage, it consists of marked fibrosis and inflammation of the walls of respiratory bronchioles with a luminal infiltrate of macrophages and large, often bizarre, giant cells that sometimes demonstrate emperipolesis (Figs. 22.26 and 22.27).[26] As the disease progresses, fibrosis may spread between bronchioles and more diffusely in the

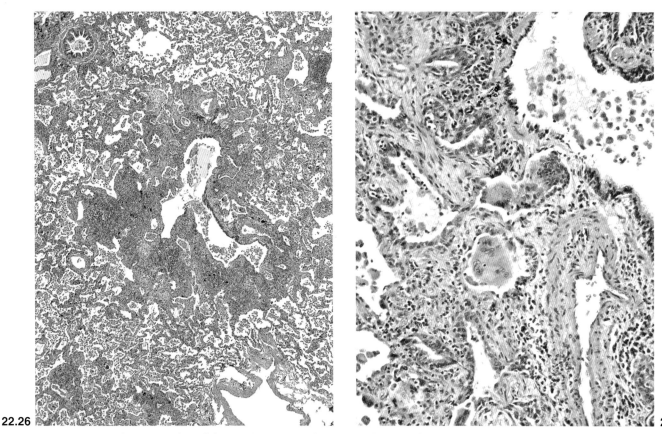

22.26   22.27

FIGURES 22.26 and 22.27. Hard metal disease. **Figure 22.26** shows a typical picture of a markedly fibrotic and inflamed respiratory bronchiole. The process is associated with numerous giant cells (**Fig. 22.27**).

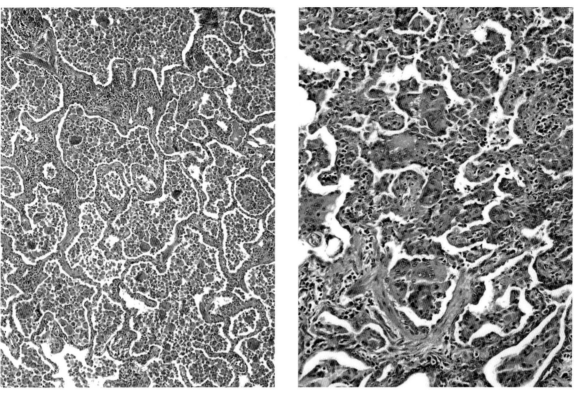

22.28   22.29

FIGURES 22.28 and 22.29. Hard metal disease mimicking DIP. At low power the process is very similar to cigarette smoke-induced DIP except for the large number of giant cells; the latter can occur in DIP but in much fewer numbers. Figure 23.29 is a high-power view from a different case in which there are numerous giant cells.

interstitium, producing a pattern that resembles desquamative interstitial pneumonia (DIP; Figs. 22.28 and 22.29, and see Chapter 8). Cigarette smoke–related DIP may have small numbers of giant cells, but not the numbers nor the sometimes bizarre forms (Fig. 22.29) seen in hard metal disease.

Hard metal disease can progress to severe diffuse fibrosis and honeycombing (Fig. 22.30) that is difficult to separate from non–dust-related ILD, unless one has a history of exposure, or there are typical bronchiolar lesions.

Silicon Carbide

Silicon carbide (carborundum) has been reported to produce a mixture of nodules with more diffuse fibrosis and a prominent alveolar macrophage response.[27] The silicon carbide particles are fibrous and form ferruginous bodies with black cores.[27]

Iron and Aluminum

When inhaled in extremely large amounts, iron and aluminum metal can produce a form of diffuse interstitial fibrosis somewhat resembling fibrotic NSIP, but with very large amounts of visible dust (Figs. 22.31 and 22.32).

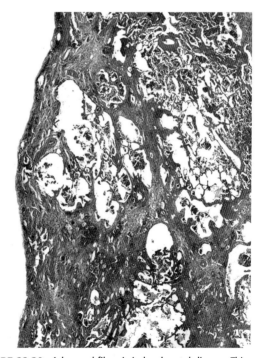

FIGURE 22.30. Advanced fibrosis in hard metal disease. This appearance is not specific and might be seen in idiopathic UIP (IPF). If there are no characteristic airway lesions (such as Figure 22.26) in the biopsy, only exposure history or analysis of the tissue for tungsten will indicate the correct diagnosis.

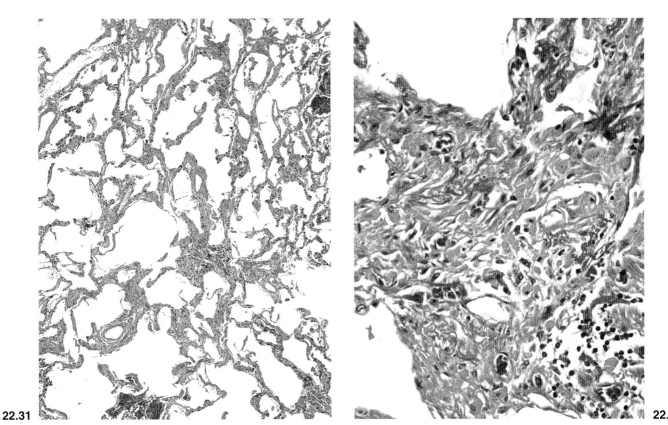

22.31   22.32

FIGURES 22.31 and 22.32. Interstitial fibrosis induced by very high exposure to aluminum dust. At low power the process mimics fibrotic NSIP. At high power (**Fig. 22.32**) macrophages loaded with silvery yellow aluminum particles are visible.

DIAGNOSTIC MODALITIES

Many pneumoconioses are diagnosed on imaging without need for a biopsy. Transbronchial biopsy is occasionally useful if it picks up a nodular or macular lesion, for example, in silicosis, but the diagnosis of conditions such as asbestosis that appear as diffuse fibrosis requires a surgical lung biopsy. The potential usefulness of cryobiopsy in this setting has yet to be demonstrated. It has been suggested that, given an appropriate history, the finding of giant cells with emperipolesis in lavage fluid can be used to support a diagnosis of hard metal disease.[25]

PROGNOSIS

Many pneumoconioses characterized by macular/nodular lesions have little functional significance and do not affect life expectancy, although there is increasing recognition that they can cause airflow obstruction.[17,28] Large PMF lesions of any cause can produce functional deficits and increased mortality. There has been a resurgence of PMF cases in coal miners, particularly young coal miners, in the Eastern United States over the last 10 years[29]; many of these patients are now coming to transplantation. Diffuse fibrosis in coal workers has a very slow course,[17] much slower than is seen with UIP. Exposure to silica increases

the risk of mycobacterial infections[30] and the presence of silicosis may increase the risk of lung cancer, although this issue is disputed.[31,32]

Asbestosis can progress to severe end-stage fibrosis, but the risk of progression is proportional to the severity of the initial radiologic changes and mild cases may stabilize. The presence of asbestosis greatly increases the risk of lung cancer, especially in cigarette smokers.[33]

REFERENCES

1. Begin R. Clinical evaluation of the patient with occupational lung disease. In: Churg A, Green FHY, eds. *Pathology of Occupational Lung Disease*. 2nd ed. Baltimore, MA: Williams and Wilkins; 1998:1–20.
2. Green FHY, Vallyathan V. Coal worker's pneumoconiosis and pneumoconiosis due to other carbonaceous dusts. In: Churg A, Green FHY, eds. *Pathology of Occupational Lung Disease*. 2nd ed. Baltimore, MA: Williams and Wilkins; 1998:129–208.
3. Englert H, Small-McMahon J, Davis K, et al. Male systemic sclerosis and occupational silica exposure-a population-based study. *Aust N Z J Med*. 2000;30:215–220.
4. Freire M, Alonso M, Rivera A, et al. Clinical peculiarities of patients with scleroderma exposed to silica: a systematic review of the literature. *Semin Arthritis Rheum*. 2015;45:294–300.
5. Gómez-Puerta JA, Gedmintas L, Costenbader KH. The association between silica exposure and development of

ANCA-associated vasculitis: systematic review and meta-analysis. *Autoimmun Rev.* 2017;12:1129–1135.

6. International Labour Organization. *Guidelines for the Use of ILO International Classification of Radiographs of Pneumoconioses.* Geneva, Switzerland: ILO; 2011.

7. Akira M. Imaging of occupational and environmental lung diseases. *Clin Chest Med.* 2008;29:117–131.

8. Expert Panel on Thoracic Imaging, Bacchus L, Shah RD, Chung JH, et al. ACR Appropriateness criteria® occupational lung diseases. *J Thorac Imaging.* 2016;31:W1–W3.

9. Chong S, Lee KS, Chung MJ, et al. Pneumoconiosis: comparison of imaging and pathologic findings. *Radiographics.* 2006;26:59–77.

10. Gaensler EA, Jederlinic PJ, Churg A. Idiopathic pulmonary fibrosis in asbestos-exposed workers. *Am Rev Respir Dis.* 1991;144:689–696.

11. Churg A, Wright JL. Small-airway lesions in patients exposed to nonasbestos mineral dusts. *Hum Pathol.* 1983; 14:688–693.

12. Wright JL, Churg A. Morphology of small-airway lesions in patients with asbestos exposure. *Hum Pathol.* 1984;15:68–74.

13. Roggli VL, Gibbs AR, Attanoos R, et al. Pathology of asbestosis—an update of the diagnostic criteria: report of the Asbestosis Committee of the College of American Pathologists and Pulmonary Pathology Society. *Arch Pathol Lab Med.* 2010;134:462–480.

14. Schneider F, Sporn TA, Roggli VL. Asbestos fiber content of lungs with diffuse interstitial fibrosis: an analytical scanning electron microscopic analysis of 249 cases. *Arch Pathol Lab Med.* 2010;134:457–461.

15. Bledsoe JR, Christiani DC, Kradin RL. Smoking-associated fibrosis and pulmonary asbestosis. *Int J Chron Obstruct Pulmon Dis.* 2014;10:31–37.

16. Terra-Filho M, Bagatin E, Nery LE, et al. Screening of miners and millers at decreasing levels of asbestos exposure: comparison of chest radiography and thin-section computed tomography. *PLoS One.* 2015;10:e0118585.

17. Cohen RA, Patel A, Green FH. Lung disease caused by exposure to coal mine and silica dust. *Semin Respir Crit Care Med.* 2008;29:651–661.

18. Brichet A, Tonnel AB, Brambilla E, et al.; Groupe d'Etude en Pathologie Interstitielle (GEPI) de la Société de Pathologie Thoracique du Nord. Chronic interstitial pneumonia with honeycombing in coal workers. *Sarcoidosis Vasc Diffuse Lung Dis.* 2002;19:211–219.

19. Arakawa H, Johkoh T, Honma K, et al. Chronic interstitial pneumonia in silicosis and mixed-dust pneumoconiosis: its prevalence and comparison of CT findings with idiopathic pulmonary fibrosis. *Chest.* 2007;131:1870–1876.

20. Gibbs AR, Pooley FD, Griffiths DM, et al. Talc pneumoconiosis: a pathologic and mineralogic study. *Hum Pathol.* 1992;23:1344–1354.

21. Gibbs AR, Craighead JE, Pooley FD, et al. The pathology of slate workers' pneumoconiosis in North Wales and Vermont. *Ann Occup Hyg.* 1988;32(Suppl. 1):273–278.

22. Landas SK, Schwartz DA. Mica-associated pulmonary interstitial fibrosis. *Am Rev Respir Dis.* 1991;144(3, pt 1):718–721.

23. Schenker MB, Pinkerton KE, Mitchell D, et al. Pneumoconiosis from agricultural dust exposure among young California farmworkers. *Environ Health Perspect.* 2009;117:988–994.

24. Nemery B, Casier P, Roosels D, et al. Survey of cobalt exposure and respiratory health in diamond polishers. *Am Rev Respir Dis.* 1992;145:610–616.

25. Adams TN, Butt YM, Batra K, et al. Cobalt related interstitial lung disease. *Respir Med.* 2017;129:91–97.

26. Churg A, Colby TV. Disease caused by metals and related compounds. In: Churg A, Green FHY, eds. *Pathology of Occupational Lung Disease.* 2nd ed. Baltimore, MA: Williams and Wilkins; 1998:77–128.

27. Massé S, Bégin R, Cantin A. Pathology of silicon carbide pneumoconiosis. *Mod Pathol.* 1988;1:104–108.

28. Rushton L. Chronic obstructive pulmonary disease and occupational exposure to silica. *Rev Environ Health.* 2007;22:255–272.

29. Stansbury RC. Progressive massive fibrosis and coal mine dust lung disease: the continued resurgence of a preventable disease. *Ann Am Thorac Soc.* 2018;15:1394–1396.

30. Cowie RL. The epidemiology of tuberculosis in gold miners with silicosis. *Am J Respir Crit Care Med.* 1994;150(5, pt 1):1460–1462.

31. Gamble JF. Crystalline silica and lung cancer: a critical review of the occupational epidemiology literature of exposure-response studies testing this hypothesis. *Crit Rev Toxicol.* 2011;41:404–465.

32. Poinen-Rughooputh S, Rughooputh MS, Guo Y, et al. Occupational exposure to silica dust and risk of lung cancer: an updated meta-analysis of epidemiological studies. *BMC Public Health.* 2016;16:1137.

33. Churg A. Neoplastic asbestos-induced disease. In: Churg A, Green FHY, eds. *Pathology of Occupational Lung Disease.* 2nd ed. Baltimore, MD: Williams and Wilkins; 1998:339–392.

Miscellaneous Forms of Interstitial Lung Disease

PULMONARY DISEASE CAUSED BY THERAPEUTIC RADIATION

Lung toxicity is seen with external radiation to the mediastinum, lung, esophagus, and chest wall (e.g., for breast carcinoma) and occasionally in patients treated with radioactive iodine for thyroid carcinoma metastatic to the lung.[1] Radiation injury depends on the volume of radiated lung tissue (the greater the volume radiated, the greater the risk of toxicity) and dose of radiation (fractionated doses are less dangerous than a single large dose).[1] Prior radio- or chemotherapy, particularly with bleomycin, may sensitize the lung to subsequent radiation,[2] and the risk of radiation-induced disease is higher in the presence of underlying infection or preexisting interstitial lung disease (ILD). Although smoking has been viewed in the past as a risk factor,[3] recent data suggest that smoking appears to be protective, perhaps because cigarette smoke induces expression of intrapulmonary antioxidants.[4] In most cases, radiation injury is confined to the area radiated, but occasionally toxicity is seen in a large area outside the radiation port[5] including the contralateral lung.

Clinical Features

Acute radiation injury (acute radiation pneumonitis) typically appears within a few weeks to a few months after radiation and can manifest as a febrile illness with accompanying shortness of breath, or in severe cases as acute respiratory distress syndrome. Radiation-induced fibrosis (chronic radiation pneumonitis) typically appears 1 year or more after completing radiation and resembles a fibrosing interstitial pneumonia. Sporadic radiation pneumonitis is less common; it can appear at any time and mimics organizing pneumonia (OP).[5]

Imaging

Radiation pneumonitis is characterized on high-resonance computed tomography (HRCT) by ground-glass opacities or consolidation involving the irradiated portions of lung and conforming to the shape of the radiation ports (Fig. 23.1).[6] Radiation fibrosis manifests as streaky

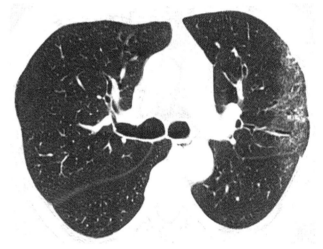

FIGURE 23.1. Radiation pneumonitis. HRCT image shows ground-glass opacities and small focal areas of consolidation in the periphery of the left lung. Note the sharp demarcation between the irradiated and the normal lung. The patient had radiation therapy to the left chest wall.

opacities, dense consolidation, volume loss, and traction bronchiectasis within the irradiated lung regions. There is typically a sharply defined edge between normal and irradiated lung, allowing distinction of radiation pneumonitis or fibrosis from other lung diseases on computed tomography (CT). Current radiation therapy techniques use multiple beams in various planes to maximize radiation to the tumor while minimizing irradiation to the adjacent lung. These may result in focal or mass-like ground-glass opacities, consolidation, or fibrosis following radiotherapy of lung tumors.[7,8]

Pathologic Features

Acute radiation injury microscopically looks like diffuse alveolar damage (Fig. 23.2 and see Chapter 4) in the acute or organizing phase. However, bizarre radiation fibroblasts may be present (Fig. 23.3), and there may also be marked vascular sclerosis, features not seen in ordinary diffuse alveolar damage. Sporadic radiation pneumonitis is not often biopsied but morphologically looks like OP (Fig. 23.4)

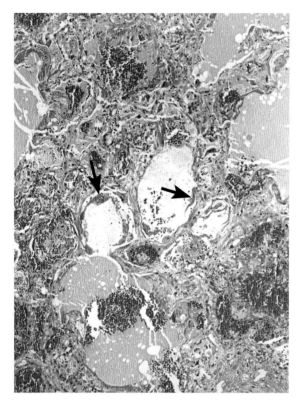

FIGURE 23.2. Acute radiation pneumonitis manifest as diffuse alveolar damage in a patient receiving therapeutic radiation for Hodgkin disease approximately 1 month before death. *Arrows* point to hyaline membranes.

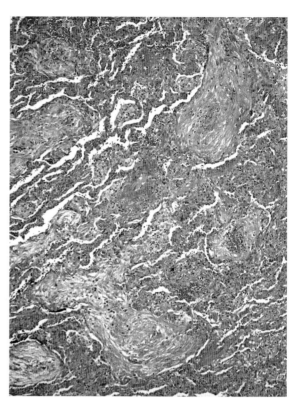

FIGURE 23.4. Sporadic radiation pneumonitis appearing as OP. OP developed 6 months after the patient completed radiation therapy for carcinoma of the breast and was present both within and outside the radiation port.

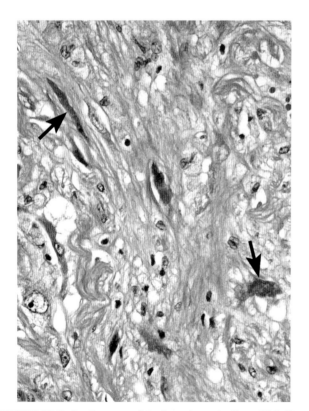

FIGURE 23.3. Another area of the lung shown in Figure 23.2. Note the bizarre radiation fibroblasts (*arrows*).

and typically occurs outside as well as inside the radiation field.[5,9,10] There are rare reports of eosinophilic pneumonia as a response to radiation.[3]

Chronic radiation injury appears as a fibrosing interstitial pneumonia. An important clue to the diagnosis is that the process in most cases is sharply localized to the radiation ports (Fig. 23.5). Some cases resemble fibrotic nonspecific interstitial pneumonia (NSIP), whereas others are more like usual interstitial pneumonia (UIP; Fig. 23.6). As opposed to typical cases of NSIP or UIP, marked elastosis mixed with the fibrosis may be present and the elastofibrotic reaction can obliterate large areas of lung parenchyma (Figs. 23.7 and 23.8). Radiation fibroblasts and vascular obliteration may also be seen (Fig. 23.9).

Radiation to the chest can also induce malignant mesotheliomas of the pleura, typically appearing fairly long (10 years or more) since completion of therapy.[11]

Prognosis

Acute radiation injury subsides in most patients[12]; however, some patients develop fatal disease.[13] Purely localized fibrosis has a good prognosis. A wide variety of therapeutic approaches including steroids, antioxidants (superoxide dismutase, genistein), and antifibrotic agents have been tried for widespread radiation-induced fibrosis, but at this point there is no consensus on treatment or outcome.[2]

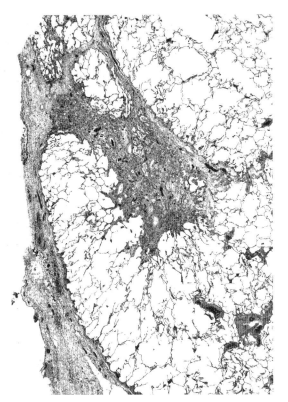

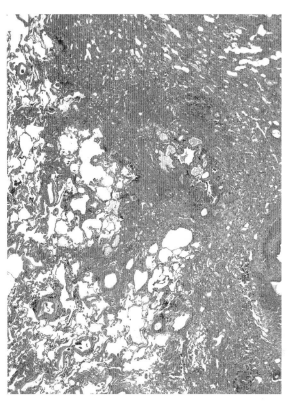

FIGURE 23.5. Chronic radiation pneumonitis. Sharply demarcated area of fibrosis at the edge of a radiation port.

FIGURE 23.6. Chronic radiation pneumonitis. Dense radiation-induced fibrosis mimicking UIP.

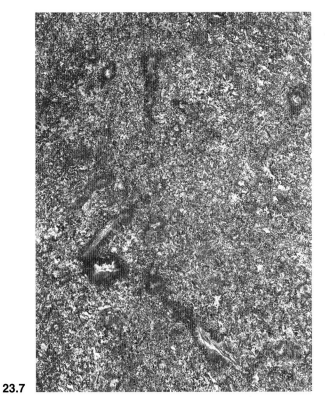

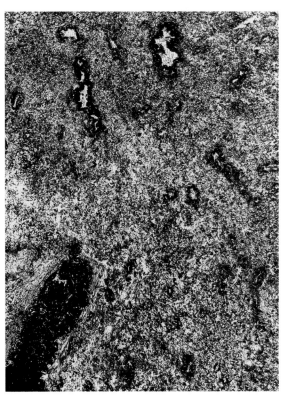

23.7

23.8

FIGURES 23.7 and 23.8. Chronic radiation pneumonitis. Higher power H&E and elastic stain views of another area from the same case as Figure 23.6. Note the extensive elastotic reaction. Although not specific, this type of fibroelastosis is very common in radiation-induced fibrosis.

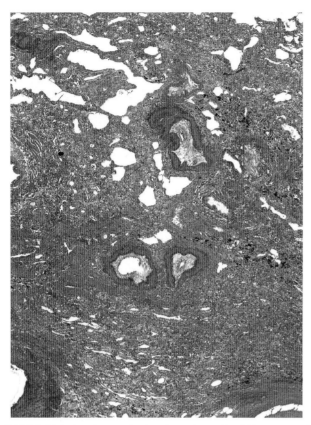

FIGURE 23.9. Nearly completely sclerosed vessels within an area of radiation-induced fibrosis. Vascular obliteration is common as a radiation reaction.

ERDHEIM–CHESTER DISEASE

Clinical Features

Erdheim–Chester disease (ECD) is a form of neoplastic histiocytosis that primarily affects the long bones, causing bone pain and radiologic osteosclerosis, but any organ can be involved. In a recent series of 73 biopsies from 42 patients,[14] disease was demonstrated in the retroperitoneum, skin, orbit, brain, lung, heart, epidural tissues, oral cavity, subcutis, and testis. Nonpulmonary manifestations include exophthalmos, diabetes insipidus, xanthelasma, and retroperitoneal fibrosis.[15] In some series, pulmonary involvement has been reported in 50% of cases.[16]

Molecular Abnormalities

ECD was traditionally regarded as a histiocytic proliferation of uncertain etiology, but the discovery of *BRAF* V600E mutations in the majority of cases along with other less common mutations (Table 23.1) has led to the designation of ECD as a histiocytic neoplasm in which there are usually genetic abnormalities in the mitogen activated protein kinase (MAPK) pathway.[14] A small proportion of cases of ECD have *PIKC3A* mutations and evidence of mTOR activation.[17] Many of the reported mutations are similar

Table 23.1
Mutations reported in ECD
BRAF V600E
MAP2K1
ARAF
MAP2K2
KRAS
NRAS
PIKC3A

to those seen in Langerhans cell histiocytosis (LCH, see Table 10.1), but the immunohistochemical properties of Erdheim–Chester histiocytes differ from those of LCH (see below) and, as opposed to LCH, Erdheim–Chester histiocytes appear to evoke an inflammatory and/or fibrotic response in many organs.

Imaging

Pulmonary involvement in ECD is usually manifested on CT by bilateral smooth thickening of the interlobular septa and interlobar fissures (Fig. 23.10).[14,18] Other common findings include poorly defined centrilobular nodules and ground-glass opacities. The pulmonary abnormalities are frequently associated with other signs of intrathoracic involvement, most commonly soft tissue infiltration around the aorta, and pleural and pericardial thickening and/or effusion. Sclerosis of the bony thorax and spine may be present.

Pathologic Features

In the lung, ECD appears as infiltrates of histiocytes that follow lymphatic routes along the bronchovascular bundles and interlobular septa and are accompanied by a variable

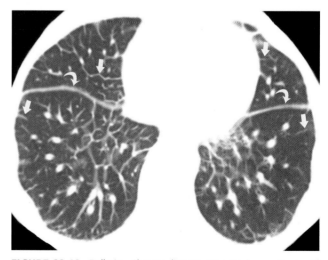

FIGURE 23.10. Erdheim–Chester disease. CT scan in a patient with pulmonary involvement in ECD shows bilateral smooth thickening of the interlobular septa (*straight arrows*) and interlobar fissures (*curved arrows*).

degree of fibrosis (Figs. 23.11 to 23.14). Although Erd-heim–Chester histiocytes have traditionally been described as xanthomatous, this is not always true, and the histiocytes can have clear or foamy to eosinophilic cytoplasm[14] (Fig. 23.14). They are CD68 (Fig. 23.15) and Factor 13a positive. In some cases, they are also S-100 positive but they are invariably CD1a negative, an important point of distinction from LCH. Most cases that harbor *BRAF* V600E mutations can be detected by BRAF V600E immunohistochemistry.[14]

Differential Diagnosis

ECD is sometimes compared to LCH (see Chapter 10), but the morphologic overlaps are actually minimal. Langerhans cells typically have grooved nuclei and never have foamy cytoplasm or very copious cytoplasm. The Langerhans cells of LCH are always S-100 and CD1a positive (see Figs. 10.29 and 10.30). Although the lesions of LCH are often centered around bronchioles, they do not involve the interlobular septa, and the lesions along the bronchovascular bundles are either cellular nodules (see Fig. 10.8) or dense scars (see Figs. 10.22 to 10.24). When LCH scars, the scars are irregular and center on the bronchovascular bundles but don't follow the interlobular septa (see Figs. 10.22 to 10.26).

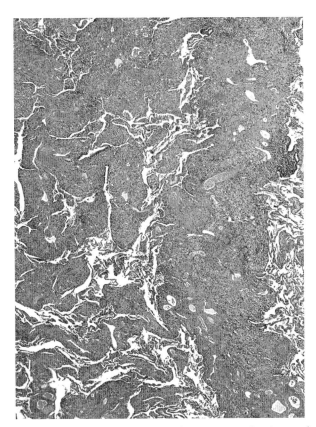

FIGURE 23.12. Medium-power view of Figure 23.11. Fibrosis extends irregularly into the lung parenchyma.

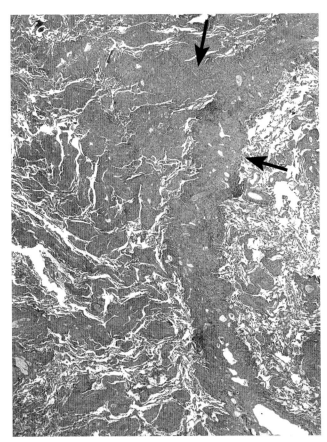

FIGURE 23.11. Low-power view of ECD. There is a fibrosing reaction that follows the interlobular septa (*arrows*). This process corresponds to the thickened interlobular septa seen in Figure 23.10.

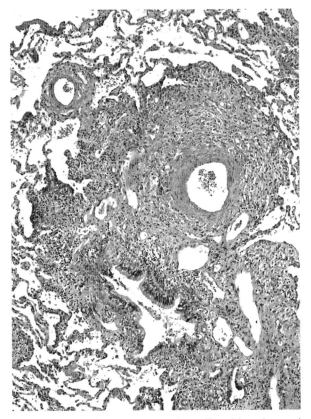

FIGURE 23.13. Higher power view of an affected bronchovascular bundle. At this magnification, histiocyte infiltration is just visible.

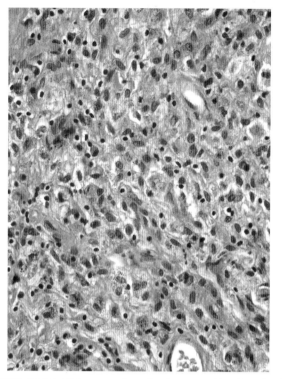

FIGURE 23.14. High-power view showing a combination of pale-staining histiocytes and fibrous tissue. In some cases, the histiocytes of ECD are eosinophilic rather than clear or foamy.

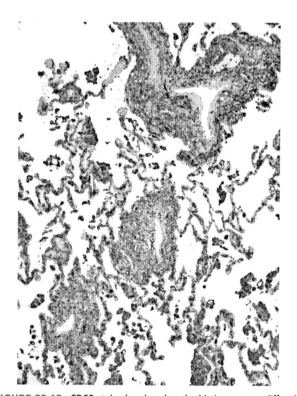

FIGURE 23.15. CD68 stain showing that the histiocytes are diffusely positive in ECD. They are also usually Factor 13a positive. These findings are in contradistinction to LCH where the Langerhans cells are CD1a positive. S-100 staining can be seen in either condition but is invariably positive in LCH and only occasionally positive in ECD.

Prognosis

The prognosis of ECD has been reported as very variable, but with an overall mortality in the literature of 60%. Some patients are asymptomatic and are detected because of bony abnormalities found on imaging. Central nervous system and cardiac involvement is associated with a poor outcome.[15] The importance of pulmonary involvement is unclear: Some authors[15] claim that it is usually of little consequence, whereas others[19] state that pulmonary involvement is usually fatal. However, the treatment picture and outcome has been changed with the use of the BRAF inhibitor vemurafenib for patients who have *BRAF* V600E mutations; in a series of 22 such patients, most stabilized and some showed regression of lesions; the 2-year progression-free survival was 86%.[20] Sirolimus plus prednisone has also been reported to be effective, at least in cases with mTOR activation,[17] and rare cases have been reported to respond to cladribine.[21]

PERIBRONCHIOLAR METAPLASIA

Clinical Features

Peribronchiolar metaplasia, sometimes called Lambertosis, is often an incidental finding on pathologic examination, and the associated specific clinical features, if any, are unclear. The lesion probably reflects bronchiolar injury of a variety of etiologies.

The only paper specifically addressing the subject of peribronchiolar metaplasia[22] reported 15 patients with clinical ILD and peribronchiolar metaplasia as the predominant finding on biopsy. Apart from a marked male predominance, there was a wide variety of clinical, functional (some obstructive, some restrictive, some mixed, some normal), and radiologic findings, and it is not clear whether peribronchiolar metaplasia per se was responsible for any of these abnormalities.

Peribronchiolar metaplasia is most often seen in association with fibrosing interstitial pneumonias, but it has become increasingly apparent that the presence of a large fraction of bronchioles with peribronchiolar metaplasia is an important clue to a diagnosis of chronic hypersensitivity pneumonitis and is helpful in separating chronic hypersensitivity pneumonitis (see Chapter 12) from collagen vascular disease–associated fibrosing interstitial pneumonias[23] and from UIP (see Chapter 6).

Imaging

The chest CT may be normal or show areas of decreased attenuation and vascularity, resulting in a mosaic pattern of attenuation on inspiratory images and air-trapping on expiratory images.[22]

Pathologic Features

Morphologically, peribronchiolar metaplasia consists of the development of ciliated bronchiolar epithelium, along with variable, but usually mild, underlying interstitial fibrosis in the alveolar walls immediately surrounding membranous and, particularly, respiratory bronchioles (Figs. 23.16 to 23.18). In some cases, small bronchiolar lumen-like structures are formed (Fig. 23.17), and occasionally there is extension of bronchiolar smooth muscle for a distance away from the bronchiole. Peribronchiolar metaplasia is occasionally found in otherwise normal lung tissue (Fig. 23.16), but is much more common in fibrosing interstitial pneumonias, particularly chronic hypersensitivity pneumonitis (see Figs. 12.35 and 12.36).

Differential Diagnosis

Considerably exaggerated forms of peribronchiolar fibrosis/metaplasia are found in the entity labeled "idiopathic bronchiolocentric interstitial fibrosis,"[24] a lesion that is probably a variant of chronic hypersensitivity pneumonitis (see Figs. 12.39 and 12.40), and in "airway-centered interstitial fibrosis,"[25] which is described elsewhere in this chapter. In both these conditions, the fibrosing process often has overlying bronchiolar metaplasia, but the fibrosis is much more diffuse than in simple peribronchiolar metaplasia/fibrosis, frequently affecting every bronchiole and sometimes linking bronchioles, or extending all the way to the pleura.

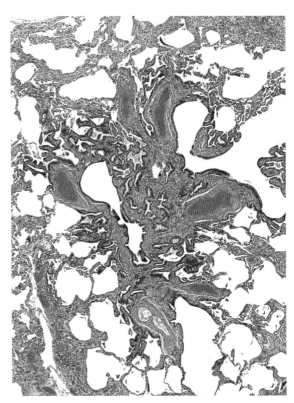

FIGURE 23.17. Peribronchiolar metaplasia in a lung with underlying fibrotic. NSIP There is fibrosis surrounding the bronchiole and forming small channels lined by metaplastic bronchiolar epithelium.

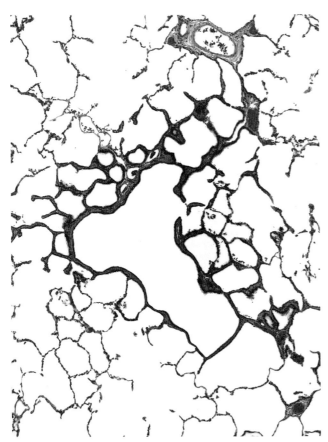

FIGURE 23.16. Peribronchiolar metaplasia. In this example, peribronchiolar metaplasia has developed in otherwise normal lung. The image shows the characteristic fine interstitial fibrosis surrounding a respiratory bronchiole.

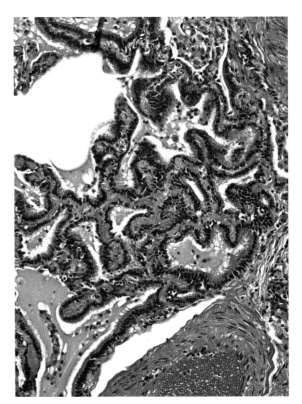

FIGURE 23.18. High-power view of another case showing peribronchiolar metaplasia with metaplastic bronchiolar epithelium covering the fibrotic alveolar walls. For additional illustrations of peribronchiolar metaplasia, see Figures 12.35 and 12.36.

Prognosis

By itself peribronchiolar metaplasia/fibrosis is usually an incidental finding that does not produce any clear-cut abnormality; in particular, despite the occasional appearance of narrow bronchiolar-like structures (Fig. 23.17), it does not produce the fixed airflow obstruction seen in constrictive bronchiolitis (see Chapter 20).

AIRWAY-CENTERED INTERSTITIAL FIBROSIS

Clinical Features

Churg et al.[25] described 12 patients with progressive shortness of breath and a widespread pattern somewhat resembling marked peribronchiolar metaplasia/fibrosis on biopsy. These patients all came from Mexico City, and they had a variety of exposures that suggested hypersensitivity pneumonitis, but none had supporting serologic evidence and only four had an increase in lavage lymphocytes. Most had a restrictive pulmonary impairment. A few subsequent cases have been described in the literature in patients with clear evidence of bird-induced hypersensitivity pneumonitis.[26,27] It is also possible that some cases represent chronic microaspiration.

The CT findings have been described in a small number of patients. The main abnormalities consist of peribronchovascular interstitial thickening, traction bronchiectasis, thickened airway walls, and surrounding fibrosis (Fig. 23.19).[25] Fibrosis may result in central peribronchial conglomerate masses.

Pathologic Features

Pathologically, airway-centered interstitial fibrosis shows a variable pattern of fibrosis that appears to start in/around membranous and respiratory bronchioles and spreads in the interstitium, often linking bronchioles or extending from the bronchioles to the pleura. The fibrosis may be fairly fine with associated overlying bronchiolar metaplasia (Fig. 23.20) and sometimes resembles an exaggerated form of peribronchiolar metaplasia or idiopathic bronchiolocentric fibrosis[24] or can form larger more diffuse blocks (Fig. 23.21).

Prognosis

In the series of Churg et al.,[25] four patients died, one progressed, and five others remained stable or improved with steroid therapy.

PLEUROPARENCHYMAL FIBROELASTOSIS

Clinical Features

Pleuroparenchymal fibroelastosis (PPFE) is an uncommon type of fibrosing interstitial pneumonia characterized by extensive elastotic pleural/subpleural scars, typically in the lung apex. Although the earliest descriptions presented PPFE as an idiopathic disease, subsequent studies

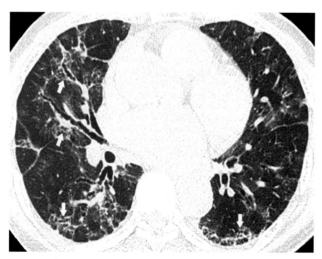

FIGURE 23.19. Airway-centered interstitial fibrosis. HRCT image shows extensive peribronchovascular fibrosis with associated traction bronchiectasis (*arrows*). These findings are easier to see on the right side in the illustrated image because several airways are cut along their long axes. At other levels similar findings could be seen on the left. Also noted are thickened airway walls, patchy ground-glass opacities, and small foci of peripheral reticulation.

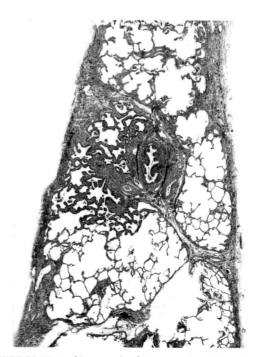

FIGURE 23.20. In this example of airway-centered interstitial fibrosis, there is fine fibrosis slightly widening the alveolar walls and extending from the bronchiole to the pleura. This pattern is similar to that seen in idiopathic bronchiolocentric interstitial fibrosis (see Chapter 12). (Reproduced with permission from Churg A, Myers J, Suarez T, et al. Airway-centered interstitial fibrosis: a distinct form of aggressive diffuse lung disease. *Am J Surg Pathol.* 2004;28:62–68.)

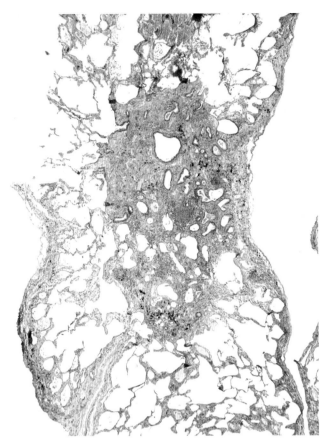

FIGURE 23.21. An example of airway-centered interstitial fibrosis in which the fibrosis forms more of a mass-like lesion around the respiratory bronchiole. Again note extension to the pleura. (Reproduced with permission from Churg A, Myers J, Suarez T, et al. Airway-centered interstitial fibrosis: a distinct form of aggressive diffuse lung disease. *Am J Surg Pathol.* 2004;28:62–68.)

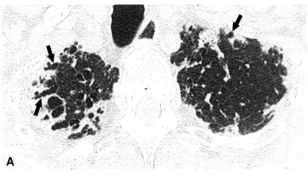
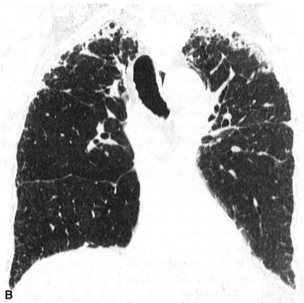

FIGURE 23.22. Pleuroparenchymal fibroelastosis. **A:** HRCT image at the lung apices demonstrates irregular bilateral pleural thickening, dense subpleural reticulation, and traction bronchiectasis (*arrows*). **B:** Coronal reformation demonstrates typical bilateral apical pleural thickening and subpleural upper lobe reticulation.

have shown a variety of associations, including bone marrow transplantation, lung transplantation, infections (aspergillus, atypical mycobacteria), autoimmune disease (rheumatoid arthritis, ankylosing spondylitis), ulcerative colitis, hypersensitivity pneumonitis, and drug reactions.[28–33] Some cases have been described in family members.[33,34] Further, a variable proportion of PPFE cases have an associated different type of ILD, most commonly UIP or hypersensitivity pneumonitis, in anywhere from 25% to 80% of cases.[28–33] Although PPFE was included as a specific form of ILD in the 2013 idiopathic interstitial pneumonia classification,[35] it appears much more likely that PPFE is a reaction pattern than one specific entity.

Imaging

The radiologic findings consist of marked apical pleural thickening associated with upper lobe subpleural reticulation, traction bronchiectasis, and volume loss with elevation of the hila.[34,36] Lower lobe fibrosis is either absent or less extensive than the upper lobe involvement (Figs. 23.22A and B).

Pathologic Features

PPFE shows fibrosis and usually marked widening of the pleura in the upper lung zones with underlying intra-alveolar fibrosis and prominent deposition of elastic tissue; the process microscopically resembles an apical cap, but is much more extensive, frequently surrounding the apical portion of the lung (Figs. 23.23 to 23.25). Vessels and airways are obliterated as well. Often the fibroelastotic process is sharply demarcated from relatively normal parenchyma (Fig. 23.24). Some, but not all, authors describe fibroblast foci at the edge of the elastotic zone.[28] Occasionally PPFE extends into the lower zones. In lung transplant recipients, PPFE is the predominant finding in the restrictive allograft syndrome,[31] and in those cases, there is extensive alveolar fibrin deposition that appears to organize into typical PPFE lesions. Granulomas were found in one-third of cases in the largest reported series (43 patients).[28]

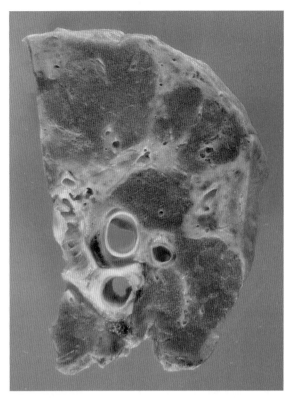

FIGURE 23.23. Gross photograph of a case of pleuroparenchymal fibroelastosis. There is a rim of fibroelastotic tissue that thickens the pleura and in places extends into the lung parenchyma. (Case Courtesy Dr. John English.)

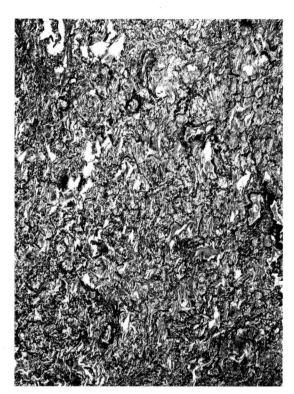

FIGURE 23.25. Elastic stain of another case of pleuroparenchymal fibroelastosis. Note the extensive elastin deposition, a pattern that is not seen in most forms of interstitial fibrosis. However, similar elastin deposition is common in radiation-induced fibrosis and in apical caps.

When present, the associated interstitial pneumonias look like UIP, subacute hypersensitivity pneumonitis, and, in the restrictive allograft syndrome cases, sometimes NSIP.[31]

Prognosis

Most reported patients have developed progressive fibrotic disease; in the series of 43 cases reported by Khiroya et al.,[28] mean survival was 30 months following biopsy.

DIFFUSE SEPTAL AMYLOIDOSIS

Clinical Features

Amyloid is a name for a variety of normally soluble proteins that, when produced in excessive amounts, tend to fold into insoluble β-pleated sheets that deposit in various organs. The most common forms of amyloidosis are listed in Table 23.2, along with specific precursor proteins and the International Society of Amyloidosis–recommended terminology.[37] Some notion of the type of amyloid, information that is important to treatment, can be obtained from immunohistochemistry for kappa and lambda chains, serum amyloid A protein, or transthyretin, but these stains can be hard to read because of protein in the serum, and analysis of paraffin-embedded material by some form of liquid chromatography/mass spectroscopy is often more accurate.[37]

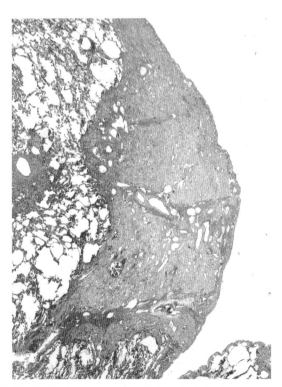

FIGURE 23.24. Pleuroparenchymal fibroelastosis. Low-power view shows a sharply demarcated mass of fibroelastic tissue thickening the pleura and extending into the underlying lung.

Table 23.2

Common forms of amyloidosis

Traditional name	International Society of Amyloidosis name	Amyloid precursor protein	Associated conditions
Primary amyloidosis	Systemic AL amyloidosis	Monoclonal immunoglobulin light chains	Plasma cell dyscrasias (MGUS, myeloma, Waldenstrom macroglobulinemia)
Secondary amyloidosis	Systemic AA amyloidosis	Apo serum amyloid A	Chronic inflammatory diseases including rheumatoid arthritis, juvenile arthritis, inflammatory bowel disease, ankylosing spondylitis, chronic infections
Senile amyloidosis	Systemic wild-type ATTR amyloidosis	Wild-type transthyretin (prealbumin)	Age
Familial amyloidosis	Systemic hereditary ATTR amyloidosis	Mutated transthyretin	Mutations in transthyretin gene
Nodular amyloid	Localized AL amyloidosis	Immunoglobulin light chain and sometimes heavy chain	MALT lymphomas, plasma cell dyscrasias, lymphocytic interstitial pneumonia

Amyloid deposition in the lung takes various morphologically different forms. In patients with nodular amyloidosis, one or more nodules are found on imaging, sometimes incidentally, and sometimes because of nonspecific pulmonary complaints such as cough, shortness of breath, or chest pain. Such patients may have associated Sjögren syndrome with or without lymphocytic interstitial pneumonia, marginal zone lymphomas, or plasmacytomas/myelomas. In nodular pulmonary amyloidosis, the amyloid light (AL) chain is usually κ rather than λ, and there is frequent codeposition of amyloid heavy chain, something that is very rare in systemic amyloidosis.[38]

In tracheobronchial amyloidosis, there may be sufficient airway narrowing to cause dyspnea, wheezing, stridor, and even spontaneous pneumothorax. The amyloid is typically AL.

Diffuse septal amyloidosis is usually a manifestation of systemic AL (λ), AA, wild-type ATTR, or mutated ATTR amyloidosis. Some patients with diffuse septal amyloidosis have cough and shortness of breath as well as a restrictive impairment, but most do not.[39] Heavy vascular deposition of amyloid may lead to pulmonary hypertension.[40] Amyloid deposits in the lung can be associated with pulmonary hemorrhage.[41]

Imaging

The most common HRCT manifestations of diffuse septal amyloidosis consist of well-defined 2 to 4 mm nodules, interlobular septal thickening, and reticular opacities in a predominantly basal and peripheral distribution.[42] Areas of consolidation and ground-glass opacities may also be present.

Pathologic Features

In diffuse septal amyloidosis, there are fine deposits of amorphous eosinophilic amyloid that slightly widen the alveolar walls, producing what at first glance can be mistaken for fine interstitial fibrosis (Figs. 23.26 to 23.28). Typically, there is no inflammatory infiltrate and the diagnosis is made on Congo red stains (Fig. 23.28). In some patients, disease that is diffuse on biopsy may nonetheless be radiologically localized.[36,39]

Small amounts of interstitial amyloid can be seen in the interstitium as well as in the vessels in senile amyloidosis (Fig. 23.29), but these interstitial deposits do not appear to produce clinically detectable abnormalities.[36]

Prognosis

Most patients with diffuse septal amyloidosis do not develop clinically significant respiratory disease; rather, the amount of septal amyloid often correlates with the amount of cardiac amyloid, and these patients may have marked cardiac impairment.[39] However, some patients die of respiratory failure.[39] If the amyloid is AL, the patient may require treatment of an underlying plasma cell dyscrasia.

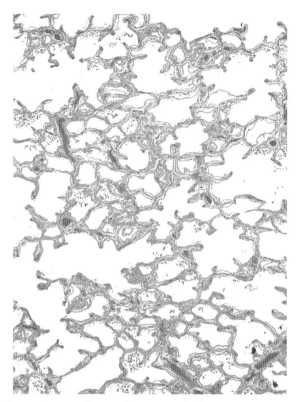

FIGURE 23.26. Diffuse pulmonary amyloidosis. Low-power view shows slightly widened alveolar walls mimicking fibrotic NSIP. Specific amyloid protein information is not available for this figure or Figures 23.27 to 23.29.

FIGURE 23.28. The same case viewed under polarized light after staining with Congo red. Note the diagnostic apple-green birefringence.

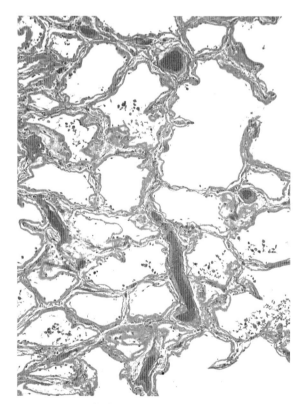

FIGURE 23.27. At higher power, deposition of amyloid is evident along the alveolar walls.

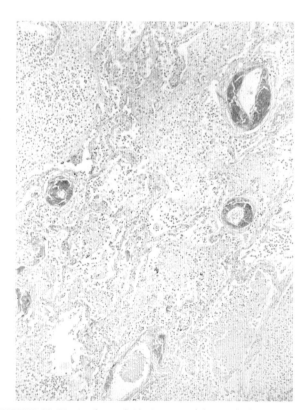

FIGURE 23.29. Senile amyloidosis. Most of the amyloid is in the vessels with little in the interstitium. This is a common finding at autopsy in the elderly and may be associated with cardiac amyloid; however, the pulmonary amyloid appears to be innocuous (Congo Red stain).

LIGHT CHAIN DEPOSITION DISEASE

In light chain deposition disease, nonamyloid immunoglobulin light chains accumulate in tissue. Light chain deposition disease is most commonly seen in Sjögren syndrome, in association with MALT lymphomas, and in patients with myeloma.[43] Light chain deposition disease can be systemic or limited to single organs. In pulmonary light chain deposition disease, amorphous material with the hematoxylin and eosin (H&E) appearance of amyloid is deposited, either in a diffuse septal pattern or as nodules.[44] However, the amorphous material does not stain with Congo red and on electron microscopy the material is granular, as opposed to the fibrillar appearance of amyloid. Mass spectroscopy techniques are useful for identifying the specific protein.[37,43]

EHLERS–DANLOS SYNDROME

Clinical Features

Vascular Ehlers–Danlos syndrome, also known as type IV Ehlers–Danlos syndrome, is an autosomal dominant condition caused by a mutation in the gene for the α chain of type III collagen. The mutation leads to collagen with low tensile strength and a tendency toward vascular rupture and organ laceration.

Imaging

The most common and life-threatening intrathoracic manifestations evident on CT are aortic aneurysm and dissection and pulmonary artery aneurysm.[45] Pulmonary manifestations are seldom seen on CT and consist mainly of bulla formation and pneumothorax.[46]

Pathologic Features

In the lung, repeated hemorrhage leads to hemosiderin deposition, OP, and parenchymal fibrous nodules that appear to represent organization of OP (Figs. 23.30 and 23.31), along with evidence of vascular disruption on elastic stains.[47] The fibrous nodules frequently ossify. Except for the evidence of hemorrhage, the morphologic picture is identical to that seen in many cases of cicatricial OP[48] (see Figs. 5.39 and 5.40).

LYSOSOMAL STORAGE DISORDERS CAUSING ILD

Gaucher disease is an autosomal recessive disorder characterized by lysosomal storage of glucosylceramide, a product of cell breakdown, because of a deficiency of glucocerebrosidase. Most patients have functional evidence of airflow obstruction, but some are restricted.[49] Microscopically, Gaucher cells with so-called "wrinkled tissue paper" cytoplasm not only infiltrate the lung either in a lymphangitic or

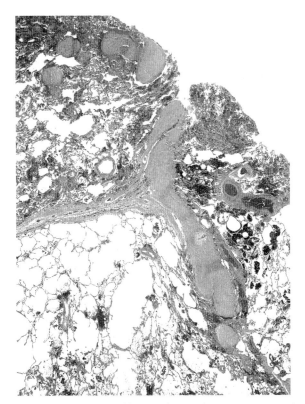

FIGURE 23.30. Vascular Ehlers–Danlos syndrome. Low-power view showing the characteristic irregular masses of fibrous tissue; these appear to represent a form of cicatricial OP (see Chapter 5), perhaps as a reaction to chronic hemorrhage.

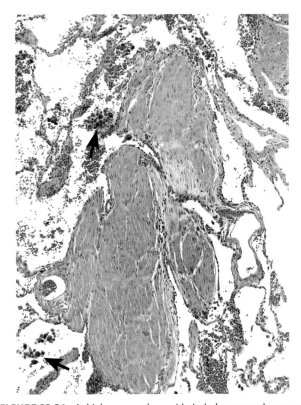

FIGURE 23.31. At higher power, hemosiderin-laden macrophages can just be discerned (*arrows*). Fibrotic masses are otherwise identical to those seen in cicatricial OP (see Chapter 5).

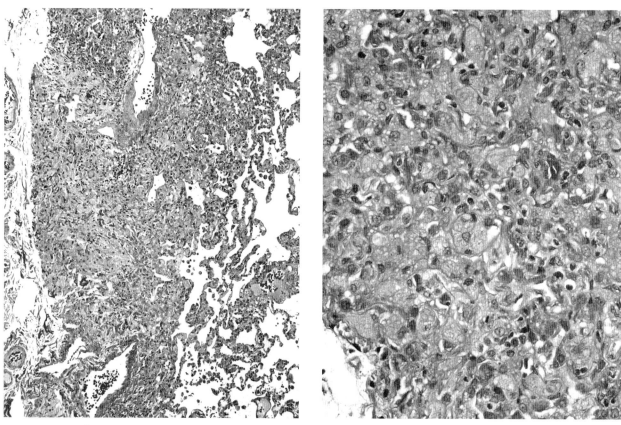

23.32

23.33

FIGURES 23.32 and 23.33. Gaucher disease. Lower power view shows expansion of the alveolar walls by an infiltrate of pale-staining histiocytes with a wrinkled appearance (Gaucher cells). These are seen better in the high-power view.

a diffuse alveolar wall pattern (Figs. 23.32 and 23.33), but can also accumulate in the alveoli and in the capillaries.[50]

Niemann–Pick disease is an autosomal recessive disorder caused by a lack of sphingomyelinase, leading to accumulation of sphingomyelin. Pulmonary accumulation of abnormal foamy histiocytes (Pick cells) is common and the patterns are similar to those seen in Gaucher disease.[51]

Hermansky–Pudlak syndrome is an autosomal recessive condition characterized by the accumulation of ceroid-filled histiocytes, oculocutaneous albinism, platelet defects, and ILD variably described as similar to UIP or to fibrotic NSIP.[52]

DIFFUSE PARENCHYMAL CALCIFICATION AND OSSIFICATION

Clinical Features

Metastatic calcification can be seen not only in the lungs in patients with abnormal calcium or phosphorus metabolism, most commonly associated with renal failure and chronic dialysis, but also in sarcoid, systemic sclerosis, following liver transplantation, hyperparathyroidism, and hypervitaminosis A and D, and in patients with tumors involving bone. In most patients with diffuse calcium deposition in the lung, calcium deposition is seen in other

organs as well. In general, patients with diffuse calcification do not have pulmonary symptoms.

Diffuse pulmonary ossification is referred to as dendriform, racemose, or branching ossification. It most commonly is seen in patients with an underlying fibrosing interstitial pneumonia. Localized or nodular ossification is usually found in patients with elevated pulmonary venous pressure, typically secondary to mitral stenosis. Ossification is also common in the densely fibrotic scars of cicatricial OP[48] (see Fig. 5.39). Neither dendriform nor nodular ossification is symptomatic.

Imaging

The HRCT manifestations of metastatic calcification usually consist of fluffy poorly defined nodular opacities measuring 3 to 10 mm in diameter in a predominantly upper lobe distribution.[53] Foci of calcification within the nodular opacities are evident on CT in only approximately 50% of cases but can be confirmed on scintigraphy using bone-imaging agents when there is high clinical suspicion and the calcification is not apparent on CT.

Fine linear or small nodular foci of calcification representing dendriform pulmonary ossification (Fig. 23.34) are seen on HRCT in up to 28% of patients with idiopathic pulmonary fibrosis and up to 8% of patients with other fibrosing

ILDs.[54] They tend to be evident in the areas with most severe fibrosis, typically in the subpleural regions of the lower lobes.

Pathologic Features

Metastatic calcification appears most often as lines of hematoxyphilic material that follow the alveolar walls (Fig. 23.35) and vessel walls. The material stains with von

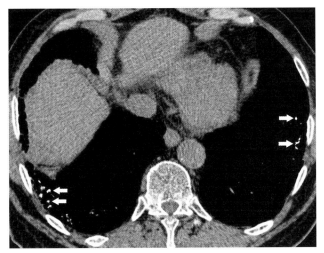

FIGURE 23.34. Pulmonary ossification. HRCT shows bilateral small nodular and linear foci of calcification (*arrows*) in the peripheral regions of the lower lobes. The patient had interstitial pulmonary ossification associated with idiopathic pulmonary fibrosis..

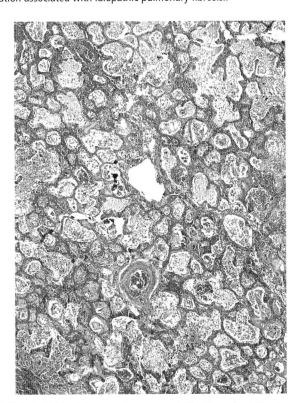

FIGURE 23.35. Diffuse pulmonary calcification. On H&E, hematoxy-philic material outlines the alveolar walls.

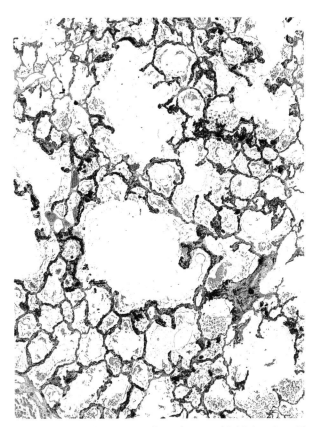

FIGURE 23.36. Calcium stain of another case highlights the widespread calcium deposition.

Kossa and other calcium stains (Fig. 23.36). Sometimes the calcium deposits expand the alveolar walls and are associated with a giant cell reaction. In other instances, the calcium appears to evoke intra-alveolar fibrosis.

Dendriform ossification appears as branching mature bone in the airspaces or in foci of interstitial fibrosis or in foci of interstitial fibrosis (Fig. 23.37).[55] In nodular ossification, the bone forms spherical nodules in the airspaces. Ossification may also be seen in the bronchial cartilages as an aging change.

DIFFUSE PULMONARY LYMPHANGIECTASIS AND DIFFUSE PULMONARY LYMPHANGIOMATOSIS

Clinical Features

Diffuse pulmonary lymphangiectasis and diffuse pulmonary lymphangiomatosis are usually seen in newborn and pediatric patients, and adult cases are extremely rare. Boland et al.[56] were able to find only 13 cases in the literature and presented 3 of their own. Lymphangiectasis is typically associated with lymphatic obstruction, usually from cardiac disease, but can be a congenital abnormality as well, whereas lymphangiomatosis is characterized by proliferating lymphatic channels and may be a neoplastic

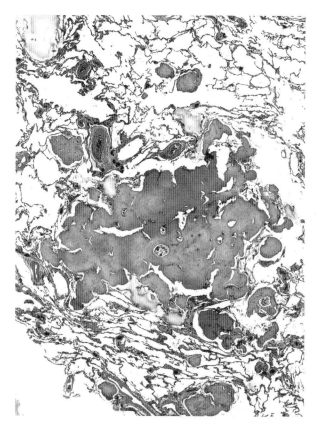

FIGURE 23.37. Dendriform ossification showing the typical pattern of irregular, somewhat branched, masses of osteoid filling airspaces.

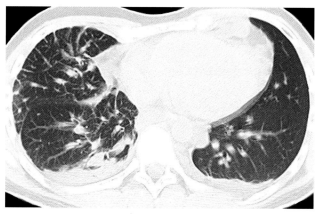

FIGURE 23.38. Diffuse pulmonary lymphangiectasis. CT image shows extensive interlobular septal thickening in the right lung, mild abnormalities in the left lung, and small bilateral pleural effusions.

a pattern that mimics Kaposi sarcoma. Lesions occur in the pleura and interlobular septa and to a lesser extent around the bronchovascular bundles. In both conditions, staining of the endothelial lining for D2-40 (podoplanin) will confirm the lymphatic nature of the vascular channels (Fig. 23.40).

process. In both conditions, lesions can be confined to the lung or can be systemic. Lymphangiectasis in adults may be associated with abnormal pulmonary function, chylous effusions, and respiratory failure.[57]

Imaging

The CT manifestations of diffuse pulmonary lymphangiectasis and lymphangiomatosis are similar, consisting of extensive interlobular septal thickening with or without associated pleural effusions (Fig. 23.38).[58]

Pathologic Feature

The pathologic separation of these entities is not entirely clear in the literature and there probably is considerable morphologic overlap. Boland et al.[56] propose that diffuse pulmonary lymphangiectasis is characterized by dilated lymphatics that follow a lymphangitic distribution (pleura, interlobular septa, bronchovascular bundles). The lymphatics typically develop fibrotic walls, which may become muscularized and can resemble pulmonary veins (Figs. 23.39 and 23.40). In lymphangiomatosis, the lymphatic channels are notionally small and anastomosing and may have areas with proliferating spindle cells in

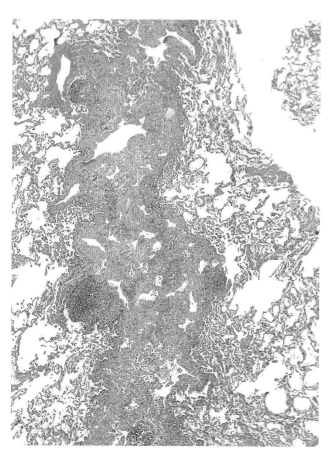

FIGURE 23.39. Diffuse pulmonary lymphangiectasis. Dilated and thick-wall lymphatic channels follow an interlobular septum.

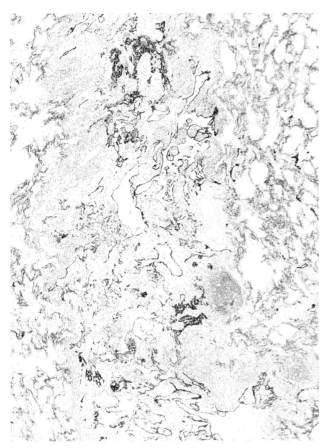

FIGURE 23.40. D2-40 stain of a section adjacent to Figure 23.39 shows that the channels have a lymphatic endothelial lining.

REFERENCES

1. Abratt RP, Morgan GW, Silvestri G, et al. Pulmonary complications of radiation therapy. *Clin Chest Med.* 2004;25:167–177.
2. Graves PR, Siddiqui F, Anscher MS, et al. Radiation pulmonary toxicity: from mechanisms to management. *Semin Radiat Oncol.* 2010;20:201–207.
3. Roden AC, Camus P. Iatrogenic pulmonary lesions. *Semin Diagn Pathol.* 2018;35:260–271.
4. Jain V, Berman AT. Radiation pneumonitis: old problem, new tricks. *Cancers (Basel).* 2018;10:E222.
5. Akita K, Ikawa A, Shimizu S, et al. Cryptogenic organizing pneumonia after radiotherapy for breast cancer. *Breast Cancer.* 2005;12:243–247.
6. Choi YW, Munden RF, Erasmus JJ, et al. Effects of radiation therapy on the lung: radiologic appearances and differential diagnosis. *Radiographics.* 2004;24:985–997.
7. Larici AR, del Ciello A, Maggi F, et al. Lung abnormalities at multimodality imaging after radiation therapy for non-small cell lung cancer. *Radiographics.* 2011;31:771–789.
8. Ghaye B, Wanet M, El Hajjam M. Imaging after radiation therapy of thoracic tumors. *Diagn Interv Imaging.* 2016;97:1037–1052.
9. Crestani B, Valeyre D, Roden S, et al. Bronchiolitis obliterans organizing pneumonia syndrome primed by radiation therapy to the breast. *Am J Respir Crit Care Med.* 1998;158:1929–1935.
10. Takigawa N, Segawa Y, Saeki T, et al. Bronchiolitis obliterans organizing pneumonia syndrome in breast conserving therapy for early breast cancer: radiation-induced lung toxicity. *Int J Radiat Oncol Biol Phys.* 2000;48:751–755.
11. Hodgson DC, Gilbert ES, Dores GM, et al. Long-term solid cancer risk among 5-year survivors of Hodgkin's lymphoma. *J Clin Oncol.* 2007;25:1489–1497.
12. Madani I, De Ruyck K, Goeminne H, et al. Predicting risk of radiation-induced lung injury. *J Thorac Oncol.* 2007;2:864–874.
13. Onishi H, Kuriyama K, Yamaguchi M, et al. Concurrent two-dimensional radiotherapy and weekly docetaxel in the treatment of stage III non-small cell lung cancer: a good local response but no good survival due to radiation pneumonitis. *Lung Cancer.* 2003;40:79–84.
14. Ozkaya N, Rosenblum MK, Durham BH, et al. The histopathology of Erdheim-Chester disease: a comprehensive review of a molecularly characterized cohort. *Mod Pathol.* 2018;31:581–597.
15. Haroche J, Arnaud L, Amoura Z. Erdheim-Chester disease. *Curr Opin Rheumatol.* 2012;24:5.
16. Brun AL, Touitou-Gottenberg D, Haroche J, et al. Erdheim–Chester disease: CT findings of thoracic involvement. *Eur Radiol.* 2010;20:2579–2587.
17. Gianfreda D, Nicastro M, Galetti M, et al. Sirolimus plus prednisone for Erdheim-Chester disease: an open-label trial. *Blood.* 2015;126:1163–1171.
18. Ahuja J, Kanne JP, Meyer CA, et al. Histiocytic disorders of the chest: imaging findings. *Radiographics.* 2015;35:357–370.
19. Veyssier-Belot C, Cacoub P, Caparros-Lefebvre D, et al. Erdheim-Chester disease. Clinical and radiologic characteristics of 59 cases. *Medicine (Baltimore).* 1996;75:157–169.
20. Diamond EL, Subbiah V, Lockhart AC, et al. Vemurafenib for BRAF V600-Mutant Erdheim-Chester disease and Langerhans cell histiocytosis: analysis of data from the histology-independent, phase 2, open-label VE-BASKET Study. *JAMA Oncol.* 2018;4:384–388.
21. Azadeh N, Tazelaar HD, Gotway MB, et al. Erdheim Chester disease treated successfully with cladribine. *Respir Med Case Rep.* 2016;18:37–40.
22. Fukuoka J, Franks TJ, Colby TV, et al. Peribronchiolar metaplasia: a common histologic lesion in diffuse lung disease and a rare cause of interstitial lung disease: clinicopathologic features of 15 cases. *Am J Surg Pathol.* 2005;29:948–954.
23. Churg A, Wright JL, Ryerson CJ. Pathologic separation of chronic hypersensitivity pneumonitis from fibrotic connective tissue disease-associated interstitial lung disease. *Am J Surg Pathol.* 2017;41:1403–1409.
24. Yousem SA, Dacic S. Idiopathic bronchiolocentric interstitial pneumonia. *Mod Pathol.* 2002;15:1148–1153.
25. Churg A, Myers J, Suarez T, et al. Airway-centered interstitial fibrosis: a distinct form of aggressive diffuse lung disease. *Am J Surg Pathol.* 2004;28:62–68.
26. Fenton ME, Cockcroft DW, Wright JL, et al. Hypersensitivity pneumonitis as a cause of airway-centered interstitial fibrosis. *Ann Allergy Asthma Immunol.* 2007;99:465–466.
27. Gaxiola M, Buendía-Roldán I, Mejía M, et al. Morphologic diversity of chronic pigeon breeder's disease: clinical features and survival. *Respir Med.* 2011;105:608–614.
28. Khiroya R, Macaluso C, Montero MA, et al. Pleuroparenchymal fibroelastosis: a review of histopathologic features and

the relationship between histologic parameters and survival. *Am J Surg Pathol.* 2017;41:1683–1689.

29. Cheng SK, Chuah KL. Pleuroparenchymal fibroelastosis of the lung: a review. *Arch Pathol Lab Med.* 2016;140:849–853.

30. Nakatani T, Arai T, Kitaichi M, et al. Pleuroparenchymal fibroelastosis from a consecutive database: a rare disease entity? *Eur Respir J.* 2015;45:1183–1186.

31. von der Thüsen JH, Vandermeulen E, Vos R, et al. The histomorphological spectrum of restrictive chronic lung allograft dysfunction and implications for prognosis. *Mod Pathol.* 2018;31:780–790.

32. von der Thüsen JH, Hansell DM, Tominaga M, et al. Pleuroparenchymal fibroelastosis in patients with pulmonary disease secondary to bone marrow transplantation. *Mod Pathol.* 2011;24:1633–1639.

33. Reddy TL, Tominaga M, Hansell DM, et al. Pleuroparenchymal fibroelastosis: a spectrum of histopathological and imaging phenotypes. *Eur Respir J.* 2012;40:377–385.

34. Frankel SK, Cool CD, Lynch DA, et al. Idiopathic pleuroparenchymal fibroelastosis: description of a novel clinicopathologic entity. *Chest.* 2004;126:2007–2013.

35. Travis WD, Costabel U, Hansell DM, et al.; ATS/ERS Committee on Idiopathic Interstitial Pneumonias. An official American Thoracic Society/European Respiratory Society Statement: update of the international multidisciplinary classification of the idiopathic Interstitial pneumonias. *Am J Respir Crit Care Med.* 2013;188:733–748.

36. Sverzellati N, Lynch DA, Hansell DM, et al. American Thoracic Society-European Respiratory Society Classification of the Idiopathic Interstitial Pneumonias: advances in knowledge since 2002. *Radiographics.* 2015;35:1849–1871.

37. Khoor A, Colby TV. Amyloidosis of the lung. *Arch Pathol Lab Med.* 2017;141:247–254.

38. Grogg KL, Aubry MC, Vrana JA, et al. Nodular pulmonary amyloidosis is characterized by localized immunoglobulin deposition and is frequently associated with an indolent B-cell lymphoproliferative disorder. *Am J Surg Pathol.* 2013;37:406–412.

39. Berk JL, O'Regan A, Skinner M. Pulmonary and tracheobronchial amyloidosis. *Semin Respir Crit Care Med.* 2002;23:155–165.

40. Eder L, Zisman D, Wolf R, et al. Pulmonary hypertension and amyloidosis—an uncommon association: a case report and review of the literature. *J Gen Intern Med.* 2007;22:416–419.

41. Shenin M, Xiong W, Naik M, et al. Primary amyloidosis causing diffuse alveolar hemorrhage. *J Clin Rheumatol.* 2010;16:175–177.

42. Czeyda-Pommersheim F, Hwang M, Chen SS, et al. Amyloidosis: modern cross-sectional Imaging. *Radiographics.* 2015;35:1381–1392.

43. Arrossi AV, Merzianu M, Farver C, et al. Nodular pulmonary light chain deposition disease: an entity associated with Sjögren syndrome or marginal zone lymphoma. *J Clin Pathol.* 2016;69:490–496.

44. Bhargava P, Rushin JM, Rusnock EJ, et al. Pulmonary light chain deposition disease: report of five cases and review of the literature. *Am J Surg Pathol.* 2007;31:267–276.

45. Chu LC, Johnson PT, Dietz HC, et al. Vascular complications of Ehlers-Danlos syndrome: CT findings. *AJR Am J Roentgenol.* 2012;198:482–487.

46. Franquet T, Giménez A, Cáceres J, et al. Imaging of pulmonary-cutaneous disorders: matching the radiologic and dermatologic findings. *Radiographics.* 1996;16:855–869.

47. Kawabata Y, Watanabe A, Yamaguchi S, et al. Pleuropulmonary pathology of vascular Ehlers-Danlos syndrome: spontaneous laceration, haematoma and fibrous nodules. *Histopathology.* 2010;56:944–950.

48. Churg A, Wright JL, Bilawich A. Cicatricial organising pneumonia mimicking a fibrosing interstitial pneumonia. *Histopathology.* 2018;72:846–854.

49. Kerem E, Elstein D, Abrahamov A, et al. Pulmonary function abnormalities in type I Gaucher disease. *Eur Respir J.* 1996;9:340–345.

50. Amir G, Ron N. Pulmonary pathology in Gaucher's disease. *Hum Pathol.* 1999;30:666–670.

51. Alymlahi E, Dafiri R. Pulmonary involvement in Niemann-Pick type B disease. *J Postgrad Med.* 2004;50:289–290.

52. Pierson DM, Ionescu D, Qing G, et al. Pulmonary fibrosis in Hermansky-Pudlak syndrome: a case report and review. *Respiration.* 2006;73:382–395.

53. Hartman TE, Müller NL, Primack SL, et al. Metastatic pulmonary calcification in patients with hypercalcemia: findings on chest radiographs and CT scans. *AJR Am J Roentgenol.* 1994;162:799–802.

54. Egashira R, Jacob J, Kokosi MA, et al. Diffuse pulmonary ossification in fibrosing interstitial lung diseases: prevalence and associations. *Radiology.* 2017;284:255–263.

55. Joines RW, Roggli VL. Dendriform pulmonary ossification. Report of two cases with unique findings. *Am J Clin Pathol.* 1989;91:398–402.

56. Boland JM, Tazelaar HD, Colby TV, et al. Diffuse pulmonary lymphatic disease presenting as interstitial lung disease in adulthood: report of 3 cases. *Am J Surg Pathol.* 2012;36:1548–1554.

57. Kadakia KC, Patel SM, Yi ES, et al. Diffuse pulmonary lymphangiomatosis. *Can Respir J.* 2013;20:52–54.

58. Raman SP, Pipavath SN, Raghu G, et al. Imaging of thoracic lymphatic diseases. *AJR Am J Roentgenol.* 2009;193:1504–1513.

Mimics of Interstitial Lung Disease

INTERSTITIAL LUNG DISEASE SECONDARY TO PULMONARY HEMORRHAGE

Clinical Features

Pulmonary hemorrhage can produce reactions that mimic interstitial lung disease (ILD). Significant pulmonary hemorrhage is seen in a variety of clinical settings, of which the most common are mechanical causes such as tumors, cavities, or bronchiectasis that typically produce localized hemorrhage. Diffuse alveolar hemorrhage (i.e., hemorrhage that is widespread in both lungs and does not have a mechanical etiology) has a strong association with underlying vasculitis, but there are numerous other causes (Table 24.1). Many of the entities in Table 24.1 produce capillaritis, but others are associated with bland hemorrhage in which the alveolar wall does not appear abnormal unless interstitial fibrosis develops.

Patients with diffuse hemorrhage commonly present with hemoptysis, but hemoptysis is absent in up to one-third of cases.[1,2] Alveolar hemorrhage can be associated with nonspecific symptoms such as fever, chest pain, cough, and dyspnea. Findings that suggest hemorrhage in the absence of hemoptysis are a falling hematocrit and low serum hemoglobin, and increasing return of red cells on serial lavage or a high percentage of hemosiderin-laden macrophages in lavage, in the presence of compatible high resolution computed tomography (HRCT) findings.[1,2]

Organizing pneumonia (OP) can be seen as a reaction to alveolar hemorrhage, but unless the patient has overt hemoptysis or other findings as described above, the clinical features are similar to OP of other etiologies.

In patients who develop widespread interstitial fibrosis from chronic hemorrhage associated with vasculitis, the process often presents as a fibrotic lung disease clinically, functionally, and radiologically,[2,3] and some of these patients never have overt hemoptysis, making the disease difficult to separate from usual interstitial pneumonia (UIP)/idiopathic pulmonary fibrosis (IPF) or nonspecific interstitial pneumonia (NSIP). Such patients often but not invariably have glomerulonephritis.[2]

Table 24.1

Nonmechanical causes of diffuse alveolar hemorrhage

- Pulmonary vasculitis
- Acute respiratory distress syndrome
- Bone marrow transplantation
- Crack cocaine inhalation
- Drug reactions
- Acute lupus pneumonitis (occasionally seen in other collagen vascular diseases)
- Radiation therapy
- Goodpasture syndrome (antiglomerular basement membrane disease)
- Coagulation disorders
- Chemical inhalation exposures (trimellitic anhydride/isocyanates)
- Cryoglobulinemia
- Henoch–Schonlein purpura
- Behçet syndrome
- Kaposi sarcoma
- Antiphospholipid antibody syndrome
- Left-sided cardiac valvular disease or failure
- Pulmonary veno-occlusive disease
- Bacterial endocarditis
- Myeloma
- Celiac disease (Lane Powell syndrome)
- Idiopathic pulmonary hemosiderosis (IPH)

Long-standing chronic hemorrhage of any cause can lead to interstitial fibrosis, but the most common cause of hemorrhage-associated fibrosis appears to be antineutrophil cytoplasmic antibodies (ANCA)-positive vasculitis. Summarizing the literature to 2017, Alba et al.[3] reported 149 patients with pulmonary fibrosis and ANCA-positive vasculitis. The vast majority had microscopic polyangiitis with MPO ANCA; a small percentage had Wegener granulomatosis (granulomatosis with polyangiitis) and PR3 ANCA. In most patients, pulmonary fibrosis preceded or appeared concomitantly with the diagnosis of vasculitis; the time interval between the diagnosis of pulmonary fibrosis and the appearance of vasculitis ranged from a few months to 12 years. The prognosis of ANCA-associated fibrosis was relatively poor, with reported numbers for 5-year survivals in various series ranging from about 30% to 60%.[3]

Interstitial fibrosis associated with chronic hemorrhage can appear in other settings including idiopathic pulmonary hemosiderosis, pulmonary veno-occlusive disease (VOD), and left-sided heart disease. Patients with VOD always have pulmonary hypertension but usually not hemoptysis. Patients with chronic hemorrhage secondary to cardiac disease may or may not have pulmonary hypertension and sometimes have small hemoptyses, but the cardiac disease usually overshadows the pulmonary disease.

Idiopathic pulmonary hemosiderosis is an uncommon cause of hemorrhage-related interstitial fibrosis that is seen mostly in children; a recent review of the English and Chinese literature from 2000 to 2015 could find only 37 reported cases in adults.[4] By definition, such patients do not have glomerulonephritis, do not have pulmonary vasculitis, and do not have ANCA or positive connective disease serology, and the diagnosis is exclusionary. A few patients have celiac disease (Lane–Hamilton syndrome) and the pulmonary hemorrhage as well as the intestinal disease is reported to respond to gluten restriction.[4–6] In the older literature, which is difficult to interpret because a significant proportion of reported patients probably did have some form of vasculitis, survival was poor, but recent patients have responded to immunosuppressive agents, suggesting that idiopathic pulmonary hemosiderosis in general may be a form of autoimmune disease.

Imaging

The HRCT findings in diffuse pulmonary hemorrhage resemble those of ILD. The computed tomography (CT) manifestations of acute pulmonary hemorrhage consist of ground-glass opacities and, less commonly, areas of consolidation (Fig. 24.1).[7] The ground-glass opacities may be focal, have a patchy distribution, or be diffuse. CT scans performed 2 to 3 days after the acute episode show a decrease in the ground-glass opacities and consolidation and presence of interlobular septal thickening and small poorly defined centrilobular nodules.[8] These findings are presumably secondary to lymphatic resorption of the blood and gradually resolve over the next 1 to 2 weeks. In patients with recurrent pulmonary hemorrhage, ground-glass opacities may be seen superimposed on a background of reticular and small nodular opacities (Fig. 24.2). CT may demonstrate the underlying cause, such as bronchiectasis and carcinoma, in patients with focal pulmonary hemorrhage.

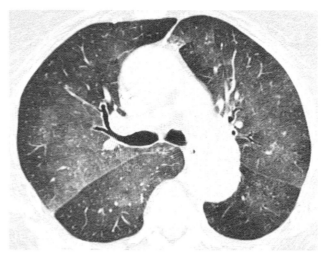

FIGURE 24.1. Diffuse pulmonary hemorrhage. HRCT image shows extensive bilateral ground-glass opacities in a patient with Goodpasture syndrome (antiglomerular basement membrane disease) and diffuse pulmonary hemorrhage.

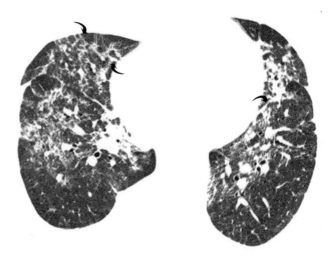

FIGURE 24.2. Recurrent pulmonary hemorrhage. HRCT image demonstrates thickening of the interlobular septa (*arrows*), small nodules, and patchy bilateral ground-glass opacities. The patient was a 45-year-old woman with Wegener granulomatosis (granulomatosis with polyangiitis) and recurrent pulmonary hemorrhage.

Pathologic Patterns of Hemorrhage and ILD-Like Reactions to Hemorrhage

Acute alveolar hemorrhage (i.e., just red cells in alveolar spaces) may be found in any of the conditions described above, but by far the most common cause of acute hemorrhage in a lung biopsy is the surgical procedure itself. Thus, absent hemoptysis or clinical evidence of hemorrhage, caution should be exercised in labeling pure acute hemorrhage as a pathologic reaction.

The presence of hemosiderin-laden macrophages indicates that the hemorrhage is real, but provides no indication of chronicity, because hemosiderin-laden macrophages

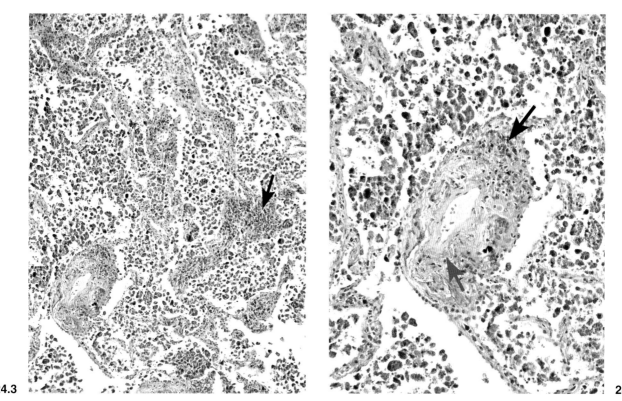

24.3   **24.4**

FIGURES 24.3 and 24.4. Low- and high-power views of chronic alveolar hemorrhage in a patient with microscopic polyangiitis leading to interstitial fibrosis. The fibrosis resembles fibrotic NSIP. Note the interstitial hemosiderin (*black arrows*), an indication that the fibrosis is secondary to hemorrhage. The vessel in **Figure 24.4** also demonstrates pale gray ferruginated elastica (*blue arrow*), another characteristic finding in chronic hemorrhage.

form in a few days and can persist for months or years. Free hemosiderin may also be present. Hemosiderin-laden macrophages need to be separated from smoker's macrophages (see Chapter 8). Both stain with iron, but in smoker's macrophages, the brown/golden pigment is finely granular and dispersed throughout the cytoplasm, producing a blush on iron stain (see Fig. 8.9), whereas hemosiderin typically appears as coarse iron-positive particles (Figs. 24.3 and 24.4).[9]

Hemorrhage can produce three different reaction patterns that mimic ILD (Table 24.1). Diffuse alveolar damage secondary to hemorrhage is morphologically no different from diffuse alveolar damage of other causes (Chapter 4) and is difficult to accurately diagnose without a good clinical/radiologic story, because diffuse alveolar damage itself sometimes causes hemorrhage. However, if diffuse alveolar damage is secondary to hemorrhage, it may be localized to only the areas with hemorrhage.

OP is a frequent reaction to hemorrhage. Because OP is a common reaction pattern after many types of insults (see Chapter 5), it is often difficult to be sure that hemorrhage is the cause of OP in a given case; however, a clue that OP is caused by hemorrhage and not a bystander is the finding of free hemosiderin or hemosiderin-laden macrophages within the granulation tissue plugs (Fig. 24.5).

Low-grade persisting hemorrhage that goes on for months or years can lead to interstitial fibrosis

Table 24.2
Pathologic reactions to hemorrhage

Diffuse alveolar damage
OP
  • Clue: hemosiderin embedded in the granulation tissue
More or less diffuse interstitial fibrosis
  • Usually NSIP-like but some cases resemble UIP
  • Seen with microscopic polyangiitis, VOD, idiopathic hemosiderosis, Wegener granulomatosis (granulomatosis with polyangiitis), and in mild forms with heart failure or mitral valvular disease
  • Clue: hemosiderin embedded in the fibrous tissue
  • Clue: iron/calcium encrustation of vessel elastic fibers

(Figs. 24.3, 24.4, 24.6, and 24.7) (Table 24.2). There are several clues to the diagnosis of hemorrhage-related fibrosis. Most such cases will have hemosiderin, free or in macrophages, in the fibrotic interstitium (Figs. 24.3 and 24.4) and often in the alveolar spaces as well (Figs. 24.3 and 24.4). Cases of fibrosis secondary to hemorrhage usually will also show iron/calcium encrustation of

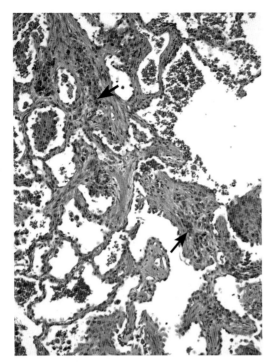

FIGURE 24.5. OP secondary to alveolar hemorrhage. The presence of hemosiderin in the granulation tissue (*arrows*) is an indication that the OP is probably a reaction to hemorrhage.

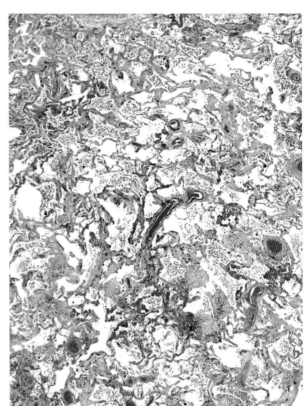

24.6

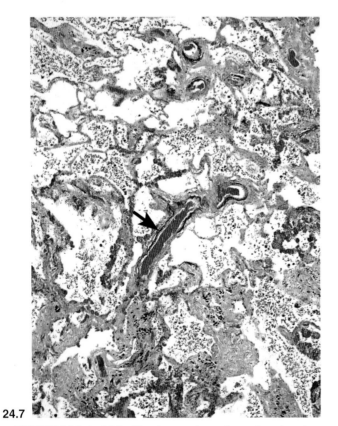

24.7

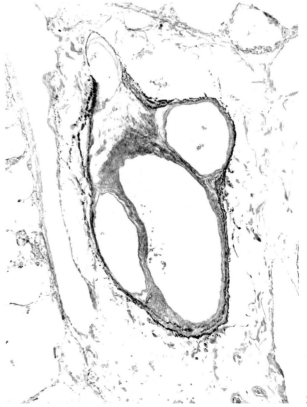

24.8

FIGURES 24.6 to 24.8. Fibrosis secondary to hemorrhage in pulmonary VOD. At low power (**Fig. 24.6**), the process resembles fibrotic NSIP, but this image is taken from a subpleural region; away from the subpleural area there was no fibrosis. The higher power view (**Fig. 24.7**) shows a vessel with ferruginated elastica (*arrow*), a marker of chronic hemorrhage. Elastic stain (**Fig. 24.8**) demonstrates a recanalized thrombus in a vein in an interlobular septum, a diagnostic finding in VOD.

vessel elastic fibers (Figs. 24.4 and 24.7), a process that has been termed "endogenous pneumoconiosis" because the encrusted elastic can resemble asbestos bodies.

In processes such as vasculitis that produce fairly widespread hemorrhage, the pattern of fibrosis typically resembles fibrotic NSIP (Chapter 7) and is present over large areas of the lung (Fig. 24.3). In contrast, in VOD and fibrosis secondary to cardiac disease, the fibrosis is usually localized to the subpleural region. The local pattern again most often resembles fibrotic NSIP (Fig. 24.6) but sometimes resembles UIP. In VOD, evidence of venous thrombosis is always present and is best detected in veins in the interlobular septa (Fig. 24.8); with time, these veins become arterialized (develop a double elastic lamina), thus mimicking pulmonary artery branches. Similar venous changes, minus thromboses, can be found in the veins in patients with heart failure or mitral valvular diseases.

NEOPLASMS PRODUCING ILD-LIKE PATTERNS: KAPOSI SARCOMA, LYMPHOMAS, LEUKEMIAS, AND LYMPHANGITIC CARCINOMA

Clinical Features

Kaposi sarcoma (KS) presents in a variety of forms including classic (elderly men, usually of Eastern European or Mediterranean origin); endemic (non-HIV related) seen in parts of Africa; associated with immunosuppressive states such as organ transplantation; and epidemic, associated with HIV infection.[10] The classic appearance is violaceous skin papules, but the disease can involve any organ. Pulmonary involvement usually is seen in patients who have disease in other sites and is nonspecific with shortness of breath, cough, fevers, night sweats, and chest pain, sometimes but not always accompanied by hemoptysis.[11,12] Tumor can often be seen on bronchoscopy as red or purple macular or papular lesions at airway bifurcations.[12]

Patients with pulmonary involvement by lymphomas can present with asymptomatic tumor masses found on imaging or with nonspecific pulmonary complaints, and sometimes have a restrictive pattern of pulmonary function if tumor has spread widely in the interstitium.

Lymphangitic carcinoma presents with the insidious onset of shortness of breath and often cough caused by submucosal endobronchial lymphatic tumor. Pulmonary function tests show a restrictive impairment with decreased diffusing capacity. Endobronchial involvement may be visible as plaque-like lesions on endoscopy. If tumor gains access to the small pulmonary artery branches, cor pulmonale may develop. The prognosis for widespread lymphangitic carcinoma is poor, with typically 3- to 6-month survivals. Statistically, lung, breast, stomach, pancreas, ovary, and prostate are the most frequent sites of origin.[13]

Imaging

The characteristic HRCT manifestations of KS consist of bilateral irregularly shaped or poorly defined nodules in a peribronchovascular distribution (Fig. 24.9).[14] The nodules are frequently surrounded by a halo of ground-glass attenuation. Other common findings include ground-glass opacities, interlobular septal thickening, peribronchovascular thickening, hilar and mediastinal lymphadenopathy, and unilateral or bilateral pleural effusions.

The CT manifestations of pulmonary lymphoma include multiple small or single or multiple large nodules, mass-like areas of consolidation, thickening of the bronchovascular sheaths and interlobular septa, and ground-glass opacities[15] (see section Lymphomas and Leukemias).

The HRCT manifestations of pulmonary leukemic cell infiltration consist mainly of bilateral thickening of the peribronchovascular sheaths and interlobular septa, a pattern that resembles that of interstitial pulmonary edema.[16] Less common findings include 3- to 10-mm-diameter nodules in a predominantly peribronchovascular distribution, ground-glass opacities, and areas of consolidation. In the vast majority of patients with leukemia, the parenchymal abnormalities seen on CT are due to pulmonary edema, infection, or hemorrhage, rather than leukemic infiltration.

The HRCT manifestations of lymphangitic carcinoma typically consist of thickening of the interlobular septa and bronchovascular bundles with preservation of normal lung architecture (see section Lymphangitic Carcinoma).[17] The thickened interlobular septa are seen in the periphery of the lung as lines extending to the pleural surface and centrally as polygonal arcades. Associated findings may include discrete nodules representing metastases, pleural effusion, and hilar or mediastinal lymph node enlargement.

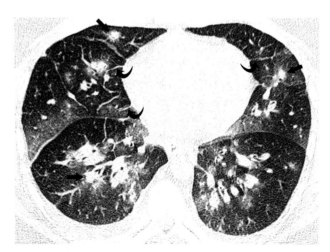

FIGURE 24.9. Kaposi sarcoma (KS). HRCT image demonstrates poorly defined nodules (*straight arrows*), thickening of the interlobular septa (*curved arrows*), peribronchovascular interstitial thickening, and patchy ground-glass opacities. The patient was a 31-year-old man with AIDS and KS.

Pathologic Features

Kaposi Sarcoma

KS (Figs. 24.9 to 24.14) can form nodules that are obviously neoplastic, but the tumor also commonly grows in a lymphangitic pattern along the bronchovascular bundles and interlobular septa, producing a pattern that looks grossly like very fine hemorrhage outlining the bronchial and pulmonary artery walls and interlobular septa (Figs. 24.10 and 24.11), with hemorrhagic discoloration of the bronchial mucosa.

Microscopically, KS can be subtle. At low power, the lymphangitic pattern of tumor often looks like hemorrhage in the walls of thickened airways and pulmonary arteries (Fig. 24.12), but at high power, this picture resolves itself into closely packed, relatively bland, spindled cells (Fig. 24.13), which may contain red cells in abortive lumina or red cells extravasated between the tumor cells. Intracellular hyaline globules are sometimes also found. In some cases, small lakes of hemorrhage form in the midst of the spindled cells, a form that has been called telangiectatic KS, and rarely the tumor has the appearance of a high-grade sarcoma.[18] KS cells are positive for CD31, variably positive for D2-40, and positive for human herpesvirus 8 (HHV8) (Fig. 24.14).

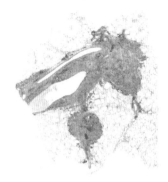

FIGURE 24.11. KS: Tumor spreads in a lymphangitic fashion around a bronchovascular bundle.

Lymphomas and Leukemias

Lymphomas, either primary or secondary, can involve the lung in three patterns: (1) as lymphoid cells in spreading in a lymphangitic pattern around the bronchovascular bundles and in the interlobular septa (Figs. 24.15 to 24.17); (2) as lymphoid cells spreading diffusely through the whole interstitium (Figs. 24.18 and 24.19); and (3) as tumor masses.

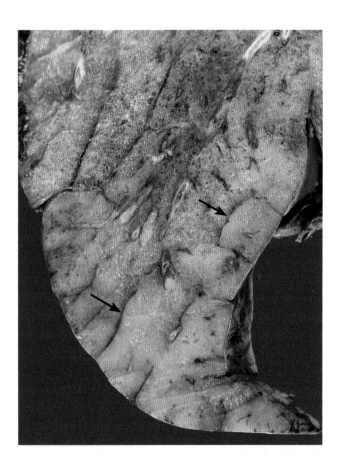

FIGURE 24.10. KS at autopsy. Tumor spreads in a lymphangitic fashion and outlines the interlobular septa (*arrows*) and bronchovascular bundles.

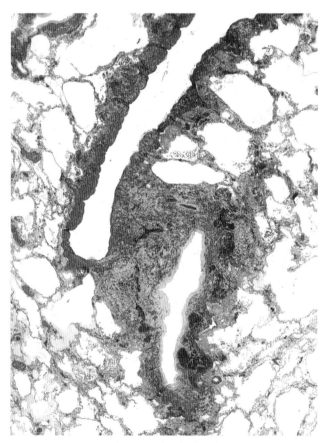

FIGURE 24.12. KS. In this example, the lymphangitic tumor appears at low power as hemorrhage in the walls of the airway and vessel.

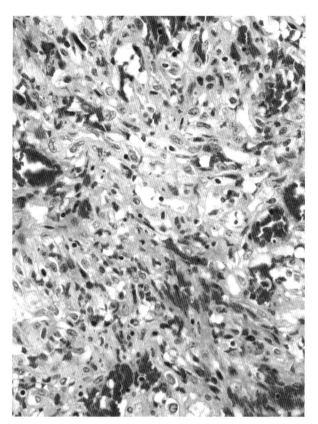

FIGURE 24.13. High power of KS showing spindle cells and extravasated red cells.

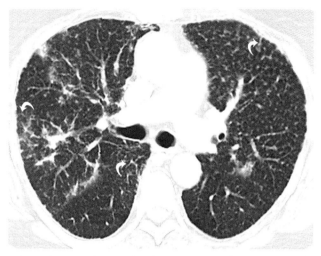

FIGURE 24.15. Pulmonary lymphoma. CT image shows numerous bilateral small nodules, bilateral thickening of the interlobular septa (*arrows*), patchy ground-glass opacities, and small foci of consolidation. The patient was a 64-year-old woman with pulmonary T-cell lymphoma following heart transplant.

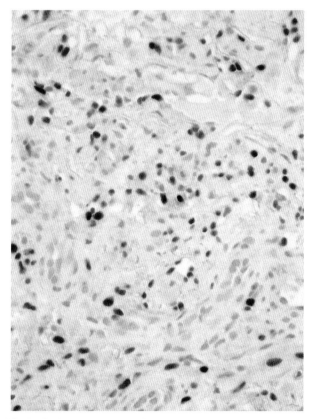

FIGURE 24.14. HHV8 staining in KS.

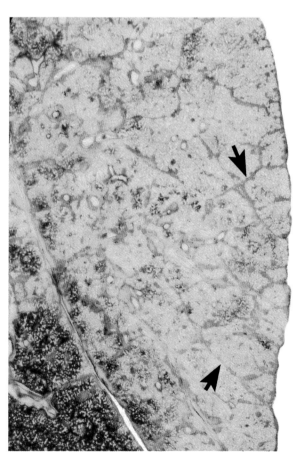

FIGURE 24.16. Gough (1-mm-thick whole lung) section showing lymphoma along the interlobular septa (*arrows*) and bronchovascular bundles, that is, in a lymphangitic distribution.

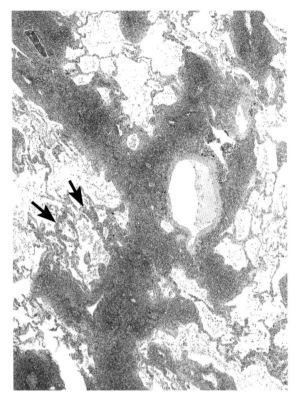

FIGURE 24.17. Lymphoma spreading in a lymphangitic fashion along the bronchovascular bundles and interlobular septa. There is also early spread into the interstitium (*arrows*).

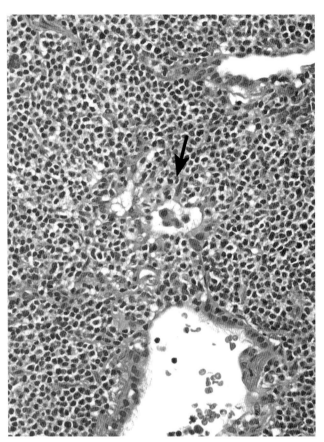

FIGURE 24.19. Another MALT lymphoma showing the monotony of the infiltrating cells and a lymphoepithelial lesion (*arrow*).

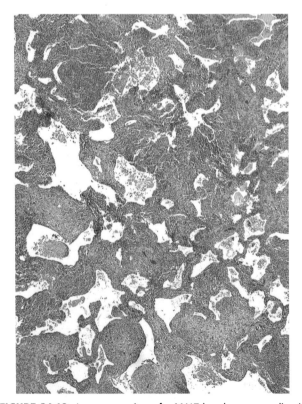

FIGURE 24.18. Low-power view of a MALT lymphoma spreading in the interstitium and widening the alveolar walls. The process mimics LIP (see Chapter 19).

High-grade lymphomas are cytologically obvious and frequently infiltrate vessels, but low-grade lymphomas with a lymphangitic distribution (Fig. 24.17) can mimic follicular bronchiolitis/lymphoid hyperplasia (Chapter 19). For diffuse low-grade lymphomas spreading through the interstitium (Fig. 24.18), the major differential diagnoses are lymphocytic interstitial pneumonia (LIP; Chapter 19), cellular NSIP (Chapter 7), and hypersensitivity pneumonitis (Chapter 11). Extranodal marginal zone (mucosa-associated lymphoid tissue, MALT) lymphomas account for about 80% of primary lung lymphoma and are typically solitary or multiple mass lesions or areas of ground-glass opacity, but spread through the interstitium is seen in a small percentage of cases (Fig. 24.18).[19]

The features of these entities are compared in Chapter 19 (Table 19.4). Most low-grade lymphomas that spread around the bronchovascular bundles or in the interstitium are cytologically monotonous (Fig. 24.19). However, residual germinal centers around bronchovascular bundles can produce a spurious appearance of a polymorphous population, and Hodgkin disease with a lymphangitic pattern can also appear polymorphous.

Lymphomas of all types typically produce a marked expansion of the interstitium, and the combination of interstitial expansion and a monotonous cell population (Figs. 24.18 and 24.19) is the most important clue to the diagnosis; immunohistochemical (Figs. 24.20 to 24.23)

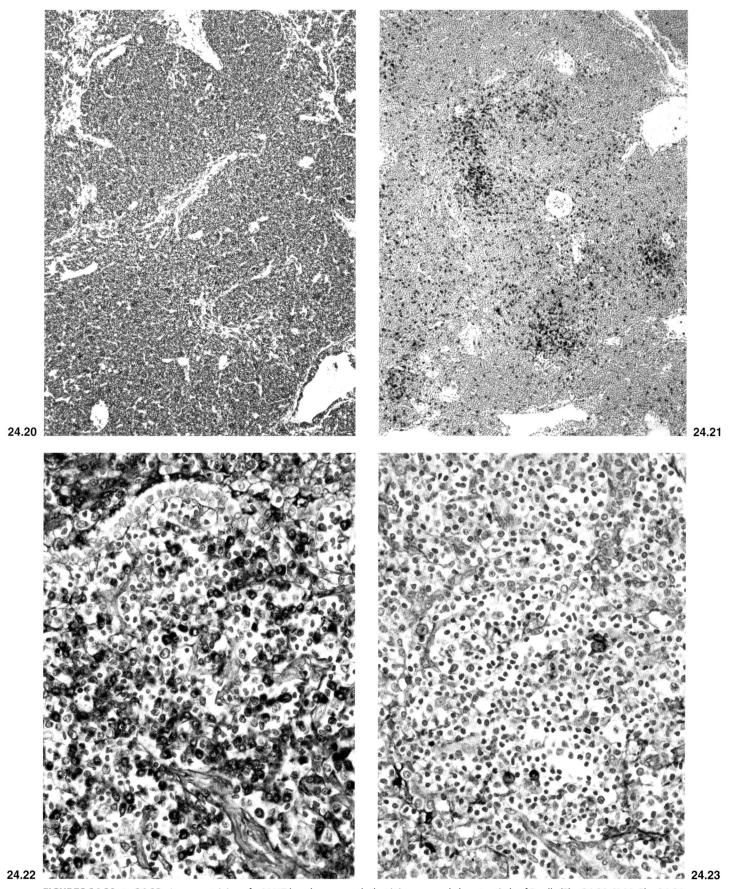

FIGURES 24.20 to 24.23. Immunostaining of a MALT lymphoma reveals that it is composed almost entirely of B cells (**Fig. 24.20** CD20; **Fig. 24.21** CD3). This example is kappa clonal (**Fig. 24.22** kappa; **Fig. 24.23** lambda). Compare the staining pattern of LIP as shown in Figures 19.17 and 19.18.

and/or molecular testing should be used to confirm the diagnosis. Primary pulmonary MALT lymphomas have BIRC3-MALT1 translocations in about 45% of cases, and this is a very specific diagnostic finding.[19,20] The interstitial expansion caused by lymphomas is generally much greater than one sees in cellular NSIP or hypersensitivity pneumonitis, but LIP can also greatly expand the interstitium to the point of loss of alveolar spaces (see Figs. 19.10 to 19.16). In lymphomas, the interstitial infiltrates may coalesce to give rise to true tumor masses. Some types of B-cell lymphomas, especially MALT lymphomas, tend to infiltrate bronchiolar epithelium, forming lymphoepithelial lesions (Fig. 24.19). Small noncaseating granulomas can be found in lymphomas but also in LIP and hypersensitivity pneumonitis.

Leukemias can also spread in the interstitium to produce a pattern of lymphangitic or diffuse interstitial infiltration. These processes are almost always very diffuse and thus mimic cellular NSIP or LIP; however, except for chronic lymphocytic leukemia, the infiltrating cells are usually cytologically atypical. Intravascular lymphoma can be more subtle, with atypical cells in vessels in the interstitium, but without marked interstitial cellularity or widening (Fig. 24.24).

Lymphangitic Carcinoma

Lymphangitic carcinoma (Figs. 24.25 to 24.29) is often grossly visible as fine white lines that outline the interlobular septa (Fig. 24.26) and create visually prominent bronchovascular bundles (Fig. 24.26). The process can

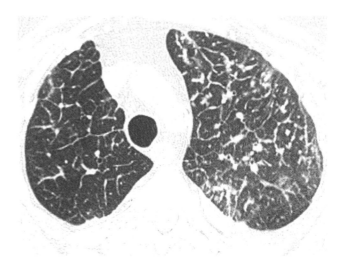

FIGURE 24.25. Lymphangitic carcinoma. HRCT shows extensive bilateral interlobular septal thickening and small pleural effusions in a patient with lymphangitic carcinoma secondary to metastatic carcinoma of the stomach.

be widespread as in Figures 24.26 and 24.27, or quite localized, particularly around primary lung cancers. Microscopically, lymphangitic carcinoma appears as individual or small groups of tumor cells that initially fill the lymphatics, that is, they are present in the visceral pleura, interlobular septa, and around the bronchovascular bundles

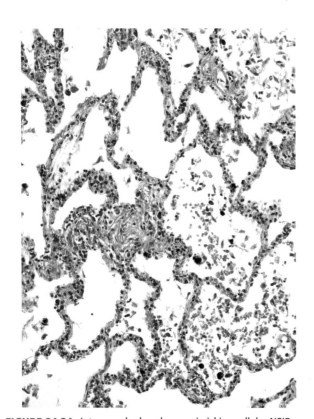

FIGURE 24.24. Intravascular lymphoma mimicking cellular NSIP.

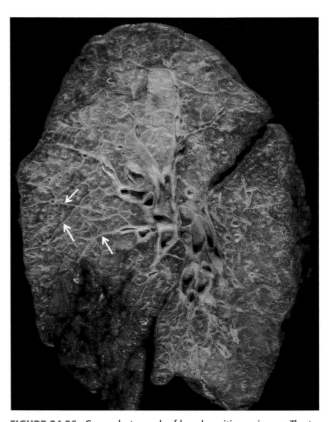

FIGURE 24.26. Gross photograph of lymphangitic carcinoma. The tumor appears as raised thickened interlobular septa (*arrows*) and bronchovascular bundles.

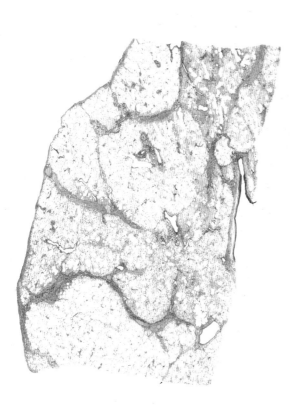

FIGURE 24.27. Lymphangitic carcinoma. Low-power view of the same case as Figure 24.26. Note the prominent, partially fibrotic, interlobular septa.

(Figs. 24.28 and 24.29). Some tumors evoke a fibrotic reaction, particularly in the interlobular septa (Fig. 24.29). With time, tumor tends to escape from lymphatics and can be found in the airspaces and/or in the vessels.

ARTIFACTUAL COLLAPSE OF THE LUNG PARENCHYMA PRODUCING A FALSE IMPRESSION OF INTERSTITIAL LUNG DISEASE

Lack of inflation of lung biopsy specimens is one of the commonest causes of processes that, at first glance, look like ILD, but are really collapse artifacts. In general, if there is clear old dense fibrosis, this separation isn't a problem, but collapse can mimic mild interstitial fibrosis or cellular NSIP (Chapter 7) (Figs. 24.30 to 24.33).

There are no hard and fast rules about how to separate collapse from mild ILD, but layers of alveolar walls stacked one on top of another represent collapse. Elastic stains can be helpful in showing the stacking. Gradual transitions from obviously normal to increasingly "fibrotic" should be examined with care, because this is a common pattern of collapse, and often one can trace individual alveolar walls into the "fibrotic" area. A very common finding is that in collapsed areas the parenchyma has airspaces with rounded "bubble" configurations (Figs. 24.32 and 24.33).

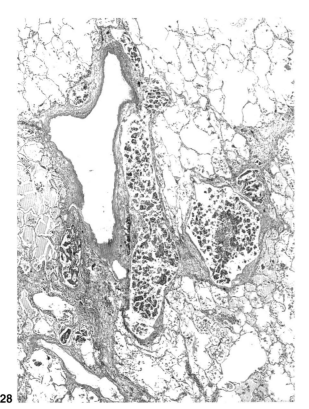

24.28

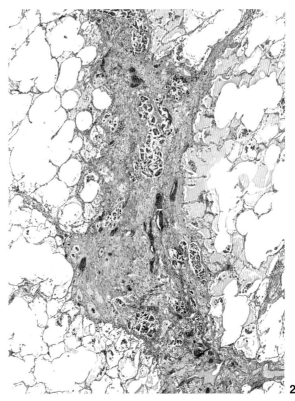

24.29

FIGURES 24.28 and 24.29. Lymphangitic carcinoma. Higher power views of the case shown in Figures 24.26 and 24.27. In **Figure 24.28**, tumor is present in lymphatics around a bronchovascular bundle; in **Figure 24.29**, tumor is present in lymphatics in an interlobular septum and has evoked a fibrotic reaction in the septum.

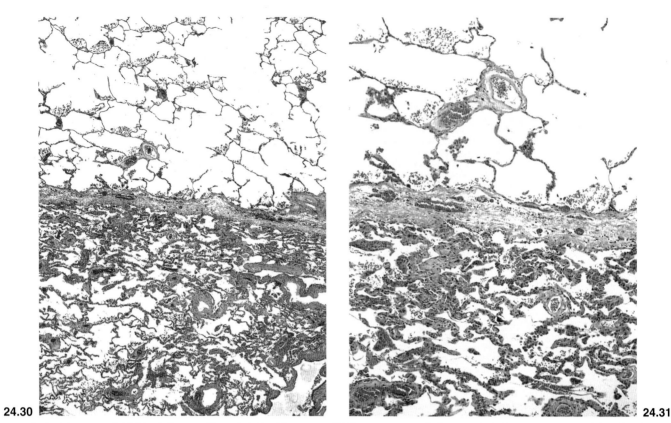

24.30   24.31

FIGURES 24.30 and 24.31. Collapse artifact mimicking ILD. Low- and high-power views of a lung in which the lobule at the top of the field has been inflated but the lobule at the bottom has not. The parenchyma in the upper portion is clearly normal, whereas the parenchyma in the lower portion is partially collapsed and mimics fine fibrotic NSIP.

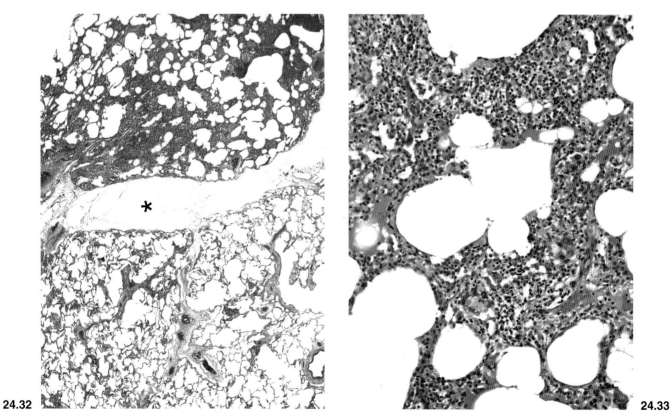

24.32   24.33

FIGURES 24.32 and 24.33. Collapse artifact mimicking ILD. Another example of a case in which one lobule has been inflated and the other is not. The parenchyma in the inflated lobule is normal, whereas that in the collapsed lobule appears to have interstitial inflammation. The rounded bubble-shaped airspaces are a hint that the parenchyma is collapsed. The interlobular septum (*) is artifactually widened as a result of inflating the biopsy.

Collapse cannot be avoided in transbronchial biopsies but inflation of surgical lung biopsies, wedge resections, and resected lobes/lungs is the best way to avoid collapse artifacts (see Chapter 3), and inflation of video-assisted thoracoscopic surgery biopsies with formalin is recommended in the latest American Thoracic Society/European Respiratory Society IPF guidelines.[21]

REFERENCES

1. Casian A, Jayne D. Management of alveolar hemorrhage in lung vasculitides. *Semin Respir Crit Care Med.* 2011;32:335–345.
2. Nasser M, Cottin V. Alveolar hemorrhage in vasculitis (primary and secondary). *Semin Respir Crit Care Med.* 2018;39:482–493.
3. Alba MA, Flores-Suárez LF, Henderson AG, et al. Interstitial lung disease in ANCA vasculitis. *Autoimmun Rev.* 2017;16:722–729.
4. Chen XY, Sun JM, Huang XJ. Idiopathic pulmonary hemosiderosis in adults: review of cases reported in the latest 15 years. *Clin Respir J.* 2017;11(6):677–681.
5. Ioachimescu OC, Sieber S, Kotch A. Idiopathic pulmonary haemosiderosis revisited. *Eur Respir J.* 2004;24(1):162–170.
6. Pacheco A, Casanova C, Fogue L, et al. Long-term clinical follow-up of adult idiopathic pulmonary hemosiderosis and celiac disease. *Chest.* 1991;99(6):1525–1526.
7. Hansell DM. Small-vessel diseases of the lung: CT-pathologic correlates. *Radiology.* 2002;225:639–653.
8. Primack SL, Miller RR, Müller NL. Diffuse pulmonary hemorrhage: clinical, pathologic, and imaging features. *AJR Am J Roentgenol.* 1995;164:295–300.
9. Tazelaar HD, Wright JL, Churg A. Desquamative interstitial pneumonia. *Histopathology.* 2011;58:509–516.
10. Antman K, Chang Y. Kaposi's sarcoma. *N Engl J Med.* 2000;343:1027.
11. Gasparetto TD, Marchiori E, Lourenço S, et al. Pulmonary involvement in Kaposi sarcoma: correlation between imaging and pathology. *Orphanet J Rare Dis.* 2009;4:18.
12. Aboulafia DM. The epidemiologic, pathologic, and clinical features of AIDS-associated pulmonary Kaposi's sarcoma. *Chest.* 2000;117:1128–1145.
13. Schwarz MI, King TE. *Interstitial Lung Disease.* 3rd ed. Hamilton, ON: BC Decker Inc; 1998.
14. Restrepo CS, Martínez S, Lemos JA, et al. Imaging manifestations of Kaposi sarcoma. *Radiographics.* 2006;26:1169–1185.
15. Lee WK, Duddalwar VA, Rouse HC, et al. Extranodal lymphoma in the thorax: cross-sectional imaging findings. *Clin Radiol.* 2009;64:542–549.
16. Koh TT, Colby TV, Müller NL. Myeloid leukemias and lung involvement. *Semin Respir Crit Care Med.* 2005;26:514–519.
17. Müller NL, Miller RR. Computed tomography of chronic diffuse infiltrative lung disease. Part 1. *Am Rev Respir Dis.* 1990;142:1206–1215.
18. Radu O, Pantanowitz L. Kaposi sarcoma. *Arch Pathol Lab Med.* 2013;137:289–294.
19. Borie R, Wislez M, Antoine M, et al. Lymphoproliferative disorders of the lung. *Respiration.* 2017;94:157–175.
20. Schreuder MI, van den Brand M, Hebeda KM, et al. Novel developments in the pathogenesis and diagnosis of extranodal marginal zone lymphoma. *J Hematopathol.* 2017;10:91–107.
21. Raghu G, Remy-Jardin M, Myers JL, et al.; American Thoracic Society, European Respiratory Society, Japanese Respiratory Society, and Latin American Thoracic Society. Diagnosis of idiopathic pulmonary fibrosis. An Official ATS/ERS/JRS/ALAT Clinical Practice Guideline. *Am J Respir Crit Care Med.* 2018;198:e44–e68.

Index

Note: Page numbers followed by *f* indicate figures; those followed by *t* indicate tables.